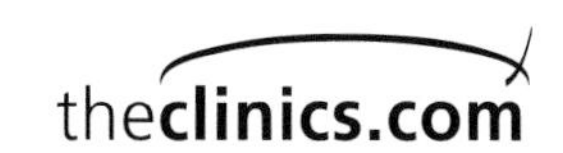

HAND CLINICS

Flexor Tendon Injuries

GUEST EDITORS
Daniel P. Mass, MD,
Craig S. Phillips, MD

May 2005 • Volume 21 • Number 2

SAUNDERS

An Imprint of Elsevier, Inc.
PHILADELPHIA LONDON TORONTO MONTREAL SYDNEY TOKYO

W.B. SAUNDERS COMPANY
A Division of Elsevier Inc.

1600 John F. Kennedy Blvd. • Suite 1800 • Philadelphia, Pennsylvania 19103

http://www.theclinics.com

HAND CLINICS
May 2005
Editor: Debora Dellapena

Volume 21, Number 2
ISSN 0749-0712
ISBN 1-4160-2661-4

Hand Clinics (ISSN 0749-0712) is published quarterly by the W.B. Saunders Company. Corporate and Editorial Offices: 1600 John F. Kennedy Blvd., Suite 1800, Philadelphia, PA 19103-2899. Accounting and Circulation Offices: 6277 Sea Harbor Drive, Orlando, FL 32887-4800. Periodicals postage paid at Orlando, FL 32862, and additional mailing offices. Subscription price is $205.00 per year (U.S. individuals), $319.00 per year (U.S. institutions), $103.00 per year (US students), $236.00 per year (Canadian individuals), $355.00 per year (Canadian institutions), $130.00 (Canadian students), $260.00 per year (international individuals), $355.00 per year (international institutions), and $130.00 per year (international students). Foreign air speed delivery is included in all *Clinics* subscription prices. All prices are subject to change without notice. POSTMASTER: Send address changes to *Hand Clinics*, W.B. Saunders Company, Periodicals Fulfillment, Orlando, FL 32887-4800. **Customer Service: 1-800-654-2452 (US). From outside the US, call 1-407-345-4000. E-mail: hhspcs@harcourt.com.**

Reprints. For copies of 100 or more, of articles in this publication, please contact the Commercial Rights Department, Elsevier Inc., 360 Park Avenue South, New York, NY 10010-1710. Tel: (212) 633-3813, Fax: (212) 462-1935, e-mail: reprints@elsevier.com

Hand Clinics is covered in *Index Medicus, Current Contents/Clinical Medicine, EMBASE/Excerpta Medica,* and *ISI/BIOMED.*

Printed in the United States of America.

GUEST EDITORS

DANIEL P. MASS, MD, Professor of Surgery, Section of Orthopaedic Surgery and Rehabilitation Medicine, Department of Surgery, University of Chicago Pritzker School of Medicine, University of Chicago Hospitals, Chicago, Illinois

CRAIG S. PHILLIPS, MD, Assistant Professor of Surgery, The University of Chicago Hospitals; Director, Hand and Upper-Extremity Surgery, Weiss Hospital, Chicago; Reconstructive Hand and Microvascular Surgery, The Illinois Bone and Joint Institute, Evanston Northwestern Healthcare, Glenview, Illinois

CONTRIBUTORS

CHRISTOPHER H. ALLAN, MD, Assistant Professor, Orthopaedics and Sports Medicine, Harborview Medical Center, University of Washington School of Medicine, Seattle, Washington

GEORGE S. ATHWAL, MD, FRCSC, Hand and Microsurgical Fellow, Hospital for Special Surgery, New York, New York

KODI K. AZARI, MD, Assistant Professor of Surgery, Associate Director of Hand Surgery Fellowship, Division of Plastic Surgery, University of Pittsburgh Medical Center, Pittsburgh, Pennsylvania

RODERICK BIRNIE, MD, MB BCh, MMed, Assistant Professor, Section of Orthopedic Surgery and Rehabilitation Medicine, The University of Chicago Hospitals, Chicago, Illinois

MARTIN I. BOYER, MD, MSc, FRCS(C), Associate Professor, Department of Orthopaedic Surgery, Washington University at Barnes-Jewish Hospital, Saint Louis, Missouri

JACK CHOUEKA, MD, Director of Hand and Upper Extremity Surgery, Department of Orthopaedic Surgery, Maimonides Medical Center, Brooklyn, New York

ROBERT W. COATS, II, MD, Hand and Upper Extremity Fellow, Section of Orthopaedic Surgery and Rehabilitation Medicine, Department of Surgery, University of Chicago Pritzker School of Medicine, University of Chicago Hospital, Chicago, Illinois

JULIO C. ECHEVARRÍA-ORÉ, MD, Attending Surgeon, Department of Orthopaedics and Traumatology, Hospital Nacional Edgardo Rebagliati Martins, Lima, Perú

KERRY FIALA, OTR/L, Hand Therapy Clinic, Occupational Therapy Department, The University of Chicago Hospitals, Chicago, Illinois

GLORIA GALLARDO, OTR/L, Hand Therapy Clinic, Occupational Therapy Department, The University of Chicago Hospitals, Chicago, Illinois

HOWARD J. GOODMAN, MD, Resident Physician, Department of Orthopaedic Surgery, Maimonides Medical Center, Brooklyn, New York

TIMOTHY G. HAVENHILL, MD, Fellow, Hand and Upper Extremity Surgery, Department of Orthopedic Surgery, Washington University School of Medicine, St. Louis, Missouri

T.C. HE, MD, PhD, Molecular Oncology Laboratory, Department of Surgery, The University of Chicago Medical Center, Chicago, Illinois

JON D. HERNANDEZ, MD, PhD, Fellow, Hand Surgery Specialists, Cincinnati, Ohio

JEFFREY LUO, MD, Orthopaedic Surgery and Rehabilitation Medicine, Department of Surgery, University of Chicago Hospitals; Molecular Oncology Laboratory, Department of Surgery, The University of Chicago Medical Center, Chicago, Illinois

PAUL R. MANSKE, MD, Professor, Orthopaedic Surgery, Washington University School of Medicine, St. Louis, Missouri

DANIEL P. MASS, MD, Professor of Surgery, Section of Orthopaedic Surgery and Rehabilitation Medicine, Department of Surgery, University of Chicago Pritzker School of Medicine, University of Chicago Hospitals, Chicago, Illinois

ROY A. MEALS, MD, Clinical Professor of Orthopaedic Surgery, University of California, Los Angeles, Los Angeles, California

VISHAL MEHTA, MD, Chief Resident, Department of Surgery, Section of Orthopaedic Surgery, The University of Chicago Hospitals, Chicago, Illinois

BRIAN A. MURPHY, MD, Hand Fellow, Department of Surgery, Section of Orthopaedic Surgery and Rehabilitation Medicine, University of Chicago, Chicago, Illinois

CRAIG S. PHILLIPS, MD, Assistant Professor of Surgery, The University of Chicago Hospitals; Director, Hand and Upper-Extremity Surgery, Weiss Hospital, Chicago; Reconstructive Hand and Microvascular Surgery, The Illinois Bone and Joint Institute, Evanston Northwestern Healthcare, Glenview, Illinois

PETER J. STERN, MD, Professor and Chairman, Department of Orthopaedic Surgery, University of Cincinnati, College of Medicine, Cincinnati, Ohio

JAMES W. STRICKLAND, MD, Clinical Professor of Orthopaedic Surgery, Indiana University Medical Center, Indianapolis; Reconstructive Hand Surgeons of Indiana, Carmel, Indiana

JIN BO TANG, MD, Professor and Chair, Department of Hand Surgery; Chair, Hand Surgery Research Center, Affiliated Hospital of Nantong University, Nantong, Jiangsu, China; Associate Professor of Surgery, Boston University School of Medicine, Boston, Massachusetts

KATHY VUCEKOVICH, OTR/L, CHT, Hand Therapy Clinic, Occupational Therapy Department, The University of Chicago Hospitals, Chicago, Illinois

SCOTT W. WOLFE, MD, Chief of the Hand Service, Clinical Director of Orthopedic Surgery, Attending Orthopedic Surgeon, Director of the Hand Surgical Fellowship, Hospital for Special Surgery, New York, New York

CONTENTS

FORTHCOMING ISSUES

August 2005

Distal Radius Fractures
Andrew P. Gutow, MD, and
David Slutsky, MD, *Guest Editors*

November 2005

Wrist Arthritis
Brian Adams, MD, *Guest Editor*

RECENT ISSUES

February 2005

Brachial Plexus Injuries in Adults
Allen T. Bishop, MD, Robert J. Spinner, MD,
and Alexander Y. Shin, MD, *Guest Editors*

November 2004

Elbow Trauma
Graham J.W. King, MD, MSc, FRCSC
Guest Editor

August 2004

Tumor of the Hand and Upper Extremity: Principles of Diagnosis and Management II
Peter M. Murray, MD,
Edward A. Athanasian, MD, and
Peter J.L. Jebson, MD, *Guest Editors*

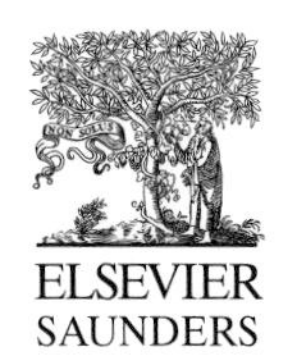

ELSEVIER
SAUNDERS

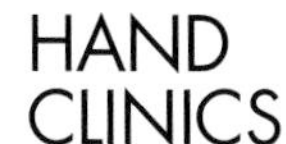

Hand Clin 21 (2005) xi–xii

Preface
Flexor Tendon Injuries

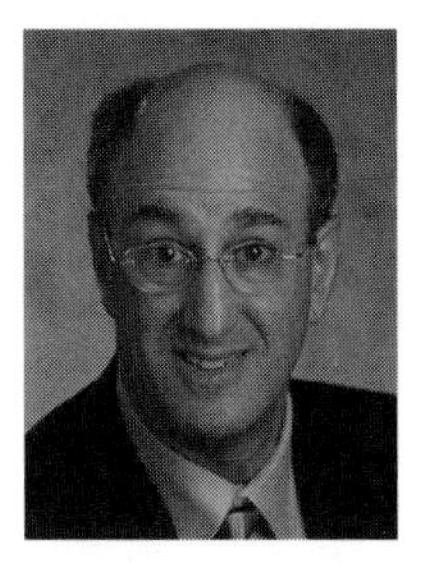

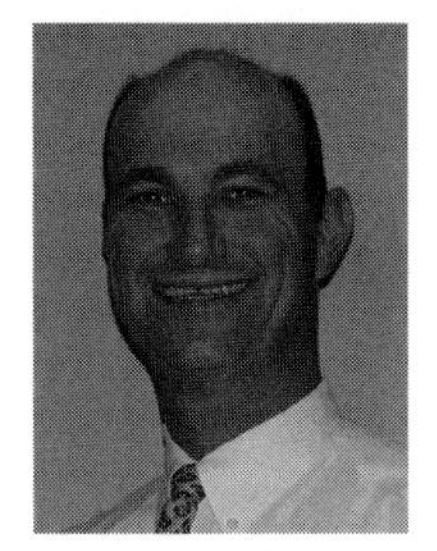

Daniel P. Mass, MD   Craig S. Phillips, MD
Guest Editors

The *Hand Clinics* debuted 20 years ago with a review on flexor tendon injuries. There have been no subsequent issues dealing with this controversial complex topic, which has produced more articles in the peer-reviewed hand literature than any other single topic. Since Sterling Bunnell's articles advocating not operating on tendons in "no-man's land," there has been ongoing debate about when and how to repair flexor tendons. The question of whether tendons heal intrinsically or require peripheral adhesions to heal is still unanswered.

Due to the unforgiving nature of flexor tendon repairs, these injuries have become the sole domain of the hand surgeon. Human flexor tendons remain unique in their anatomy (micro- and macroscopic), biomechanics, intimacy with the fibro-osseous sheath, and proximity to the neurovascular structures of the digit, as well as the response to trauma and their ability to heal through both extrinsic and intrinsic healing. The dichotomy of regaining tendon strength and gliding while avoiding adhesions or rupture after repair remains an intellectual and technical challenge today, 76 years after Bunnell advocated removing the flexor tendon from the digit and grafting the defect after zone II injury. Due to average functional outcomes, considerable research has emerged over the last 15 years directed toward identifying the "ideal zone II flexor tendon repair," often overwhelming and confusing the treating surgeon. The goal of this issue of the *Hand Clinics* is to combine long-standing dogma with recent advances associated with flexor tendon repair in all zones to increase understanding of these often complex problems. The diverse content of this issue includes 15 articles encompassing the history of flexor tendon repairs, tendon/pulley biomechanics, the most recent suture techniques, and the ability to alter the flexor tendon milieu through molecular manipulation in an effort to enhance healing and functional outcomes associated with flexor tendon repairs.

The literature is filled with recommendations for flexor tendon repair, yet evidence-based outcome studies are still lacking. Clinical studies have been primarily case reports or small series with no comparison groups. Intellectual understanding and technical detail are paramount when optimizing function after restoring flexor tendon continuity, yet they are useless when not combined with an appropriate, well-supervised postoperative rehabilitation course. For this reason we have included an article highlighting the different postoperative protocols after flexor tendon repair.

The insight afforded by the individual authors of this issue provides a concise yet thorough overview of all injuries to the flexor tendon system.

It is with pride that this anniversary issue be dedicated to those who have spent many hours

0749-0712/05/$ - see front matter
doi:10.1016/j.hcl.2005.01.002

attempting to solve the mysteries associated with improving results after flexor tendon repair.

Daniel P. Mass, MD
Section of Orthopaedic Surgery and Rehabilitation Medicine
University of Chicago Pritzker School of Medicine
University of Chicago Hospitals
5841 South Maryland Avenue, MC 3079
Chicago, IL 60637, USA

E-mail address: dmass@surgery.bsd.uchicago.edu

Craig S. Phillips, MD
Reconstructive Hand and Microvascular Surgery
The Illinois Bone and Joint Institute
Evanston Northwestern Healthcare
Glenview, IL USA

E-mail address: handphillips@hotmail.com

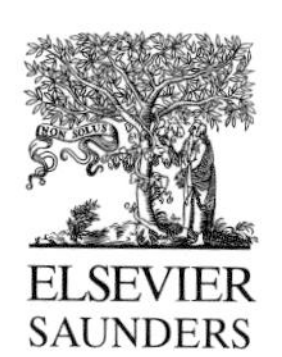
ELSEVIER
SAUNDERS

Hand Clin 21 (2005) 123–127

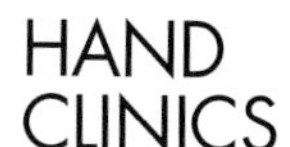
HAND
CLINICS

History of Flexor Tendon Repair

Paul R. Manske, MD

Orthopaedic Surgery, Washington University School of Medicine, One Barnes-Jewish Hospital Plaza, Suite 11300, West Pavilion, St. Louis, MO 63110, USA

The first issue of *Hand Clinics* published 20 years ago was devoted to flexor tendon injuries. This was most appropriate, because no subject in hand surgery has sparked more interest or discussion. That inaugural issue included excellent presentations on the basic science of tendon injuries (anatomy, biomechanics, nutrition, healing, adhesions) and the clinical practice of tendon repair. Of interest, there was no presentation on the fascinating history of flexor tendon surgery. It is most appropriate, therefore, that this current update of the flexor tendon begins with a historical review of the evolution of flexor tendon repair.

The treatment of injured tendons dates to antiquity. Hippocrates and other ancient physicians did not recognize the tendon as a distinct structure. They observed a white slender cord entering the fleshy substance of skeletal muscle that they knew to be nerve. The muscle was seen to terminate in a similar whitish cord-like structure that they did not distinguish from the nerve entering the muscle; they used the term "neuron" to identify this terminating structure, not recognizing it as a tendon. Several investigators [1–3] mistakenly assigned this erroneous anatomic observation to Galen and used it to explain Galen's written admonition to physicians not to suture tendons. Although Galen had written that pricking the tendon would lead to twitching and convulsions, the recent writings of Siegel [4] make clear that Galen understood the anatomic differences between nerve and tendon and the different functions of muscle and tendon. Muscle actively contracts, whereas the tendon moves passively; the tendon's attachment to the bone results in movement of the distal part.

E-mail address: manskep@wustl.edu

Galen's error in advising not to suture tendons was more subtle [4]. In his anatomic dissections of skeletal muscles, he observed that nerve and ligament fibers became progressively smaller and finer on entering the muscle tissue. He concluded that in the course of fetal development, these fine ligament and nerve fibers were woven together within the muscle and fused to form the terminating tendon. The tendon thus was sensitive to pricking because it was composed in part of nerve fibers, and therefore the advice not to prick tendons with sutures. Not withstanding this admonition, there is evidence from Galen's other writings that suggest that he did, in fact, repair injured tendons in his role as physician to the gladiators. According to Kuhn's translation, Galen wrote, "I found one of the gladiators called horseman with a transverse division of the tendon on the anterior surface of the thigh, the lower part being separated from the upper, and without hesitation I brought them together with suture."

Galen was a prolific writer and had a profound impact on shaping medical concepts and practices for more than 1500 years. His extensive medical treatises were translated first into Arabic and subsequently into Latin. Undoubtedly they influenced Avicenna, the great Muslim physician–philosopher of the eleventh century who succeeded Hippocrates and Galen as an important medical writer. Although Avicenna is described [1–3,5–7] as the first surgeon to advocate suturing of tendons, he undoubtedly was aware of Galen's scientific dissections and his clinical practices as physician to the gladiators. As reported in Gratz's interesting treatise [5], Avicenna's tendon repair concepts were adopted subsequently by several European surgeons in the fourteenth to sixteenth centuries. Despite these reports of successful

0749-0712/05/$ - see front matter
doi:10.1016/j.hcl.2004.03.004

tenorrhaphy, however, Galen's precepts based on his anatomic dissections predominated and tendon repair was not practiced universally. Gratz [5] reported that Meekren performed the first experimental study in 1682 that directly challenged Galen's concept; he crushed tendon fibers (presumably the Achilles tendon of the dog) and did not observe pain, twitching, or convulsions in the animal. It was not until Von Haller performed similar experimental studies in 1752, however, investigating the irritability and sensibility of various body tissues, including tendon, that the coup de grace was finally rendered to the dictum against tendon suture.

In 1767, John Hunter performed the first experimental study investigating the tendon healing process [7]. He noted that the canine Achilles tendon healed by formation of callus, similar to that seen in healing bone. As reported by Mason and Shearon [7], Hunter's study was followed by numerous others that attempted to define the morphologic changes associated with tendon repair, the contribution to tendon healing by extrinsic fibroblasts and the intrinsic components of the tendon, and the effect of tension and motion at the repair site. These questions are remarkably similar to experimental questions and studies of recent times.

For the most part, these early studies were performed primarily on the Achilles and other paratenon covered tendons and did not specifically consider flexor tendons, which are in a distinctly different anatomic environment within the synovial lined flexor digital sheath. The specific investigation of flexor tendon healing within the digital sheath began early in the twentieth century. Around 1920, Bier [8] and Saloman [9,10] noted poor tendon healing following suture of canine flexor tendons. Saloman attributed this poor response to an inhibitory hormone in the synovial fluid and to the paucity of cells capable of proliferation within the tendon. Saloman advocated leaving a defect in the tendon sheath at the time of repair to permit contact between the repaired tendon and the subcutaneous tissue. Hueck [11], however, noted that healing was poor whether the sheath was left open or sutured closed.

At this same time, Bunnell [12,13] and Garlock [14] recognized the clinical occurrence of restrictive adhesions at the flexor tendon laceration site within the digit. Bunnell used the term "No Man's Land" (NML) to describe this region where the flexor tendon passed through the digital sheath. The historical derivation of the term No Man's Land dates to its description in the fourteenth century of a plot of land outside the city of London used for executions. Bunnell encountered the term in his World War I experience in France when it was used to describe the strip of devastated lands between the front line trenches of the two opposing armies where soldiers ventured with extreme caution. Similarly, Bunnell advised surgeons to be cautious when repairing tendons within this region in the digital sheath. According to Boyes (JH Boyes, personal communication), Bunnell used the term No Man's Land to describe this region as early as 1934; the term was written for the first time in the second edition (1948) of his text *Surgery of the Hand* [15]. Bunnell outlined rigid conditions that must be present to perform flexor tendon repair within the digital sheath [16]; these included the use of stainless steel suture, an admonition to repair only the profundus tendon, and postoperative immobilization of the wrist in flexion to prevent the involved muscle from contracting too forcefully and separating the ends of the sutured tendon. Of interest, Bunnell also noted that the flexed wrist position still allowed sufficient motion to "stimulate growth and lessen adhesions while physiological union is occurring"; it is apparent that Bunnell was aware of the importance of motion and tension on tendon healing.

In 1940, Mason also advised similar specific conditions for repairing acutely lacerated flexor tendons within the digital sheath. These included never repairing both tendons, wide excision of the overlying sheath, and adequate elimination of all contaminates from the wound [17].

Despite the establishment of the concept and conditions for primary repair of lacerated flexor tendons within the digital sheath by these two well respected hand surgeons, the predominant opinion during the first half of the twentieth century was that primary repair of flexor tendons in No Man's Land should be discouraged in preference to tendon grafting. In 1947, Boyes noted that primary flexor tendon repair in the critical No Man's Land area usually failed because of infection, excessive scarring, and flexion contracture caused by poorly placed incisions [18]. Because of the generally unsatisfactory results, his preferred treatment was tendon grafting [19]. Boyes' opinion regarding the poor results following primary flexor tendon repair also was held by numerous other investigators [20–22].

Because of the great interest in tendon grafting throughout the first half of the twentieth century, few experimental studies investigated the mechanism of flexor tendon healing within the digital sheath. The tendon was believed to be an avascular structure [23–25] with low metabolic activity [25–28] with minimal healing potential. Consequently the reparative cells were believed to be derived not from the tendon itself, but rather from the extrinsic fibroblasts that migrate from the peripheral tissues and attach to the surface of the injured tendon, as noted in the extensive writings of Potenza [29–34] and Peacock [35–37]. These fibrous adhesions thus were considered to be an integral and essential component of the healing process.

Despite the prevalent concept of Boyes and others that repair of flexor tendons within the digital sheath leads to poor results, a few surgeons with specialized interest in hand surgery began to publish reports indicating that reasonable success could be obtained following flexor tendon suture. In 1950, Siler [38] reported 62% excellent and good results of tendon repair in No Man's Land. In 1956, Posch reported 87% satisfactory results [39]. These early reports were supported further by subsequent publications in the early 1960s that also reported good results [40–42]. It was the 1967 presentation "Primary Repair of Flexor Tendons in No Man's Land" by Kleinert, Kutz, et al at the annual meeting of the American Society for Surgery of the Hand [43], however, that proved to be the turning point in establishing the practice of primary repair of flexor tendons among hand surgeons. Although their report of good and excellent results following primary flexor tendon repair initially generated a great deal of controversy, discussion, and disbelief, in time primary repair supplanted tendon grafting as the treatment of choice for acute flexor tendon lacerations.

The emerging popularity of this clinical practice stimulated numerous experimental studies of the tendon's potential role in the healing process. Several investigators determined that diffusion of nutrients is an effective source of flexor tendon nutrition within the digital sheath [44–50], thereby obviating the specific need for tendon vascularization. Matthews and Richards [51–54] observed "rounding off" and healing of lacerated stumps of rabbit flexor tendons within the intact digital sheath in the absence of peripheral adhesions, and McDowell and Snyder [55] made similar observations in canine flexor tendons. The experimental studies of Lindsay and associates are particularly important [55–57]. These in vivo histologic studies in chickens described the flexor tendon's cellular response to injury. Initially the epitenon cells proliferate and migrate to the laceration site, followed several days later by a similar proliferation and migration of endotenon cells from within the substance of the tendon. The cells subsequently bridged the laceration site and in time formed mature collagen bundles. Furthermore, this cellular response took place in the presence or absence of the tendon sheath, which Lindsay believed contributed minimally to the repair response.

The ingenious "in situ tissue culture" studies of Lundborg et al [58–61] demonstrated healing of lacerated flexor tendon segments when placed within the synovial environment of the knee joint. Lundborg together with Katsumi and Tajima [62] also observed complete healing when the lacerated tendon segment was isolated in a synthetic membrane pouch placed in a subcutaneous pocket of the back or abdomen of the rabbit. Although these studies strongly supported the concept that flexor tendon healing was an intrinsic process, the results were challenged theoretically and experimentally by Potenza and Herte [63] and by Chow [64], who demonstrated in a similar experimental model that extrinsic synovial cells could "seed" on to nonviable tendon segments, therefore again suggesting that extrinsic cells were the source of healing. Subsequent in vitro organ culture studies by Manske, Lesker, Gelberman et al [6,65–69] in the mid 1980s demonstrated healing of lacerated flexor tendon segments of several different experimental animals when placed in an extracorporeal tissue culture environment in the complete absence of extrinsic cells, thereby conclusively establishing the tendon's intrinsic capacity to heal.

As a result of these studies that established that peripheral adhesions are not essential to the healing process, clinicians and investigators began to devise various methods and techniques to minimize adhesions and to enhance the tendon's response to injury. These include mobilizing the tendon at the repair site and applying tension to the healing cells, and enhancing the strength of the repair with heavier suture material, multiple suture strands, and various core and peripheral suture configurations. These are the subject of the pages that follow in this issue of the *Hand Clinics*. Nevertheless, hand surgeons of today are indebted to the many twentieth century clinicians and investigators who were instrumental in establishing the concept that because the flexor tendon has the intrinsic capacity to participate in the repair process in the absence of peripheral adhesions, primary repair of injured flexor tendons is the preferred treatment.

References

[1] Adamson JE, Wilson JN. The history of flexor-tendon grafting. J Bone Joint Surg 1961;43A: 709–16.

[2] Schneider JH. The history of flexor tendon suture. In: Flexor tendon injuries. Boston: Little Brown and Co; 1985. p. 1–4.

[3] Kleinert HE, Spokevicius S, Papas NH. History of flexor tendon repair. J Hand Surg 1995;20A(Suppl): S48–52.

[4] Siegel RE. Galen on psychology, psychopathology, and function and diseases of the nervous system. Basel: S. Karger; 1973. p. 53–62.

[5] Gratz CM. The history of tendon suture. Med J Rec 1928;127:156–7; 213–5.

[6] Manske PR, Gelberman RH, Lesker PA. Flexor tendon healing. Hand Clin 1985;1:25–34.

[7] Mason ML, Shearon CG. The process of tendon repair. An experimental study of tendon suture and tendon graft. Arch Surg 1932;25:615–92.

[8] Bier A. Beobachtungen über Regeneration beim Menschen, Deutsche med. Wehnschr 1917;43:705, 833, 865, 897, 925, 1025, 1057, 1121, 1249.

[9] Salomon A. Klinische und experimentelle Untersuchungen über Heilung von Schnenverletzungen insbesondere innerhalb der Sehnenscheiden, Arch. F. klin. Chir 1924;129:397.

[10] Salomon A. Ueber den Ersatz grosser Sehnendefekte durch Regeneration, Arch. F. klin. Chir 1919; 113:30.

[11] Hueck H. Ueber Sehnenregeneration innerhalb echter Sehnenscheiden, Arch. F. klin. Chir 1923; 127:137.

[12] Bunnell S. Repair of tendons in the fingers and description of two new instruments. Surg Gynecol Obstet 1918;26:103–10.

[13] Bunnell S. Repair of tendons in the fingers. Surg Gynecol Obstet 1922;35:88–97.

[14] Garlock JH. Repair of wounds of the flexor tendons of the hand. Ann Surg 1926;83:111–22.

[15] Bunnell S. Surgery of the hand. 2nd edition. Philadelphia: JB Lippincott; 1948. p. 627.

[16] Bunnell S. Primary repair of severed tendons: the use of stainless steel wire. Am J Surg 1940;47: 502–16.

[17] Mason ML. Primary and secondary tendon suture. A discussion of the significance of technique in tendon surgery. Surg Gyn Obstet 1940;70:392–402.

[18] Boyes JH. Immediate vs. delayed repair of the digital flexor tendons. Ann West Med Surg 1947;1: 145–52.

[19] Boyes JH. Flexor tendon grafts in the fingers and thumb. J Bone Joint Surg 1950;32A:489–99.

[20] Hauge MF. The results of tendon suture of the hand. Act Orthop Scandinavica 1955;24:258–70.

[21] Van't Hof A, Heiple KG. Flexor-tendon injuries in the finger and thumb: a comparative study. J Bone Joint Surg 1958;40A:256–61.

[22] Boyes JH. Discussion of Van't Hof, Heiple paper. J Bone Joint Surg 1958;40A:262–322.

[23] Rau E. Die Gefassversorgung der Sehnen. Anatomische Hefte 1914;50:679–91.

[24] Dychno A. Zur Frage uber die Blutversorgung der Sehnen. Anat Anz 1936;82:282–91.

[25] Edwards DAW. The blood supply and lymphatic drainage of the tendon. J Anat 1946;80:147–52.

[26] Neuberger A, Slack HGB. The metabolism of collagen from liver, bone, skin and tendon in the normal rat. Biochem J 1953;53:47–52.

[27] White NB, Ter-Pogossian MM, Stein AH. A method to determine the rate of blood flow in long bone and selected soft tissues. Surg Gynecol Obstet 1964;119: 535–40.

[28] Peacock EE. A study of the circulation in normal tendons and healing grafts. Ann Surg 1959;149: 415–28.

[29] Potenza AD. Effect of associated trauma on healing of divided tendons. J Trauma 1962;2:175–84.

[30] Potenza AD. Tendon healing within the flexor digital sheath in the dog. J Bone Joint Surg 1962;44A: 49–64.

[31] Potenza AD. Critical evaluation of flexor-tendon healing and adhesion formation within artificial digital sheaths: an experimental study. J Bone Joint Surg 1963;45A:1217–33.

[32] Potenza AD. Prevention of adhesions to healing digital flexor tendons. JAMA 1964;187:99–103.

[33] Potenza AD. Mechanisms of healing of digital flexor tendons. Hand 1969;1:40–1.

[34] Potenza AD. Concepts of tendon healing and repair. In: American Academy of Orthopaedic Surgeons: symposium on tendon surgery in the hand. St. Louis: CV Mosby; 1975. p. 18–47.

[35] Peacock EE. Fundamental aspect of wound healing relating to the restoration of gliding function after tendon repair. Surg Gynecol Obstet 1964;119: 241–50.

[36] Peacock EE. Biological principles in the healing of long tendons. Surg Clin N Am 1965;45:461–76.

[37] Peacock EE. Repair of tendons and restoration of gliding function. In: Surgery and biology of wound repair. Philadelphia: WB Saunders; 1970.

[38] Siler VE. Primary tenorrhaphy of the flexor tendons in the hand. J Bone Joint Surg 1950;32A:218–24.

[39] Posch JL. Primary tenorrhaphies and tendon grafting procedures in the hand. AMA Arch Surg 1956; 73:609–24.

[40] Carter SJ, Mersheimer WL. Deferred primary tendon repair: results in 27 cases. Ann Surg 1966;164: 913–6.

[41] Lindsay WK, McDougall EP. Direct digital flexor tendon repairs. Plast Reconstr Surg 1960;26:613–21.
[42] Verdan CE. Primary repair of flexor tendons. J Bone Joint Surg 1960;42A:647–57.
[43] Kleinert HE, Kutz JE, Ashbell TS, Martinez E. Primary repair of lacerated flexor tendons in "No Man's Land" [abstract]. J Bone Joint Surg 1967; 49A:577.
[44] Manske PR, Bridwell K, Lesker PA. Nutrient pathways to flexor tendons of chickens using tritiated proline. J Hand Surg 1978;3:352–7.
[45] Manske PR, Bridwell K, Whiteside LA, et al. Nutrition of flexor tendon in monkeys. Clin Orthop 1978; 136:294–8.
[46] Manske PR, Lesker PA. Nutrient pathways of flexor tendons in primates. J Hand Surg 1982;7:436–47.
[47] Manske PR, Lesker PA. Comparative nutrient pathways to the flexor profundus tendons in zone II of various experimental animals. J Surg Res 1983;34: 83–93.
[48] Manske PR, Lesker PA. Flexor tendon nutrition. Hand Clin 1985;1:13–24.
[49] Lundborg G, Holm S, Myrhage R. The role of the synovial fluid and tendon sheath for flexor tendon nutrition. Scand J Plast Reconstr Surg 1980;14: 99–107.
[50] Hooper G, Davies R, Tuthill P. Blood flow and clearance in tendons. J Bone Joint Surg 1984;66B: 441–3.
[51] Matthew P. The fate of isolated segments of flexor tendons within the digital sheath. Br J Plast Surg 1976;28:216–24.
[52] Matthews P, Richards H. The repair potential of digital flexor tendons. J Bone Joint Surg 1974;56B: 618–25.
[53] Matthews P, Richards H. The repair reaction of flexor tendon within the digital sheath. Hand 1975; 7:27–9.
[54] Matthews P, Richards H. Factors in the adherence of flexor tendons after repair. J Bone Joint Surg 1976;58B:230–6.
[55] Lindsay WK, Thomson HG. Digital flexor tendons: an experimental study (part I). The significance of each compartment of the flexor mechanism in tendon healing. Br J Plast Surg 1959;12:289–316.
[56] Digital flexor tendon: an experimental study (part II). The significance of a gap occurring at the line of suture. Br J Plast Surg 1960;13:1–9.
[57] Lindsay WK, McDougall EP. Digital flexor tendons: an experimental study (part III). The fate of autogenous digital flexor tendon grafts. Br J Plast Surg 1961;13:293–304.
[58] Lundborg G. Experimental flexor tendon healing without adhesion formation—a new concept of tendon nutrition and intrinsic healing mechanisms. Hand 1976;8:235–8.
[59] Lundborg G, Hansson HA, Rank F, et al. Superficial repair of severed flexor tendons in synovial environment—an experimental study on cellular mechanisms. J Hand Surg 1980;5: 451–61.
[60] Lundborg G, Rank F. Experimental intrinsic healing of flexor tendons based upon synovial fluid nutrition. J Hand Surg 1978;3:21–31.
[61] Lundborg GN, Rank F. Experimental studies on cellular mechanisms involved in healing of animal and human flexor tendon in synovial environment. Hand 1980;12:3–11.
[62] Katsumi M, Tajima T. Experimental investigation of healing process of tendons with or without synovial coverage in or outside of synovial cavity. J Niigata Med Assoc 1981;95:532–67.
[63] Potenza AD, Herte MC. The synovial cavity as a "tissue culture in situ"—science or nonsense. J Hand Surg 1982;7:196–9.
[64] Chow SP, Hooper G, Chan CW. The healing of freeze-dried rabbit flexor tendon in a synovial fluid environment. Hand 1983;15:136–42.
[65] Manske PR, Gelberman RH, Vande Berg J, et al. Flexor tendon repair: morphological evidence of intrinsic healing in vitro. J Bone Joint Surg 1984; 66A:385–96.
[66] Manske PR, Lesker PA. Histological evidence of flexor tendon repair in various experimental animals. An in vitro study. Clin Orthop 1984;182: 353–60.
[67] Manske PR, Lesker PA. Biochemical evidence of flexor tendon participation in the repair process—an in vitro study. J Hand Surg 1984;9B:117–20.
[68] Gelberman RH, Manske PR, Vande Berg JS, et al. Flexor tendon healing in vitro: comparative histologic study of rabbit, chicken, dog and monkey. J Orthop Res 1984;2:39–48.
[69] Russell JE, Manske PR. Collagen synthesis during primate flexor tendon repair in vitro. J Orthop Res 1990;8:13–20.

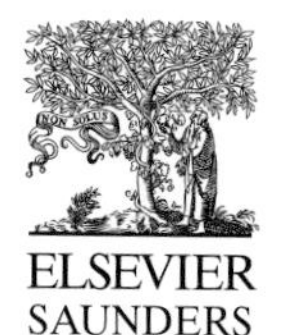

ELSEVIER
SAUNDERS

Hand Clin 21 (2005) 129–149

HAND
CLINICS

Biomechanics of the Flexor Tendons

Howard J. Goodman, MD*, Jack Choueka, MD

Maimonides Medical Center, Department of Orthopaedic Surgery, 927 49th Street, Brooklyn, NY 11219, USA

"The finger knows more than the surgeon."
—Paul W. Brand

An understanding of the biomechanics of the flexor tendon system is essential to proper evaluation and treatment of disorders of the upper extremity. The flexor tendons are essentially cables that transmit forces developed by muscle contraction in the forearm to the fingers, moving and stabilizing the joints. The versatility of the human hand—its ability to perform precise manipulation and forceful grasping—stems from the organization of the flexor tendons and their ability to generate varying degrees of force at different locations.

This discussion of the biomechanics of the digital flexor tendons begins with a review of their molecular and cellular composition and structure, their organization within the hand in the complex pulley system, and the way their relationship to the joints and bones of the hand governs organized movement. This article concludes with a discussion of physiologic and pathologic conditions that affect flexor tendon function and of clinical biomechanics as it applies to tendon transfers and flexor tendon repair.

Tendon anatomy

The biomechanic properties of tendon arise from its molecular organization, morphology, and cellular arrangement. As in nature's axiom, "Form begets function and function begets form," the makeup of a tendon implies its purpose. Tendon consists of cellular and noncellular elements. The cellular component is predominantly made up of fibroblasts, spindle-shaped cells whose role is the production of collagen and reorganization of the extracellular matrix, which consists primarily of water (60%–80% of the wet weight), collagen (86% of dry weight), proteoglycans (1%–5% of dry weight), and elastin (2% of dry weight) [1,2].

The major component of the extracellular matrix is collagen. Type I collagen, the most prominent type in tendon, is formed by three polypeptide chains linked by covalent and hydrogen bonds. The collagen molecule is organized with complementary acidic and basic amino acids, which impart strength to the structure of the tendon. Crosslinking varies along a tendon's length, lending itself to different mechanical properties. At the musculotendinous junction and the tendon–bone junction there is less crosslinking and more cellularity than in the central portion of the tendon, with the highest strength in the middle portion of the tendon, followed by the tendon–bone insertion, and the least strength at the muscle–tendon junction [3–5].

The micro-architecture of tendon is shown in Fig. 1. Five crosslinked collagen molecules form a microfibril, groups of which join to make subfibrils, which then combine to form larger fibrils [6]. Fibrils are closely packed in parallel bundles with proteoglycans and water to make up the nonorganic matrix. Proteoglycans and glycosaminoglycans, like collagen, are extremely hydrophilic, consisting of several long carbohydrates linked to a central protein structure.

Tendon fascicles are bound together with the endotenon, a loose connective tissue that provides a route for vessels and nerves. The whole tendon is encased in a synovial membrane, the epitenon, which produces the synovial fluid that assists in tendon gliding and provides nutrition to cells.

* Corresponding author.
E-mail address: hjg@alumni.upenn.edu
(H.J. Goodman).

doi:10.1016/j.hcl.2004.11.002

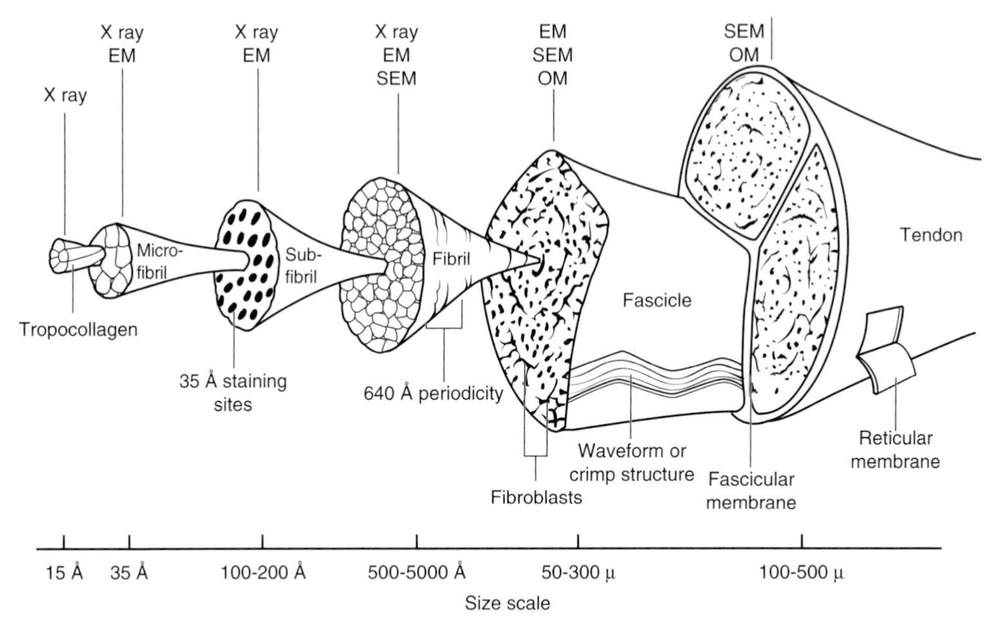

Fig. 1. Microarchitecture of collagen. Collagen molecules are arranged in progressively larger strands, coalescing into the structure of tendon. *Used with permission from* Woo S, An KN, Frank C, et al. Anatomy, biology, and biomechanics of tendon and ligament. In: Buckwalter JA, Einhorn TA, Simon SR, editors. Orthopaedic basic science. 2nd edition. St. Louis: American Academy of Orthopaedic Surgeons; 2000 (*Adapted from* Kastelic J, Baer E. Deformation in tendon collagen. In: Vincent JFV, Currey JD, editors. The mechanical properties of biologic materials. Cambridge, England: Cambridge University Press; 1980. p. 397–435; with permission).

Mechanical properties of tendon

As implied by its name—derived from the Latin *tendere*, "to stretch"—the tendon serves to conduct tension. Collagen is primarily responsible for this property: its stress–strain curve is virtually identical to that of tendon. Collagen's structure—parallel fibers with strong crosslinks—is ideal for tension bearing. The mechanical properties of tendon are revealed by analysis of its stress–strain curve (Fig. 2). This curve has three regions: a toe region with the beginning ramp, a linear region, and a failure region. The toe region, the initial loading phase, is attributed on the molecular level to the uncrimping of collagen and grossly to tendon tightening before stress sets in. The linear region shows a constant elongation (or strain) for a given load (or stress). This slope, or ratio of stress to strain, represents a fundamental property of tendon: its Young's modulus of elasticity. The final region includes areas of irreversible changes, including the yield point (the point at which the material begins elongating with a decrease in load) and the failure point (the point at which the material's integrity breaks down). The total area under the stress–strain curve is the total energy absorbed in the test.

The Young's modulus of human tendon ranges from 1200–1800 Mpa, with ultimate strength ranging from 50–150 MPa. Ultimate strain, the deformation at which the material fails, has been calculated to range in human tendon as an increase of 9%–35% of initial length [5].

Time-dependent factors

Simple linear analysis of tendon mechanics neglects its rate- and time-dependent properties, most important, its viscoelasticity. The two major parameters of viscoelasticity are creep and stress relaxation. Creep is the time-dependent elongation of tissue under a constant load characterized by an initial large elongation followed by elongation in smaller increments. Stress relaxation is the concomitant decrease in load exhibited as the tissue is subjected to constant elongation. Monleon et al analyzed the viscoelastic behavior of flexor tendons in the human hand and confirmed its viscoelastic relationship, with the stress–strain

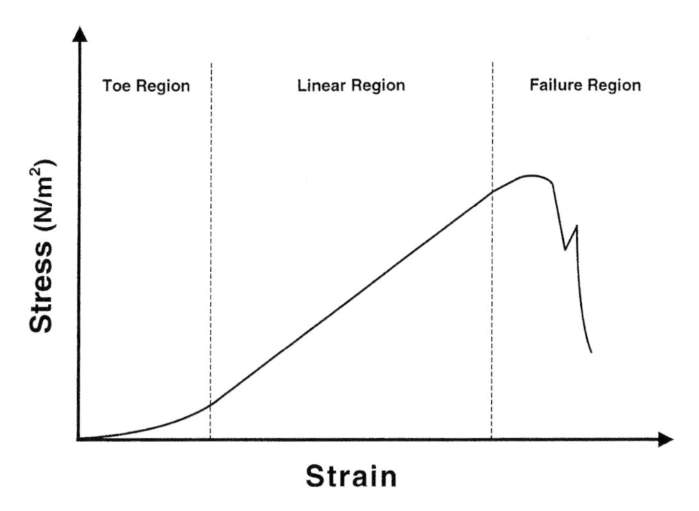

Fig. 2. A stress–strain curve representative of a tendon's response to mechanical testing. Note the ramping toe region at the beginning of the curve. (*Adapted from* Woo S, An KN, Frank C, et al. Anatomy, biology, and biomechanics of tendon and ligament. In: Buckwalter JA, Einhorn TA, Simon SR, editors. Orthopaedic Basic Science. 2nd edition. St. Louis: American Academy of Orthopaedic Surgeons; 2000; with permission).

relationship dependent on recent loading history [5,7].

The viscoelastic properties of tendon may be visualized by use of a schematic in which the elastic property is represented as a spring, with displacement directly proportional to force, and the viscous property as a dashpot, which, depending on the rate of applied force, increases resistance to motion (Fig. 3).

The mechanical behavior of tendon changes over the course of repeated loads. During cycling, there is a tendency for creep to continue elongating the tissue and, during unloading, for friction to prevent the tissue from returning to its original length. As shown in Fig. 4, over time there is progressively less difference between the successive amounts of elongation. Note also the disparity between the upswing (loading) and downswing (unloading) of each cycle. This area between the limbs of the cycle is termed *hysteresis* and represents the energy absorbed by the tissue within each cycle [5].

Several other factors—behavioral, physiologic, and pathologic—may affect the mechanical properties of tendon. Exercise promotes collagen synthesis and influences the length of collagen fibrils, increasing the tendon's strength [8,9]. Animal studies have demonstrated that exercise results in increased collagen concentration, increased tendon weight, increased maximum stress, and a decrease in maximum strain [10]. Although the long-term effects of exercise on tendon seem to be positive, individuals may experience periods of weakness in the course of training that require rest to allow the tendon to adapt morphologically [11]. By the same token, stress-shielding experiments have shown that periods of immobilization result in decreases in tendon modulus of elasticity and

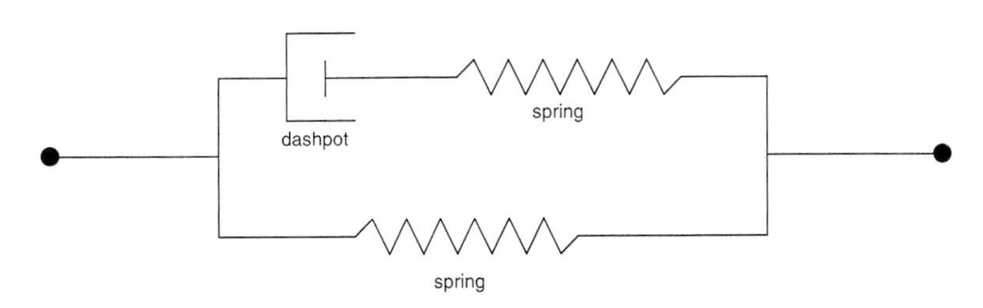

Fig. 3. Kelvin's model of viscoelastic properties. The spring represents the elastic component and the dashpot the viscous component.

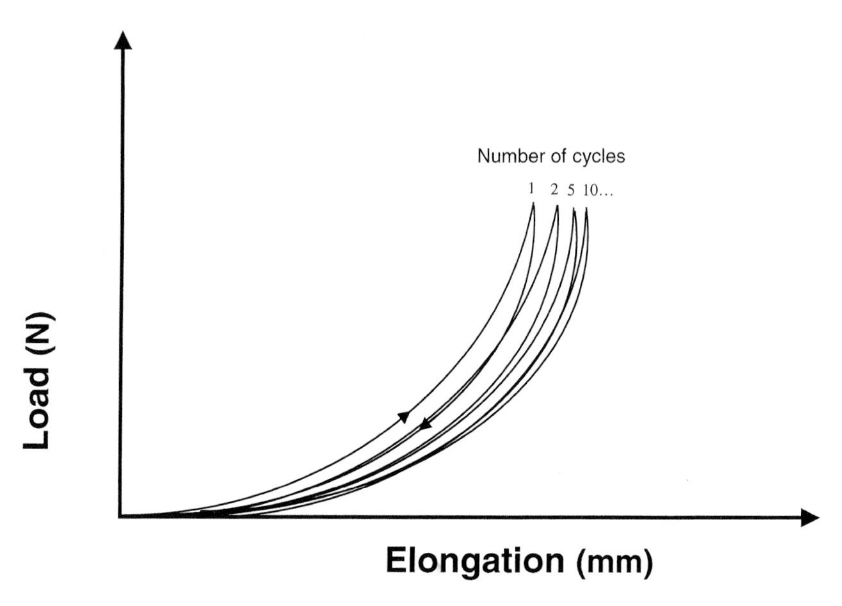

Fig. 4. Tendon response to cyclic loading showing change based on recent cycles and hysteresis. (*Adapted from* Woo S, An KN, Frank C, et al. Anatomy, biology, and biomechanics of tendon and ligament. In: Buckwalter JA, Einhorn TA, Simon SR, editors. Orthopaedic basic science. 2nd edition. St. Louis: American Academy of Orthopaedic Surgeons; 2000; with permission.).

tensile strength; the longer the duration of immobilization, the greater the decrease [12,13].

Patient age also may contribute to tendon quality. Tendon cross-sectional area increases until skeletal maturity; consequently, the elastic modulus of tendon is highest at maturity and declines in old age [14,15]. The crimp angle also decreases with age, reflected by a decrease in the toe region of the stress–strain curve [16]. Aging is accompanied by decreased tendon collagen, proteoglycan, and water content, resulting in the tendon becoming smaller, weaker, and more prone to injury.

Disease states such as diabetes affect tendon health. One in vivo study demonstrated a glucose-induced increase in collagen crosslinking. When compared with normal tendon, tendon that had been treated with a glucose solution exhibited an increase in maximum load, elastic modulus, energy-to-yield, toughness, and significantly less deformation than the control subjects [17].

The effect of external modalities used to augment tendon healing has been evaluated in several animal models with varying results. Studies of healing rabbit tendons reported increased strength using ultrasound and electrical stimulation [18–20]; similar studies performed on chicken tendon using pulsed electromagnetic fields reported decreased strength and increased peritendinous adhesions [21].

Dynamics of flexor tendons

Flexor tendons transmit force from the muscle belly to the finger to produce motion. Excursion, the distance that the tendon slides along its path, is limited by how much the muscle to which it is attached can be shortened. Brand has coined three terms, variants of *excursion*, to clarify the relationship of the muscle–tendon unit [22]: *potential excursion* is the resting fiber length of a muscle independent of connective tissue restraints, *required excursion* is the maximum excursion required of a muscle in situ, and *available excursion* is the maximum excursion of a muscle when freed from its insertion [23]. Excursion of a tendon can be affected adversely by extrinsic factors, such as contractures and adhesions, and enhanced by exercise or stretching. Wehbe and Hunter studied 48 hands in vivo and found a mean excursion of 32 mm (range, 15–43 mm) for the flexor digitorum profundus (FDP) and of 24 mm (range, 14–37 mm) for the flexor digitorum superficialis (FDS). Wrist motion increased the excursion to 50 mm and 49 mm for the FDP and FDS, respectively [24].

The distance the tendon lies from the joint moderates the force acting on it. This distance, the moment arm, determines the leverage that the tendon can exert on the joint. The total moment of the tendon on the joint is the product of tension and moment arm (Fig. 5). As the moment arm increases—as the tendon is farther away from the joint—less tension is required to move the joint. Anatomic constraints place limitations on the moment arm, however, which allows a balance between force generation and movement, a concept discussed later with regard to pulley biomechanics. With the moment arm kept constant, the independent variable is tension. Although tension may vary in response to muscle strength, the tension throughout the segments of the tendon cannot be changed. Tension seen by one part of the tendon is constant throughout the whole tendon. To change the force and torque seen by each joint crossed by a single tendon, therefore, the moment arm for the different joints must vary. This indeed happens: the FDP has a different moment arm at each joint it crosses: 1.25 cm at the wrist, 1.0 cm at the metacarpophalangeal (MCP) joint, and 0.75 cm and 0.5 cm, respectively, at the proximal and distal interphalangeal (PIP and DIP) joints. This allows different amounts of torque to be delivered by one tendon to each joint, increasing the moment seen at the more proximal, larger joints.

The relationship between excursion, joint motion, and moment arm is best understood using the geometric concept of the radian (Fig. 6). A radian is a unit of angular measure equal to the angle formed along the circumference of a circle by an arc equal to its radius, and is 57.29°. When a joint moves through 1 radian of arc, the excursion and moment arms are equal. This permits the precise calculation of excursion for a known moment arm and joint motion. For instance, the MCP joint has a normal arc of 90° or 1.57 radians. To move the joint through its full range of motion, the FDP (with a known moment arm of 1 cm) must have an excursion of 1.57 cm (1.0 cm × 1.57 radians). This also allows for calculation of motion loss in pathologic conditions such as loss of pulleys. Pulley loss leads to increased moment arms; with excursion of the muscle fixed, it leads to a predictable loss of motion. An increase in moment arm from 1.0 to 1.5 cm results in a loss of joint motion of 30° [25].

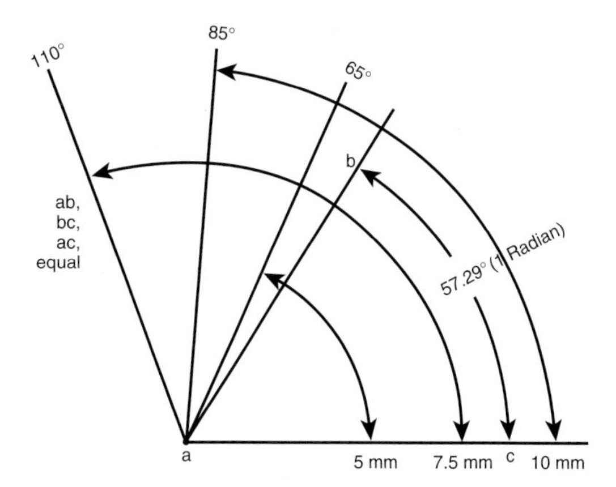

Fig. 6. The concept of radians as they relate to joint motion and excursion. (*From* Doyle JR. Palmar and digital flexor tendon pulleys. Clin Orthop 2001;383: 84–96; with permission).

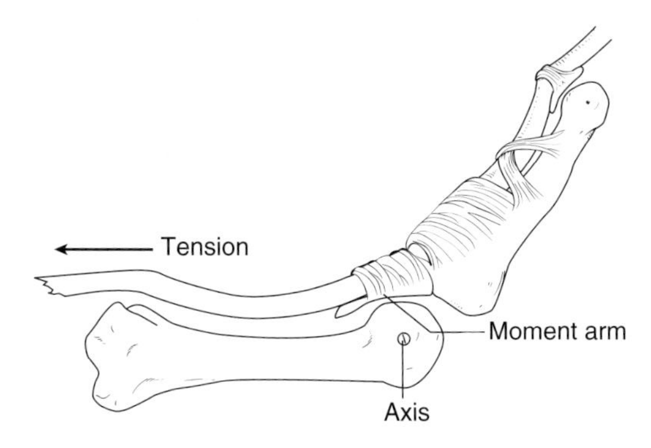

Fig. 5. Moment seen by a joint from a tendon, which is based on the force in that tendon and its moment arm. (*From* Brand PW, Hollister AM. Clinical mechanics of the hand. 3rd edition. St. Louis: Mosby; 1999; with permission.)

Biomechanics of the flexor pulley system

Maintaining a short moment arm of the flexor tendons allows conversion of the limited excursion of the flexor tendons to the large joint motions needed for functional hand and finger motion. This system allows a 3-cm flexor tendon excursion to translate into an arc of motion of 260°. The pulley mechanism sacrifices force for efficiency. By keeping moment arms smaller, the pulleys decrease some of the available force for joint movement but make it easier for precise control of the fingers. Absence of the pulleys would lead to bowstringing of the tendons, and although this would lead to greater moment arm and force transmission across a particular joint, the range of motion of that joint would be markedly decreased

(Fig. 7). The ability to straighten the fingers would be limited, leading to joint contractures.

Lin hypothesized that normal pulleys play an important role in the initiation of PIP flexion [26]. By maintaining the flexor tendons along the bony architecture, tension on the tendon produces a three-point pressure system with anteriorly directed pressure on the pulleys and posteriorly directed pressure on the condyles, with the net effect of flexing the digit.

The biomechanic effects of the pulleys on tendon and finger motion have been studied from a variety of perspectives, including studying the effects of sequential pulley sectioning on bowstringing, examining tendon excursion and tendon pulley angle, and measuring gliding resistance and work efficiency [27–39]. This variation in approach makes comparisons between studies difficult. For example, whereas Peterson et al found the A2 pulley to be the most important pulley for flexor tendon function [32], Rispler et al found that absence of the A4 pulley produced the largest changes in efficiency [40]. They agreed, however, that retaining A2, A3, and A4 pulley was necessary to preserve work and excursion efficiency.

Components of the flexor pulley system

The flexor pulley system of the hand spans the transverse carpal ligament, the palmar aponeurosis (PA) pulley, and finally the digital fibro-osseous canal, the last of which is the most complex and sensitive and therefore has received the most attention.

Transverse carpal ligament

It has been suggested that the transverse carpal ligament, besides being a roof for the carpal tunnel, also serves as a flexor pulley [25]. Kline and Moore found increased requirements for excursion of the FDS and FDP on ligament transection by 20% and 25%, but only with the wrist in flexion [41]. This was partially substantiated by Netcher et al, who found that a significant difference in excursion was required at 60° of flexion and 30° of extension [42,43]. Grip strength weakness immediately following carpal tunnel release may be the result of loss of this pulley mechanism; there have been reports of return to preoperative strength taking up to 3 months and of ligament reconstruction increasing postoperative grip and pinch strength [44,45].

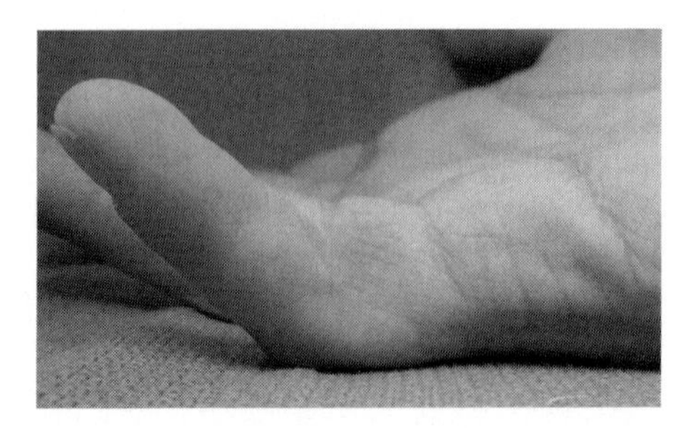

Fig. 7. Loss of pulleys resulting in bowstringing.

Palmar aponeurosis pulley

The PA pulley, described originally by Manske and Lesker in 1983, is found proximal to the A1 pulley (approximately 1.0 cm proximal to the MCP joint) [46]. Manske and Lesker described a tunnel around the flexor tendons in this region formed by the transverse fascicular fibers and paratendinous bands of the PA. Dolye in 1990 argued that its function warrants inclusion as an integral part of the flexor tendon pulley system [47]. Phillips and Mass in 1996 confirmed the biomechanic importance of this pulley by showing that sectioning of the PA pulley in combination with either or both proximal annular pulleys decreases excursion efficiency [48]. Sectioning of the PA pulley alone did not affect any efficiency parameters. This is consistent with Manske and Lesker's finding that finger range of motion can be maintained with preservation of the PA pulley and sectioning of either the A1 or A2 pulleys.

Digital fibro-osseous canal

Current nomenclature for the pulley system was established in 1975 by Doyle and Blythe, who described four annular and three cruciate pulleys [49]. A fifth annular pulley was later identified distal to the A4 pulley. The A1, A3, and A5 pulleys are located over the MP, PIP, and DIP joints, respectively, with dorsal attachments to the volar plates. The A2 and A4 pulleys are located over the length of the proximal and middle phalanges, respectively, and span a much larger distance than other pulleys, with stouter bony attachments to their respective bones (Fig. 8). The A2 and A4 pulleys, which offer significantly tighter constraint over a larger distance, are most important in preventing bowstringing and loss of joint motion [32,39,50]. Their preservation during tendon surgery is a well accepted concept,

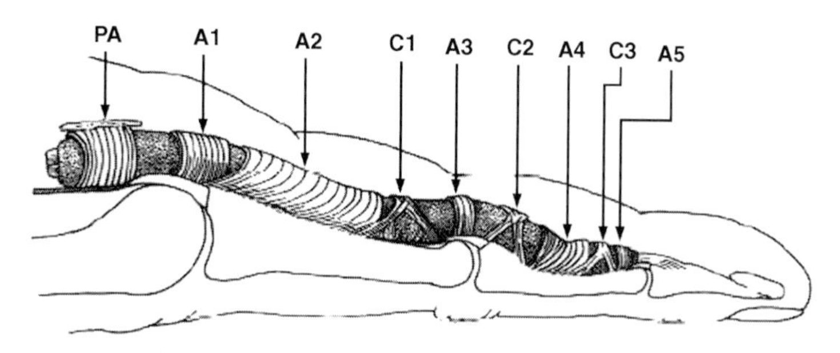

Fig. 8. The digital pulley system. (*From* 1996 Regional Review Courses in Hand Surgery [review course syllabus]. American Society for Surgery of the Hand, Englewood, CO 1996; with permission).

although partial excision of up to 75% has been shown to have small but significant effects on angular rotation, capable of maintaining strength sufficient to withstand physiologic tendon loads [36,51].

The A3 pulley has recently been the subject of several articles. Zhao et al proposed that the major function of the A3 pulley is to reduce tendon pulley gliding resistance through the A2 pulley by decreasing the angle of attack of the flexor tendons during flexion [35]. Tang and Xie in 2001 found that excision of the A3 pulley alone has little effect on bowstringing and tendon excursion and that the surrounding sheath, including the cruciate pulleys—and especially the proximal section up to the A2 pulley—offers more resistance to bowstringing [52]. It has been hypothesized that the insignificant effect of the A3 pulley on PIP moment arm is a result of its attachment to the volar plate, which moves away from the joint axis of rotation on flexion [53].

The three cruciate pulleys are located distal to the A2, A3, and A4 pulleys. Little attention has been given to their biomechanic role in finger function. Lin et al evaluated them anatomically and found that although they are in fact cruciate (x-shaped) 60%–70% of the time, they otherwise have only a single oblique component [26]. It has been suggested that the cruciate pulleys modulate force transmission during finger flexion. Tang et al found that sectioning the area between the A3 and A2 pulleys, including the C1 pulley, has a greater impact on bowstringing than sectioning the A3 alone [52]. Clinical observation reveals that during finger flexion the cruciate pulleys collapse to form a single annular band similar in appearance to the other annular pulleys (Fig. 9). This accordion-like collapse of the cruciate pulleys seems to be the mechanism by which the pulley system maintains consistent adherence to the flexor tendons throughout the range of motion of the finger. The biomechanic implications of this phenomenon have yet to be investigated, but it suggests a greater role for the cruciate pulleys during flexion and a possible role in maintaining the dynamic structure of the entire system.

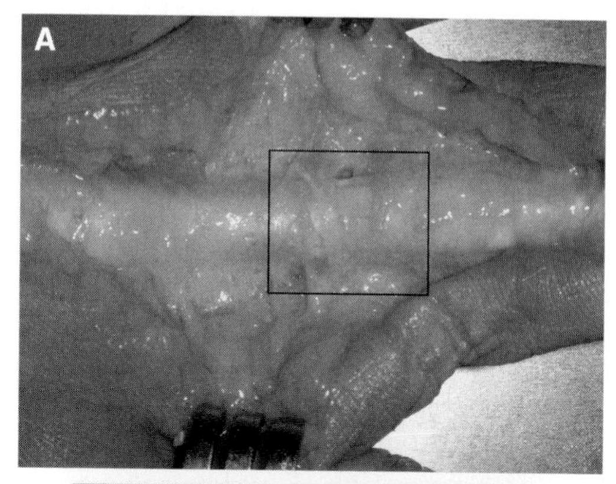

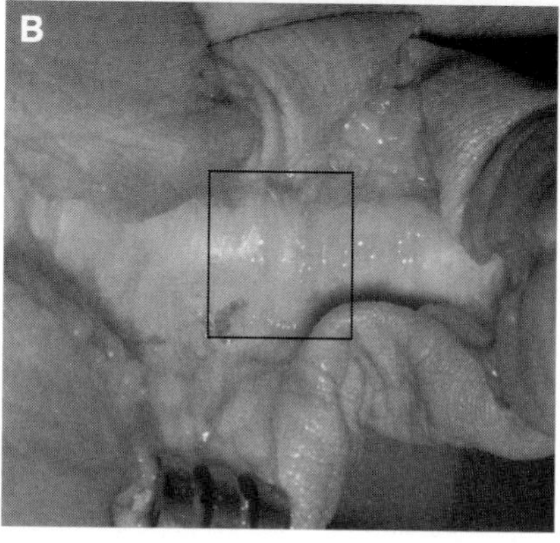

Fig. 9. (*A*) The C2 cruciate pulley in extension. (*B*) Its collapse to an annular form on flexion.

Pulley biomechanics and rock climbing

Flexor tendon and pulley biomechanics has particular significance in rock climbing injuries, 20% of which involve the flexor pulley system [54]; as many as 26% of elite rock climbers demonstrate clinical bowstringing [55]. The high load seen by the flexor tendons are almost exclusive to this sport, as the climber's full body weight may need to be supported by the distal phalanges alone. Of the two main grips used by climbers, the crimp and slope grips, the crimp grip, characterized by up to 100° of PIP flexion and DIP hyperextension, is favored by nearly 90% of climbers (Fig. 10). The advantage of the crimp grip is that it brings the middle phalanx away from the ledge, preventing injury to the skin. Schweizer found that the crimp grip produces a significant amount of FDP bowstringing at the PIP, placing stress on the distal portion of the A2 pulley [56]. This approaches maximum sheath strengths [26], which helps to explain the high incidence of sheath injuries and bowstringing in this population [57–62]. Biomechanic analysis of the A2 taping technique often used by rock climbers to prevent pulley ruptures was found to be minimally effective in relieving force on the A2 pulley and not at all effective in preventing pulley rupture [63].

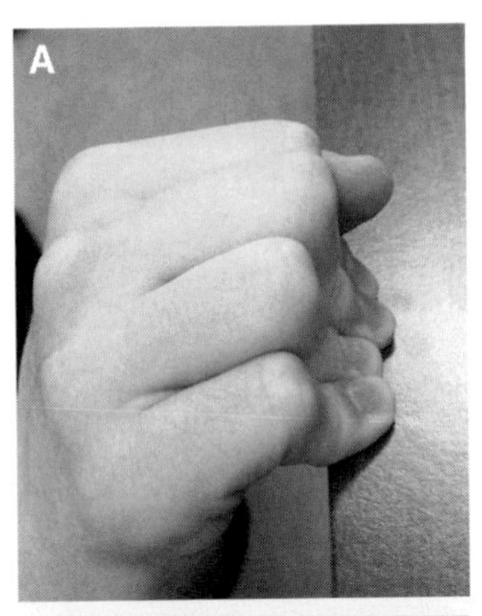

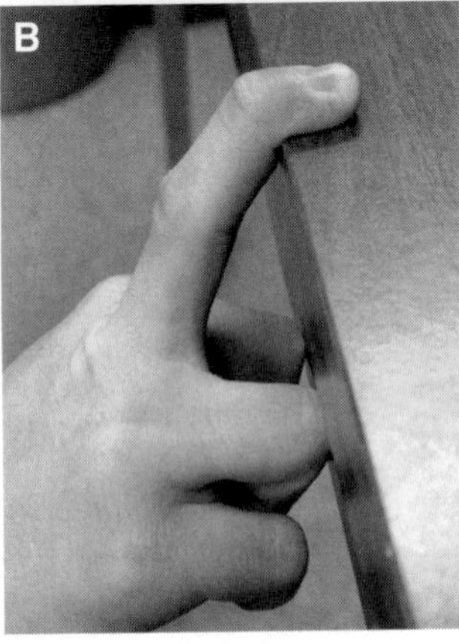

Fig. 10. The crimp (*A*) and slope (*B*) grips used in rock climbing.

Finger-moving tendons

Flexor digitorum profundus

The workhorse of the extrinsic finger flexion system is the FDP; accordingly, most of the literature on flexor tendons is devoted to its physiology, especially to the treatment of the injuries it sustains. The FDP is the only tendon with the ability to flex all three joints of the finger; in doing so, it provides most of the finger's strength [22].

The FDP muscle originates from the proximal medial and anterior surfaces of the ulna and the ulnar half of the interosseous membrane, and occasionally from the radius just distal to the radial tuberosity. As the single muscle belly travels distally in the forearm, it separates into an ulnar and a radial bundle. At the musculotendinous junction, the radial bundle forms the profundus tendon of the index finger, and the ulnar bundle forms the remaining three tendons. The muscles of the ulnar bundle are difficult to separate, and their interconnectedness continues into their tendinous portion. Fibers of cross-connection that occur at the level of the carpal tunnel make the tendons even more interdependent. They run through the carpal tunnel in a straight transverse row deep to the superficialis tendons and provide the insertion to the lumbricals as they course along the metacarpals. At this point, further interconnectedness of the third, fourth, and fifth tendons occurs as the two ulnar lumbricals are bipennate, each with origins from two FDP tendons. The FDP tendons then enter into the flexor sheath together with the FDS. As the superficialis tendons separate just proximal to the chiasm of Camper, the FDP flows through it, running along the middle phalanx to its insertion along the volar part of the distal phalanx. By crossing the MCP, PIP, and DIP joints, the FDP has a moment arm on each of them and can exert torque, thereby flexing them.

The mechanism by which the FDP produces flexion differs at each joint. At the DIP, flexion occurs by direct insertion into the distal phalanx.

At the PIP joint, flexion is implemented by other means. Because the FDP has a moment arm on the PIP, by shortening it exerts a flexing force. A secondary factor in flexion is the spiral oblique retinacular ligament, a fibrous link between the flexor sheath and the extensor tendon. As it passes the PIP, the oblique retinacular ligament lies volar to the axis of rotation; thus, with DIP flexion, tension is created in the spiral oblique retinacular ligament, flexing the PIP [22,53].

Although the ability of the FDP to flex the MCP joint may seem obvious, its role in the initiation of MCP flexion has been debated [64–68]. Without a direct attachment of an extrinsic flexor to the proximal phalanx, an alternative mechanism is needed—possibly translation of forces from the annular and cruciform pulley system attached to the phalanges [69] or propagation of moments created at the DIP and PIP joints. Kamper et al, using a computer simulation, found that with a passive joint torque the extrinsic flexors are capable of flexing all three finger joints [70]. Without this passive joint torque, simultaneous shortening of the FDP and FDS caused the finger to collapse into PIP flexion and slight MCP and DIP extension [53].

The tendon of the FDP has been studied in detail, and its mechanical properties have been found to vary along its length. Its vascular supply is from its dorsal surface; this part of the tendon has been found to be stronger, characterized by less collagen crosslinking and a larger cross-sectional area. This is significant when repairing the tendon, and it might be more prudent to place the core sutures in the more dorsal portion of the tendon. This has been substantiated experimentally by Soejima with the mean failure load of the dorsally placed sutures being 26.5% greater than those on the palmar side [71].

The FDP tendon has different shapes at different locations along its length [72]. At the MCP joint it is more or less oval, becomes triangular at the mid-proximal phalanx level (apex volar), and then continues to divide (with a volar groove) into two bundles (Fig. 11). These radial and ulnar bundles are separated but connected by the endotenon. Understanding this bundle anatomy can improve accuracy in partial laceration size assessment. It was long the consensus that lacerations involving more than 50% of the tendon's cross-sectional area warrant repair. Hariharan et al challenged this 50% rule by

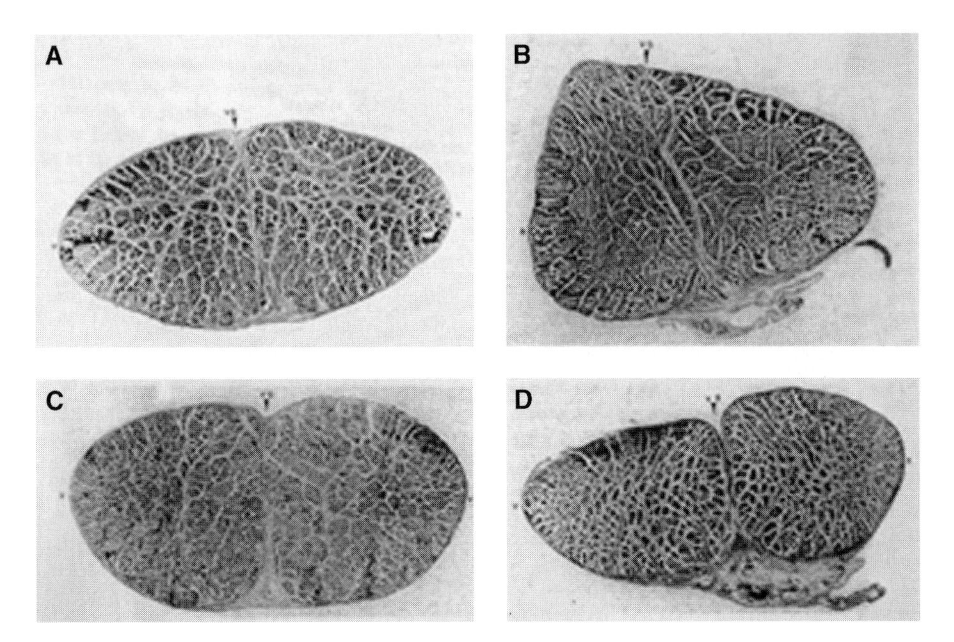

Fig. 11. Cross-sections of the FDP at different points along its course. (*A*) MCP joint (*B*) midpoint between MCP and PIP joint. (*C*) PIP joint (*D*) midpoint between PIP and DIP joint. VG, volar groove; R, radial side of the tendon; U, ulnar side of the tendon. (*From* Grewal R, Sotereanos DG, Rao U, Herndon JH, Woo SL. Bundle pattern of the flexor digitorum profundus tendon in zone II of the hand: a quantitative assessment of the size of a laceration. J Hand Surg [Am] 1996;21(6):978–83; with permission).

testing lacerations of 50% and 75%. They found that the threshold for failure of even a 75% laceration was higher than physiologic load levels for active unresisted motion, and thus questioned the need for primary repair of these injuries [73].

The force evident in the FDP has been hotly disputed, because it serves as the basis for the needed repair strength on tendon injury. Greenwald et al performed a dynamic analysis of the tendon using a specialized testing platform to test load, excursion, grip strength, pinch strength, and joint angle for loads up to 75 N [74]. They found that excursion was greatest at full fist with flexion of all three joints and flexion of the wrist with excursion of a medium-sized middle finger FDP tendon being approximately 6.0 cm (half of which was for wrist flexion); there was no plastic deformation of the tendons at these loads.

Flexor digitorum superficialis

Although often relegated to a secondary role, the FDS is a vital part of the flexor system, a fact that becomes most evident in its absence. In contrast to the FDP, which has one muscle belly, the FDS has four independent muscles. The tendons of the FDS enter into the carpal canal arranged as a square, with the index and little finger lying side-by-side, deep to the tendons of the middle and ring fingers. Lying superficial to the profundus tendons, the FDS tendons have a larger moment arm at the wrist and MCP joint. Each tendon then splits toward the base of the proximal phalanx, allowing the profundus tendon between them, rejoining at Camper's chiasm before splitting again to insert on the sides of the proximal part of the middle phalanx. Throughout this terminal course, they lie closer to the bone, giving it a smaller moment arm than the profundus, at the PIP joint. Furthermore, as the PIP joint flexes, the two terminal side branches of the superficialis can bowstring, adding to their moment arm and their effective flexing power.

Although the FDP, having more tension at its disposal, is the primary finger flexor, the FDS becomes more active as more force is needed. Different fingers use different proportions of FDP/FDS in flexion, related to the various strengths of the FDS muscles rather than to the strength of the FDPs. The middle finger FDS is approximately 75% stronger than those of the ring or index finger, and the little finger superficialis has only half of the latter's strength. This is evident in the relative ratio that each finger uses of the two tendons: the index FDS contributes approximately 28% to total tension, whereas in the middle finger 50% of the load is borne by its superficialis [22].

The FDS has four muscle bellies, making it possible to flex each PIP independently. Because the FDP has only one muscle belly, clinical testing for FDS function in individual fingers is possible. By holding three of the four digits in extension, the function of the conjoined FDP is eliminated, and any flexion of the PIP is the result of FDS contraction. The absence of the FDS can be tested with the DIP extension test [75]. Normally, when performing precision pinch with PIP flexion, the DIP hyperextends. Without the FDS, the FDP cannot simultaneously sustain PIP flexion and DIP hyperextension, leading to flexion of both joints.

Because the FDP can flex all finger joints, the superficialis tendon can be sacrificed as a donor for tendon transfers. Because of its length, strength, excursion, and ability to change direction, the FDS is considered an ideal candidate for transfers in certain situations. Its loss, however, is not without potential consequence. Without the insertion on the proximal part of the middle phalanx, the "superficialis minus finger" can develop, with loss of balance at the PIP leading to a hyperextension deformity. A compensatory DIP flexion deformity ensues as the FDS attempts to maintain tension along its length, which can lead to a swan-neck deformity. To avoid this deformity, the harvest can be done at the MCP joint, proximal to the A2 pulley. Potential pitfalls with harvest from this area include tendon scarring of the proximal stump, which can lead to PIP flexion contractures. This also has been shown to decrease the efficiency of the FDP tendon compared with loss distal to the A2 pulley [27].

The contribution of the FDS to finger balance and the inability of the FDP alone to control all three joints were eloquently illustrated by Brand using simple mechanics and moment arm analysis [22]. Because of increasing moment arms with the more proximal joints and because tension along the tendon must remain constant, the force generated by the FDP to resist a load at the fingertip is sufficient to prevent hyperextension at the DIP joint but not at the more proximal joints. Addition of the FDS provides the necessary tension at the PIP joint. Both tendons together are still incapable of controlling the MCP joint; this is where the flexion role of the intrinsics enters.

Lumbricals

The lumbricals have the unique distinction of having a moving origin and insertion. The origin of the lumbricals is along the FDP tendon as it courses along the metacarpal shaft. Each lumbrical remains volar and radial as it crosses the MCP joint. It then combines with tendon fibers from the interossei and inserts along the border of the radial lateral band of the extensor mechanism along the length of the proximal phalanx [65]. A recent study has shown that, although the origin of lumbricals is invariably on the FDP, they may be uni- or bipennate and that the insertion varies from the extensor tendon to the volar plate or even bone itself [76].

One would expect the lumbrical, by maintaining an axis of rotation volar to the MCP and dorsal to the PIP, to flex the MCP and extend the PIP joint. To flex the MCP, however, it must pull on the profundus with the same force that it exerts, negating its own effect on the MCP. Additionally, as it contracts, it pulls the FDP closer to the joint axis, lessening its moment arm, pulling it distally, and decreasing its flexion. The FDP therefore may function more efficiently without the lumbrical [77,78]. A cadaveric study demonstrated that without any FDP flexion, less than 5 N of lumbrical flexion brought the finger from rest to the intrinsic plus position. This demonstrates that besides PIP extension, the lumbrical alone can flex the MCP joint [77–79].

The role of the lumbrical at the IP joint is less controversial. Lumbrical contractions cause relaxation of the FDP and extend the IP joint by inserting on the radial lateral band of the extensor tendon, which lies dorsal to the axis of rotation of the joint. This is true regardless of MCP position.

It has been suggested that the lumbricals play a role in the closing sequence of the digits and in monitoring the rate of hand closure during grip [77,80]. Because of the moving origin and insertion of the lumbricals, biomechanic modeling of their behavior has been difficult. Wells and Ranney developed a method of loading the lumbrical in a cadaver hand based on a bicycle brake concept and demonstrated that without any other restraints, the index finger lumbrical moves the finger from the claw position to neutral to the intrinsic plus position [81].

Leijnse used a kinematic model of the lumbricals to demonstrate that they lie in an ideal position to provide fast movement and may be important to the musician [80]. He later evaluated the size of the lumbrical and found it to be most efficient, with increasing size becoming redundant [82].

The lumbrical plus finger nicely illustrates how loss of one part of the flexor system can lead to imbalance of function throughout the finger. In the case of lacerations to the FDP in an area distal to the origin of the lumbrical, a paradoxic extension of the digit may occur with attempted flexion. As the FDP loses its insertion it can act only through the remaining lumbrical, which, through its attachment on the lateral band, causes extension (Fig. 12).

Models of flexor tendon function

Mathematical and computer modeling has vastly improved understanding of the mechanical complexities of the human hand. Landsmeer's pioneering mathematical models have been substantiated by numerous studies. More recently, computer-generated models have yielded more insights into the mechanics of the hand. Although limitations exist, including variations in the size of individuals' hands, and disregard for sheath mechanics, modeling has still advanced understanding [83]. Clinically, biomechanic modeling has been used to elucidate forces in the FDP tendon and has helped determine necessary strengths for flexor tendon repairs [84,85]. Lieber et al have also demonstrated the ability of intraoperative modeling to evaluate the functional effects of tendon transfer surgery [83,86].

Landsmeer developed three models for the possible displacement of the tendon's path around the joint (Fig. 13) [87–89]. According to his first model, elegant in its simplicity, the tendon is securely maintained against the articular surfaces

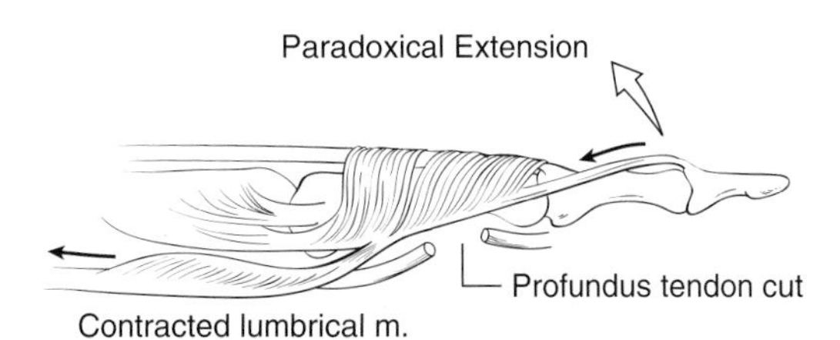

Fig. 12. The "lumbrical plus" finger, with a lacerated FDP pulling only on the lumbrical, causing paradoxic extension. (*From* 1996 Regional Review Courses in Hand Surgery [review course syllabus]. American Society for Surgery of the Hand, Englewood, CO 1996; with permission).

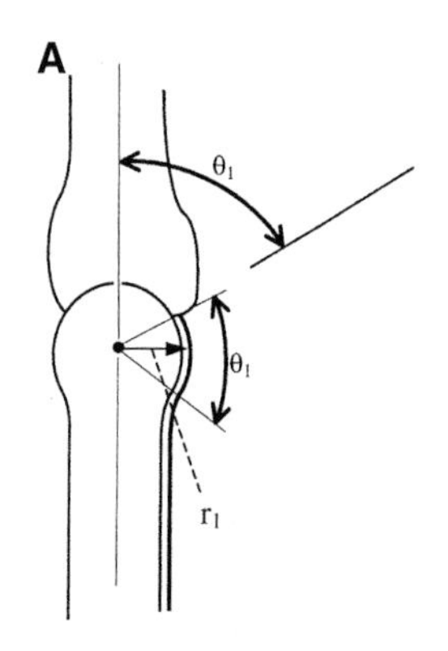

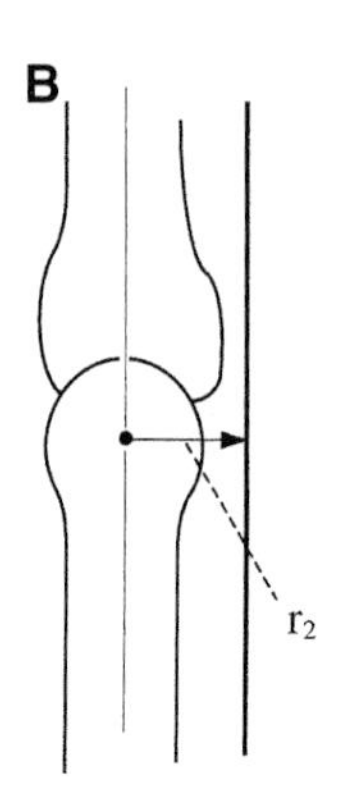

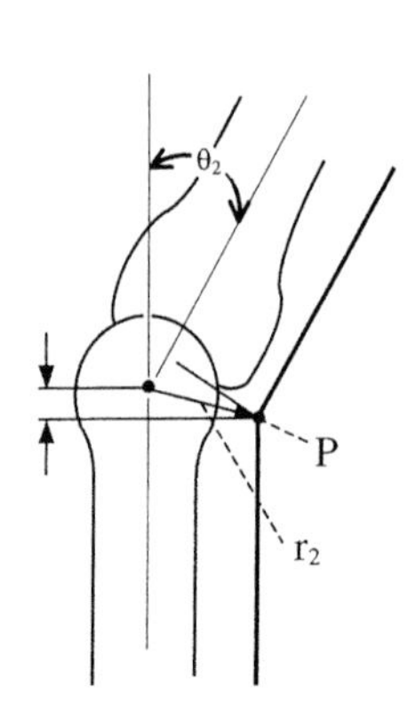

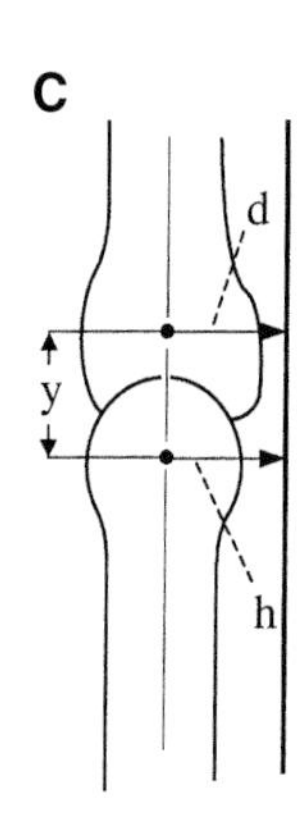

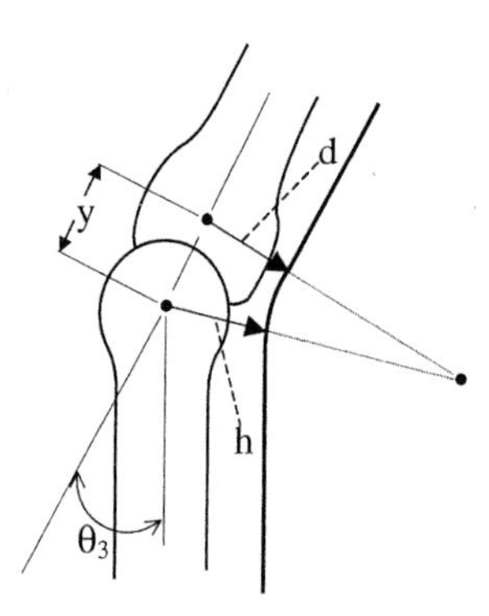

Fig. 13. Landsmeer's three models of finger tendon function. (*A*) First model. (*B*) Second model. (*C*) Third model. (*Adapted from* Armstrong TJ, Chaffin DB. An investigation of the relationship between displacements of the finger and wrist joints and the extrinsic finger flexor tendons. *J Biomech* 1978;11(3):119–28; with permission).

of the joints and the moment arm remains unchanged at all angles. Displacement of the tendon in this case is rendered as $x = r_1\theta_1$, where r_1 is the moment arm and the distance from the axis to the joint surface and θ_1 is the arc of motion through which the joint travels.

Landsmeer's second model takes into account anatomic considerations: the tendon is kept at a specified constant distance from the joint and phalanges. On joint motion, there is no bowstringing; rather, the tendon is constrained at a fixed geometric point *P*. The displacement of the tendon is described as $x = 2r_2\sin(\theta_2/2)$, where r_2 again is the moment arm, being the distance from the joint axis to the bending point *P* of the tendon.

Landsmeer's third model allows for physiologic bowstringing. As θ_3 increases, so does the moment arm. As the tendon arcs and shortens, a new variable is introduced: *y*, the distance along the axis of the bone at which the tendon begins to bowstring. This has been estimated at the proximal end of the A4 pulley. The displacement by the tendon at any angle of rotation is then

$$x = \theta_3 d + y(2 - \theta_3\tan\{\theta_3/2\}),$$

where *d* is the original distance of the tendon to the axis of rotation (equal to the distance from the tendon to the center of the bone at point *y*). As the moment arm also changes with the angle, it is described as

$$h = y\left[\frac{1 - \cos(\theta_3/2)}{\sin(\theta_3/2)}\right] + d.$$

At angles of $\theta_3 \leq 40°$

Landsmeer believed that his first model was almost equivalent to his third model. Armstrong measured the physiologic displacement of the tendons relative to the angles created (at individual joints) of $\leq 80°$ and found that the experimental data correlated best with Landsmeer's first model and that r_1 differed by hand size [83].

Although these early models accounted for force only in a straight path, advanced models have greater analytic flexibility. Thompson developed a multi-joint model based on the idea that as each point on a phalanx is moved, its new position can be calculated by a transformation matrix in three dimensions. The tendon's course is described by a combination of multiple elements, including straight segments inside pulleys, curved segments between pulleys, and divergent segments such as the insertion of the FDS. By linking these paths together (like sections of track in a model train set), Thompson's model linked the properties of each path to a whole, allowing calculation of tendon excursion for any given joint motion. Comparison of the results of this analysis with data for excursion and joint position from previous studies revealed an error of less than 10% [90].

Several other models have combined kinematic, computer, and radiographic modalities to simulate forces and stresses on other forearm muscles and the flexors [80,91,92]. Fowler and Nicol created a model using MRI to obtain moment arms and tendon lines of action in three dimensions. Results using their model agreed with other studies that measured tendon force in the hand [84,93–95].

Clinical applications

Biomechanics of flexor tendon repairs

Most biomechanic studies on the digital flexor tendons focus on the repair and rehabilitation of flexor tendon injuries, mostly in zone II. Long labeled a surgical "No Man's Land," zone II flexor tendon lacerations are now almost always considered for primary repair. Outcomes in function and motion remain less than ideal, and so the search for a better repair and rehabilitation protocol continues. Such a repair should maximize intrinsic healing while limiting extrinsic healing and adhesion formation, be strong enough to prevent rupture and gapping during an early motion rehabilitation program, and yet be technically feasible for routine use.

The biomechanics of tendon healing and repair has been the source of considerable debate for almost a century. The importance of early motion and prevention of adhesion formation was discussed by Konrad Biesalski in 1910, Erich Lexer in 1912, and Leo Mayer in 1916 [96]. Mayer also published a series of articles elaborating the role of the digital sheath, tendon nutrition, and blood supply, and stressing the importance of tendon sheath motion [97,98]. In the early 1920s Sterling Bunnell set forth the essential principles of hand surgery, including atraumatic technique, preservation of the pulley system, and avoidance of infection, all aimed at limitation of scar formation [99,100]. Although Bunnell's use of the term "No Man's Land" to describe zone II lacerations was long taken to imply that these injuries should be considered off-limits for surgery [101], it was Bunnell himself who in 1940 established the conditions needed for primary flexor tendon repair and described how motion stimulates growth and minimizes adhesions [102]. The misunderstanding over the term caused a reluctance for primary flexor tendon repair in zone II for many years, perhaps curtailing the advancement of flexor tendon surgery [103].

According to the timeline for tendon healing established by Mason and Allen in 1941, tensile force reaches its lowest level on postoperative day 5 and only returns to its immediate postoperative level by postoperative day 19 [104]. This observation led many to believe that a 3-week waiting period of immobilization is necessary to prevent rupture. Kleinert and Duran, however, later demonstrated that passive or active unresisted motion yields better results than immobilization [105,106], and Gelberman in a series of articles demonstrated the ability of tendons subjected to early passive motion to heal with few adhesions and scar formation [107–112].

Tendon healing proceeds through three phases: inflammation, proliferation, and remodeling. It starts with the migration of peripheral cells and proliferation of external capillaries. The tendon edges then can unite with the help of these surrounding tissues, with the final stage of remodeling occurring with motion. Beyond these basic facts, two broad theories of tendon repair have long competed for legitimacy. The extrinsic theory, first put forward by Potenza and Peacock, holds that tendons in and of themselves are inert and require external factors for healing, that the synovial sheath is the sole requisite for healing, and that the tendon itself plays no role in its own repair [113–117].

According to the second, intrinsic theory, the tendon has inherent healing capabilities. Lundberg showed that, even when isolated from its synovium, the tendon exhibits end encapsulation [118–121]. Becker was the first to illustrate that tendon fibroblasts contribute to repair by producing collagen; he created a hole in chicken tendon and added a plasma clot, which resulted in tendon cell migration and proliferation and subsequent collagen synthesis [122]. Manske later argued that direct (perfusion) and indirect (diffusion) nutrient pathways are important to tendon healing. He demonstrated that diffusion is not only as effective as perfusion, but can even provide necessary support in the absence of a perfusing vessel [123–126]. Mass substantiated this finding by demonstrating the intrinsic healing capabilities of human tendons in vitro [127,128].

It is likely that tendon heals by way of intrinsic and extrinsic mechanisms. Current repair techniques and rehabilitation protocols must take a balanced approach by controlling rigid adhesions and providing enough strength to permit motion to stimulate diffusion. Although early motion is necessary, it is attended by the risk for rupture. Even given the decrease in tensile strength postoperatively, current methods of surgical repair provide sufficient strength to start early active motion while paying attention to reducing adhesions and increasing synovial diffusion. As hand surgeons approach the limits of their ability to control gap formation, tendon excursion, and force during rehabilitation, further progress in tendon repair may require controlling the biologic factors associated with healing on the cellular and molecular levels. Treatments of this type include injection of progenitor cells and manipulation of DNA with gene therapy [129–131]. Studies have investigated the insertion of DNA coding for wanted proteins into healing tendons. For example, PDGF-B has been shown to enhance angiogenesis and matrix formation [132,133]. Unwanted proteins have also been investigated, such as pp125FAK, whose overexpression may induce adhesion formation [134].

Testing methods

Numerous methodologies have been used to test flexor tendon repairs, in humans and animals, including single load-to-failure tests and cyclic testing, and testing in linear and curvilinear modes. Unfortunately a lack of uniformity among these studies has resulted in wide ranging results that make comparisons difficult.

In vitro linear loading to failure is an extra-anatomic testing method that tests the tendon in isolation. It allows for testing large numbers of tendons and allows direct visualization of the tendon during testing so that gap formation is measured easily. It ignores the physiologic loading and environment of the tendon, sheath mechanics, and the effects of the post-repair milieu. Gripping of the tendon in the linear testing machine has been problematic because of slippage, which could produce erroneously increased strain measurements. This has been used in human and animal tendons. Testing can be performed cyclically and single load to failure. In vitro linear loading test's major use has been in direct comparison of various primarily to compare suture methods [135–139].

Curvilinear testing leaves the tendon within the intact hand [140–142]. During finger motion a variety of forces are applied to the tendon, including tension on the dorsal surface, compression on the volar surface, and frictional forces within the sheath. An example of a curvilinear testing apparatus is seen in Fig. 14. The disadvantage of curvilinear testing is that it cannot be used to visually examine tendon during the loading cycle, and thus gap measurements are difficult to assess.

The greatest limitation of biomechanic testing in the cadaveric human hand model is that it can only provide information on the immediate post-repair state; it cannot simulate the healing environment. Because ruptures, gapping, and adhesion formation usually occur days or weeks after surgery, their effects on the repair can only be assumed or extrapolated from animal models.

Tendon forces

Successful tendon surgery is predicated on the repaired tendon's ability to withstand the forces of early motion. Although there are many studies about obtaining a strong repair, there are few biomechanic studies of forces in the human flexor profundus tendon, and those few are mutually inconsistent in methodology. Mathematical and spatial analyses [84,85], direct measures in vivo [143,144], and in vitro cadaveric studies [136] have all been performed with great variability and little correlation among them. The studies most often quoted in the hand literature are those of Urbaniak [143] and Schuind [144], who found flexor tendon forces ranging from 9–22 N. Although performed on tendons in vivo, neither study accounted for changes in biomechanics after

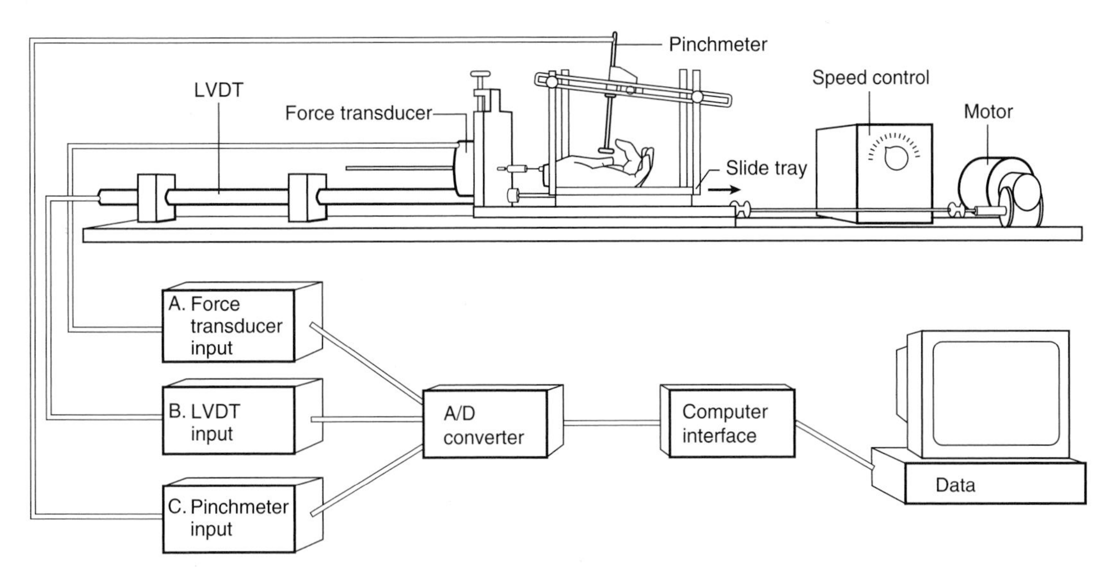

Fig. 14. Curvilinear, cyclical testing apparatus used to replicate natural tendon motion. LVDT, linear variable differential transformer. (*From* Choueka J, Heminger H, Mass DP. Cyclical testing of zone II flexor tendon repairs. J Hand Surg [Am] 2000;25(6):1127–34; with permission).

repair, including decreased gliding ability, edema, and postoperative pain. Additional limitations include calculated (as opposed to directly measured) forces and lack of external controls, as sedated and anesthetized patients were asked to apply the forces.

Several studies have based treatment regimens on Urbaniak and Schuind's values. Savage postulated that, based on the known decrease in repair strength postoperatively, initial repair strengths to permit active motion should be in the vicinity of 75 N [137]. Much recent research has been aimed at developing the strongest repair to allow active motion postoperatively. These studies include use of multistrand repairs, locking sutures, changing location of repair, various suture calibers and sizes, tendon splints and grafts, and even metallic implants [145–150]. Unfortunately, because repairs and techniques become increasingly complex, the attendant disadvantages multiply, such as increased operative time, cost, expertise, and manipulation of the tendon, the last of which has been shown to increase adhesion formation [111,151].

Although certain in vitro techniques and methods clearly result in superior strength, clinical results show that rupture rates with an active motion protocol remain low regardless of the technique used [137,145,152–166]. Clinical in vivo studies of the Kessler repair with a known strength of 20–30 N have reported rupture rates of only 3%–9% [152]. If 75 N or more strength were needed, one would expect a 100% rupture rate with this weaker repair. Intrinsic tendon forces thus may have been overestimated. Choueka et al tested this theory in an in vitro study using a curvilinear model to evaluate the tendon forces experienced during a simulated active rehabilitation protocol. In vitro forces in tendons were found to range from 2.4–3.8 N, which is 3 to nearly 10 times less than values previously reported in vivo. To satisfy the forces from in vitro tests, two-strand repairs with initial strengths of 25 N thus may be acceptable for initiating early motion protocols [167]. Based on the in vivo forces seen by Schuind [144] and Urbaniak [143] and the known decreases in repair strength ranging from 60%–80% [104,143], however, a multistrand repair (such as was found with the four-strand locking cruciate repair) would satisfy all criteria.

References

[1] Kannus P, Jozsa L, Natri A, Jarvinen M. Effects of training, immobilization and remobilization on tendons. Scand J Med Sci Sports 1997;7(2):67–71.

[2] Jozsa L, Kannus P. Histopathological findings in spontaneous tendon ruptures. Scand J Med Sci Sports 1997;7(2):113–8.

[3] Thomopoulos S, Williams GR, Gimbel JA, Favata M, Soslowsky LJ. Variation of biomechanical, structural, and compositional properties along the

tendon to bone insertion site. J Orthop Res 2003;21(3):413–9.
[4] Okuda Y, Gorski JP, An KN, Amadio PC. Biochemical, histological, and biomechanical analyses of canine tendon. J Orthop Res 1987;5(1):60–8.
[5] Woo S, An KN, Frank C, et al. Anatomy, biology, and biomechanics of tendon and ligament. In: Buckwalter JA, Einhorn TA, Simon SR, editors. Orthopaedic basic science. 2nd edition. St. Louis: American Academy of Orthopaedic Surgeons; 2000.
[6] Kastelic J, Galeski A, Baer E. The multicomposite structure of tendon. Connect Tissue Res 1978;6(1):11–23.
[7] Monleon Pradas M, Diaz Calleja R. Nonlinear viscoelastic behaviour of the flexor tendon of the human hand. J Biomech 1990;23(8):773–81.
[8] O'Brien M. Functional anatomy and physiology of tendons. Clin Sports Med 1992;11(3):505–20.
[9] Patterson-Kane JC, Wilson AM, Firth EC, Parry DA, Goodship AE. Exercise-related alterations in crimp morphology in the central regions of superficial digital flexor tendons from young thoroughbreds: a controlled study. Equine Vet J 1998;30(1):61–4.
[10] Woo SL, Gomez MA, Woo YK, Akeson WH. Mechanical properties of tendons and ligaments. II. The relationships of immobilization and exercise on tissue remodeling. Biorheology 1982;19(3):397–408.
[11] Lin TW, Cardenas L, Soslowsky LJ. Biomechanics of tendon injury and repair. J Biomech 2004;37(6):865–77.
[12] Yamamoto E, Hayashi K, Yamamoto N. Effects of stress shielding on the transverse mechanical properties of rabbit patellar tendons. J Biomech Eng 2000;122(6):608–14.
[13] Yamamoto N, Ohno K, Hayashi K, Kuriyama H, Yasuda K, Kaneda K. Effects of stress shielding on the mechanical properties of rabbit patellar tendon. J Biomech Eng 1993;115(1):23–8.
[14] Cherdchutham W, Becker C, Smith RK, Barneveld A, van Weeren PR. Age-related changes and effect of exercise on the molecular composition of immature equine superficial digital flexor tendons. Equine Vet J Suppl 1999;(31):86–94.
[15] Cherdchutham W, Becker CK, Spek ER, Voorhout WF, van Weeren PR. Effects of exercise on the diameter of collagen fibrils in the central core and periphery of the superficial digital flexor tendon in foals. Am J Vet Res 2001;62(10):1563–70.
[16] Patterson-Kane JC, Firth EC, Goodship AE, Parry DA. Age-related differences in collagen crimp patterns in the superficial digital flexor tendon core region of untrained horses. Aust Vet J 1997;75(1):39–44.
[17] Reddy G. Glucose-mediated in vitro glycation modulates biomechanical integrity of the soft tissues but not hard tissues. J Orthop Res 2003;21:738–43.
[18] Gum SL, Reddy GK, Stehno-Bittel L, Enwemeka CS. Combined ultrasound, electrical stimulation, and laser promote collagen synthesis with moderate changes in tendon biomechanics. Am J Phys Med Rehabil 1997;76(4):288–96.
[19] Enwemeka CS, Rodriguez O, Mendosa S. The biomechanical effects of low-intensity ultrasound on healing tendons. Ultrasound Med Biol 1990;16(8):801–7.
[20] Enwemeka CS. The effects of therapeutic ultrasound on tendon healing. A biomechanical study. Am J Phys Med Rehabil 1989;68(6):283–7.
[21] Robotti E, Zimbler AG, Kenna D, Grossman JA. The effect of pulsed electromagnetic fields on flexor tendon healing in chickens. J Hand Surg [Br] 1999;24(1):56–8.
[22] Brand PW, Hollister AM. Clinical mechanics of the hand. 3rd edition. St. Louis: Mosby; 1999.
[23] Freehafer AA, Peckham PH, Keith MW. Determination of muscle–tendon unit properties during tendon transfer. J Hand Surg [Am] 1979;4(4):331–9.
[24] Wehbe MA, Hunter JM. Flexor tendon gliding in the hand. Part I. In vivo excursions. J Hand Surg [Am] 1985;10(4):570–4.
[25] Doyle JR. Palmar and digital flexor tendon pulleys. Clin Orthop 2001;383:84–96.
[26] Lin GT, Amadio PC, An KN, Cooney WP. Functional anatomy of the human digital flexor pulley system. J Hand Surg [Am] 1989;14(6):949–56.
[27] Tang JB, Xu Y, Chen F. Impact of flexor digitorum superficialis on gliding function of the flexor digitorum profundus according to regions in zone II. J Hand Surg [Am] 2003;28(5):838–44.
[28] Tang JB. The double sheath system and tendon gliding in zone 2C. J Hand Surg [Br] 1995;20(3):281–5.
[29] Walbeehm ET, McGrouther DA. An anatomical study of the mechanical interactions of flexor digitorum superficialis and profundus and the flexor tendon sheath in zone 2. J Hand Surg [Br] 1995;20(3):269–80.
[30] Zhao C, Amadio PC, Momose T, Zobitz ME, Couvreur P, An KN. Remodeling of the gliding surface after flexor tendon repair in a canine model in vivo. J Orthop Res 2002;20(4):857–62.
[31] Zhao C, Amadio PC, Zobitz ME, An KN. Resection of the flexor digitorum superficialis reduces gliding resistance after zone II flexor digitorum profundus repair in vitro. J Hand Surg [Am] 2002;27(2):316–21.
[32] Peterson WW, Manske PR, Bollinger BA, Lesker PA, McCarthy JA. Effect of pulley excision on flexor tendon biomechanics. J Orthop Res 1986;4(1):96–101.

[33] Savage R. The mechanical effect of partial resection of the digital fibrous flexor sheath. J Hand Surg [Br] 1990;15(4):435–42.
[34] Paillard PJ, Amadio PC, Zhao C, Zobitz ME, An KN. Pulley plasty versus resection of one slip of the flexor digitorum superficialis after repair of both flexor tendons in zone II: a biomechanical study. J Bone Joint Surg [Am] 2002;84A(11): 2039–45.
[35] Zhao CF, Amadio PC, Berglund L, An KN. The A3 pulley. J Hand Surg [Am] 2000;25(2):270–6.
[36] Mitsionis G, Fischer KJ, Bastidas JA, Grewal R, Pfaeffle HJ, Tomaino MM. Feasibility of partial A2 and A4 pulley excision: residual pulley strength. J Hand Surg [Br] 2000;25(1):90–4.
[37] Tang JB, Wang YH, Gu YT, Chen F. Effect of pulley integrity on excursions and work of flexion in healing flexor tendons. J Hand Surg [Am] 2001; 26(2):347–53.
[38] Tomaino M, Mitsionis G, Basitidas J, Grewal R, Pfaeffle J. The effect of partial excision of the A2 and A4 pulleys on the biomechanics of finger flexion. J Hand Surg [Br] 1998;23(1):50–2.
[39] Hume EL, Hutchinson DT, Jaeger SA, Hunter JM. Biomechanics of pulley reconstruction. J Hand Surg [Am] 1991;16(4):722–30.
[40] Rispler D, Greenwald D, Shumway S, Allan C, Mass D. Efficiency of the flexor tendon pulley system in human cadaver hands. J Hand Surg [Am] 1996;21(3):444–50.
[41] Kline SC, Moore JR. The transverse carpal ligament. An important component of the digital flexor pulley system. J Bone Joint Surg [Am] 1992;74(10): 1478–85.
[42] Netscher D, Lee M, Thornby J, Polsen C. The effect of division of the transverse carpal ligament on flexor tendon excursion. J Hand Surg [Am] 1997; 22(6):1016–24.
[43] Netscher D, Dinh T, Cohen V, Thornby J. Division of the transverse carpal ligament and flexor tendon excursion: open and endoscopic carpal tunnel release. Plast Reconstr Surg 1998;102(3): 773–8.
[44] Netscher D, Mosharrafa A, Lee M, et al. Transverse carpal ligament: its effect on flexor tendon excursion, morphologic changes of the carpal canal, and on pinch and grip strengths after open carpal tunnel release. Plast Reconstr Surg 1997;100(3): 636–42.
[45] Gellman H, Kan D, Gee V, Kuschner SH, Botte MJ. Analysis of pinch and grip strength after carpal tunnel release. J Hand Surg [Am] 1989; 14(5):863–4.
[46] Manske PR, Lesker PA. Palmar aponeurosis pulley. J Hand Surg [Am] 1983;8(3):259–63.
[47] Doyle JR. Anatomy and function of the palmar aponeurosis pulley. J Hand Surg [Am] 1990;15(1): 78–82.
[48] Phillips C, Mass D. Mechanical analysis of the palmar aponeurosis pulley in human cadavers. J Hand Surg [Am] 1996;21(2):240–4.
[49] Doyle JR, Blythe W. The finger flexor tendon sheath and pulleys: anatomy and reconstruction. In: Hunter JM, Schneider LH, editors. AAOS Symposium on Tendon Surgery in the Hand. St. Louis: CV Mosby; 1975. p. 81–7.
[50] Peterson WW, Manske PR, Kain CC, Lesker PA. Effect of flexor sheath integrity on tendon gliding: a biomechanical and histologic study. J Orthop Res 1986;4(4):458–65.
[51] Mitsionis G, Bastidas JA, Grewal R, Pfaeffle HJ, Fischer KJ, Tomaino MM. Feasibility of partial A2 and A4 pulley excision: effect on finger flexor tendon biomechanics. J Hand Surg [Am] 1999; 24(2):310–4.
[52] Tang JB, Xie RG. Effect of A3 pulley and adjacent sheath integrity on tendon excursion and bowstringing. J Hand Surg [Am] 2001;26(5):855–61.
[53] Idler RS. Anatomy and biomechanics of the digital flexor tendons. Hand Clin 1985;1(1):3–11.
[54] Schoffl V, Hochholzer T, Winkelmann HP, Strecker W. Pulley injuries in rock climbers. Wilderness Environ Med 2003;14(2):94–100.
[55] Rohrbough JT, Mudge MK, Schilling RC. Overuse injuries in the elite rock climber. Med Sci Sports Exerc 2000;32(8):1369–72.
[56] Schweizer A. Biomechanical properties of the crimp grip position in rock climbers. J Biomech 2001;34(2):217–23.
[57] Marco RA, Sharkey NA, Smith TS, Zissimos AG. Pathomechanics of closed rupture of the flexor tendon pulleys in rock climbers. J Bone Joint Surg [Am] 1998;80(7):1012–9.
[58] Bollen SR. Soft tissue injury in extreme rock climbers. Br J Sports Med 1988;22(4):145–7.
[59] Bollen SR. Injury to the A2 pulley in rock climbers. J Hand Surg [Br] 1990;15(2):268–70.
[60] Bollen SR. Upper limb injuries in elite rock climbers. JR Coll Surg Edinb 1990;35(6 Suppl): S18–20.
[61] Bollen SR, Gunson CK. Hand injuries in competition climbers. Br J Sports Med 1990;24(1):16–8.
[62] Bollen SR, Wright V. Radiographic changes in the hands of rock climbers. Br J Sports Med 1994; 28(3):185–6.
[63] Schweizer A. Biomechanical effectiveness of taping the A2 pulley in rock climbers. J Hand Surg [Br] 2000;25(1):102–7.
[64] Long C II. Intrinsic–extrinsic muscle control of the fingers. J Bone Joint Surg [Am] 1968;50A:973–84.
[65] Zancolli E. Structural and dynamic bases of hand surgery. 2nd edition. Philadelphia: JB Lippincott Co.; 1979.
[66] Moore KL, Dalley AF II. Clinically oriented anatomy. Philadelphia: Lippincott Williams & Wilkins; 1999.

[67] Snell R. Clinical anatomy for medical students. Philadelphia: Lippincott Williams & Wilkins; 2000.
[68] Darling W, Cole WK, Miller GF. Coordination of index finger movements. J Biomech 1994;27: 479–91.
[69] Bejjani F, Landsmeer JMF. Biomechanics of the hand. In: Nordin M, Frankel VH, editors. Basic biomechanics of the musculoskeletal system. Philadelphia: Lea & Febiger; 1989. p. 275–304.
[70] Kamper DG, George Hornby T, Rymer WZ. Extrinsic flexor muscles generate concurrent flexion of all three finger joints. J Biomech 2002;35(12): 1581–9.
[71] Soejima O, Diao E, Lotz JC, Hariharan JS. Comparative mechanical analysis of dorsal versus palmar placement of core suture for flexor tendon repairs. J Hand Surg [Am] 1995;20(5):801–7.
[72] Grewal R, Sotereanos DG, Rao U, Herndon JH, Woo SL. Bundle pattern of the flexor digitorum profundus tendon in zone II of the hand: a quantitative assessment of the size of a laceration. J Hand Surg [Am] 1996;21(6):978–83.
[73] Hariharan JS, Diao E, Soejima O, Lotz JC. Partial lacerations of human digital flexor tendons: a biomechanical analysis. J Hand Surg [Am] 1997; 22(6):1011–5.
[74] Greenwald D, Shumway S, Allen C, Mass D. Dynamic analysis of profundus tendon function. J Hand Surg [Am] 1994;19(4):626–35.
[75] Dogan T, Celebiler O, Gurunluoglu R, Bayramicli M, Numanoglu A. A new test for superficialis flexor tendon function. Ann Plast Surg 2000;45(1):93–6.
[76] Eladoumikdachi F, Valkov PL, Thomas J, Netscher DT. Anatomy of the intrinsic hand muscles revisited: part II. Lumbricals. Plast Reconstr Surg 2002; 110(5):1225–31.
[77] Ranney D, Wells R. Lumbrical muscle function as revealed by a new and physiological approach. Anat Rec 1988;222(1):110–4.
[78] Ranney DA. Some aspects of lumbrical function. J Hand Surg [Br] 1988;13(4):483–4.
[79] Ranney DA, Wells RP, Dowling J. Lumbrical function: interaction of lumbrical contraction with the elasticity of the extrinsic finger muscles and its effect on metacarpophalangeal equilibrium. J Hand Surg [Am] 1987;12(4):566–75.
[80] Leijnse JN, Kalker JJ. A two-dimensional kinematic model of the lumbrical in the human finger. J Biomech 1995;28(3):237–49.
[81] Wells RP, Ranney DA. Lumbrical length changes in finger movement: a new method of study in fresh cadaver hands. J Hand Surg [Am] 1986;11(4): 574–7.
[82] Leijnse JN. Why the lumbrical muscle should not be bigger–a force model of the lumbrical in the unloaded human finger. J Biomech 1997;30(11–12):1107–14.
[83] Armstrong TJ, Chaffin DB. An investigation of the relationship between displacements of the finger and wrist joints and the extrinsic finger flexor tendons. J Biomech 1978;11(3):119–28.
[84] Fowler NK, Nicol AC. Interphalangeal joint and tendon forces: normal model and biomechanical consequences of surgical reconstruction. J Biomech 2000;33(9):1055–62.
[85] Lotz JC, Hariharan JS, Diao E. Analytic model to predict the strength of tendon repairs. J Orthop Res 1998;16(4):399–405.
[86] Lieber RL, Friden J. Intraoperative measurement and biomechanical modeling of the flexor carpi ulnaris-to-extensor carpi radialis longus tendon transfer. J Biomech Eng 1997;119(4):386–91.
[87] Landsmeer JM. Anatomical and functional investigations on the articulation of the human fingers. Acta Anat (Basel) 1955;25(Suppl 24):1–69.
[88] Landsmeer JM. A report on the coordination of the interphalangeal joints of the human finger and its disturbances. Acta Morphol Neerl Scand 1958; 2(1):59–84.
[89] Landsmeer JM. The kinetic apparatus of the human finger; anatomical structure and functional significance. Ned Tijdschr Geneeskd 26 1952; 96(17):1039–41.
[90] Thompson DE, Giurintano DJ. A kinematic model of the flexor tendons of the hand. J Biomech 1989; 22(4):327–34.
[91] Leijnse JN. A graphic analysis of the biomechanics of the massless bi-articular chain. Application to the proximal bi-articular chain of the human finger. J Biomech 1996;29(3):355–66.
[92] Freund J, Takala EP. A dynamic model of the forearm including fatigue. J Biomech 2001;34(5): 597–605.
[93] Fowler NK, Nicol AC, Condon B, Hadley D. Method of determination of three dimensional index finger moment arms and tendon lines of action using high resolution MRI scans. J Biomech 2001; 34(6):791–7.
[94] Fowler NK, Nicol AC. Functional and biomechanical assessment of the normal and rheumatoid hand. Clin Biomech (Bristol, Avon) 2001;16(8): 660–6.
[95] Fowler NK, Nicol AC. Measurement of external three-dimensional interphalangeal loads applied during activities of daily living. Clin Biomech (Bristol, Avon) 1999;14(9):646–52.
[96] Kleinert JM, McGoldrick FM, Papas NH. Concepts that changed flexor tendon surgery. In: Mackin EJ, editor. Tendon and nerve surgery in the hand: A third decade. St. Louis: Mosby-Year Book, Inc.; 1997. p. 307–13.
[97] Mayer L. The physiologic method of tendon transplantation. Surg Gynecol Obstet 1916;22: 182–92.
[98] Mayer L. Repair of severed tendons. Am J Surg 1938;12:714.
[99] Bunnell S. Repair of tendons in the fingers. Surg Gynecol Obstet 1922;35:88–97.

[100] Bunnell S. Reconstructive surgery of the hand. Surg Gynecol Obstet 1924;39:259–74.
[101] Bunnell S. Surgery of the hand. 2nd edition. Philadelphia: JB Lippincott; 1948.
[102] Bunnell S. Primary repair of severed tendons. The use of stainless steel wire. Am J Surg 1940;47: 502–16.
[103] Newmeyer WL III, Manske PR. No man's land revisited: the primary flexor tendon repair controversy. J Hand Surg [Am] 2004;29(1):1–5.
[104] Mason M, Allen HS. The rate of healing of tendons: an experimental study of tensile strength. Ann Surg 1941;113:424–59.
[105] Kleinert HE, Cash SL. Management of acute flexor tendon injuries in the hand. Instr Course Lect 1985; 34:361–72.
[106] Kleinert HE, Spokevicius S, Papas NH. History of flexor tendon repair. J Hand Surg [Am] 1995; 20(3 Pt 2):S46–52.
[107] Gelberman RH, Boyer MI, Brodt MD, Winters SC, Silva MJ. The effect of gap formation at the repair site on the strength and excursion of intrasynovial flexor tendons. An experimental study on the early stages of tendon-healing in dogs. J Bone Joint Surg [Am] 1999;81(7):975–82.
[108] Gelberman RH, Siegel DB, Woo SL, Amiel D, Takai S, Lee D. Healing of digital flexor tendons: importance of the interval from injury to repair. A biomechanical, biochemical, and morphological study in dogs. J Bone Joint Surg [Am] 1991;73(1): 66–75.
[109] Gelberman RH, Nunley JA Jr, Osterman AL, Breen TF, Dimick MP, Woo SL. Influences of the protected passive mobilization interval on flexor tendon healing. A prospective randomized clinical study. Clin Orthop 1991;264:189–96.
[110] Gelberman RH, Woo SL, Amiel D, Horibe S, Lee D. Influences of flexor sheath continuity and early motion on tendon healing in dogs. J Hand Surg [Am] 1990;15(1):69–77.
[111] Gelberman RH, Manske PR. Factors influencing flexor tendon adhesions. Hand Clin 1985;1(1): 35–42.
[112] Gelberman RH, Vandeberg JS, Manske PR, Akeson WH. The early stages of flexor tendon healing: a morphologic study of the first fourteen days. J Hand Surg [Am] 1985;10(6 Pt 1):776–84.
[113] Potenza AD. Tendon healing within the flexor digital sheath in the dog. Am J Orthop 1962;44A: 49–64.
[114] Peacock EE Jr. Biological principles in the healing of long tendons. Surg Clin N Am 1965;45: 461–76.
[115] Peacock EE Jr. Fundamental aspects of wound healing relating to the restoration of gliding function after tendon repair. Surg Gynecol Obstet 1964;119:241–50.
[116] Potenza AD. Critical evaluation of flexor-tendon healing and adhesion formation within artificial digital sheaths. J Bone Joint Surg [Am] 1963;45: 1217–33.
[117] Potenza AD. Prevention of adhesions to healing digital flexor tendons. JAMA 1964;187: 187–91.
[118] Lundborg G, Rank F. Experimental intrinsic healing of flexor tendons based upon synovial fluid nutrition. J Hand Surg [Am] 1978;3(1):21–31.
[119] Lundborg G, Rank F. Experimental studies on cellular mechanisms involved in healing of animal and human flexor tendon in synovial environment. Hand 1980;12(1):3–11.
[120] Lundborg G, Holm S, Myrhage R. The role of the synovial fluid and tendon sheath for flexor tendon nutrition. An experimental tracer study on diffusional pathways in dogs. Scand J Plast Reconstr Surg 1980;14(1):99–107.
[121] Lundborg G, Rank F, Heinau B. Intrinsic tendon healing. A new experimental model. Scand J Plast Reconstr Surg 1985;19(2):113–7.
[122] Becker H, Graham MF, Cohen IK, Diegelmann RF. Intrinsic tendon cell proliferation in tissue culture. J Hand Surg [Am] 1981;6(6):616–9.
[123] Manske PR, Gelberman RH, Vande Berg JS, Lesker PA. Intrinsic flexor-tendon repair. A morphological study in vitro. J Bone Joint Surg [Am] 1984;66(3):385–96.
[124] Manske PR, Bridwell K, Whiteside LA, Lesker PA. Nutrition of flexor tendons in monkeys. Clin Orthop 1978;136:294–8.
[125] Manske PR, Lesker PA. Nutrient pathways of flexor tendons in primates. J Hand Surg [Am] 1982;7(5): 436–44.
[126] Manske PR, Lesker PA. Flexor tendon nutrition. Hand Clin 1985;1(1):13–24.
[127] Mass DP, Tuel R. Human flexor tendon participation in the in vitro repair process. J Hand Surg [Am] 1989;14(1):64–71.
[128] Mass DP, Tuel RJ. Intrinsic healing of the laceration site in human superficialis flexor tendons in vitro. J Hand Surg [Am] 1991;16(1):24–30.
[129] Awad HA, Butler DL, Boivin GP, et al. Autologous mesenchymal stem cell-mediated repair of tendon. Tissue Eng 1999;5(3):267–77.
[130] Young RG, Butler DL, Weber W, Caplan AI, Gordon SL, Fink DJ. Use of mesenchymal stem cells in a collagen matrix for Achilles tendon repair. J Orthop Res 1998;16(4):406–13.
[131] Smith RK, Korda M, Blunn GW, Goodship AE. Isolation and implantation of autologous equine mesenchymal stem cells from bone marrow into the superficial digital flexor tendon as a potential novel treatment. Equine Vet J 2003; 35(1):99–102.
[132] Nakamura N, Horibe S, Matsumoto N, et al. Transient introduction of a foreign gene into healing rat patellar ligament. J Clin Invest 1996;97(1):226–31.
[133] Nakamura N, Shino K, Natsuume T, et al. Early biological effect of in vivo gene transfer of

platelet-derived growth factor (PDGF)-B into healing patellar ligament. Gene Ther 1998;5(9):1165–70.
[134] Lou J, Kubota H, Hotokezaka S, Ludwig FJ, Manske PR. In vivo gene transfer and overexpression of focal adhesion kinase (pp125 FAK) mediated by recombinant adenovirus-induced tendon adhesion formation and epitenon cell change. J Orthop Res 1997;15(6):911–8.
[135] Sanders DW, Milne AD, Dobravec A, MacDermid J, Johnson JA, King GJ. Cyclic testing of flexor tendon repairs: an in vitro biomechanical study. J Hand Surg [Am] 1997;22(6):1004–10.
[136] Choueka J, Heminger H, Mass DP. Cyclical testing of zone II flexor tendon repairs. J Hand Surg [Am] 2000;25(6):1127–34.
[137] Savage R. In vitro studies of a new method of flexor tendon repair. J Hand Surg [Br] 1985;10(2):135–41.
[138] Lee H. Double loop locking suture: a technique of tendon repair for early active mobilization. Part II: clinical experience. J Hand Surg [Am] 1990;15: 953–8.
[139] Mass DP, Tuel RJ, Labarbera M, Greenwald DP. Effects of constant mechanical tension on the healing of rabbit flexor tendons. Clin Orthop 1993;296: 301–6.
[140] Williams RJ, Amis AA. A new type of flexor tendon repair. Biomechanical evaluation by cyclic loading, ultimate strength and assessment of pulley friction in vitro. J Hand Surg [Br] 1995;20(5): 578–83.
[141] Pruitt DL, Manske PR, Fink B. Cyclic stress analysis of flexor tendon repair. J Hand Surg [Am] 1991; 16(4):701–7.
[142] Pruitt DL, Tanaka H, Aoki M, Manske PR. Cyclic stress testing after in vivo healing of canine flexor tendon lacerations. J Hand Surg [Am] 1996;21(6): 974–7.
[143] Urbaniak J, Cahill J, Mortenson R. Tendon suturing methods: analysis in strength. In: Hunter J, Schneider L, editors. American Academy of Orthopaedic Surgeons Symposium on Tendon Surgery in the Hand. St. Louis: Mosby; 1975. p. 70–80.
[144] Schuind F, Garcia-Elias M, Cooney WP III, An KN. Flexor tendon forces: in vivo measurements. J Hand Surg [Am] 1992;17(2):291–8.
[145] Silfverskiold KL, May EJ. Flexor tendon repair in zone II with a new suture technique and an early mobilization program combining passive and active flexion. J Hand Surg [Am] 1994;19(1): 53–60.
[146] Papandrea R, Seitz WH Jr, Shapiro P, Borden B. Biomechanical and clinical evaluation of the epitenon-first technique of flexor tendon repair. J Hand Surg [Am] 1995;20(2):261–6.
[147] Diao E, Hariharan JS, Soejima O, Lotz JC. Effect of peripheral suture depth on strength of tendon repairs. J Hand Surg [Am] 1996;21(2):234–9.
[148] Wada A, Kubota H, Hatanaka H, Miura H, Iwamoto Y. Comparison of mechanical properties of polyvinylidene fluoride and polypropylene monofilament sutures used for flexor tendon repair. J Hand Surg [Br] 2001;26(3):212–6.
[149] Taras JS, Raphael JS, Marczyk SC, Bauerle WB. Evaluation of suture caliber in flexor tendon repair. J Hand Surg [Am] 2001;26(6):1100–4.
[150] Moneim MS, Firoozbakhsh K, Mustapha AA, Larsen K, Shahinpoor M. Flexor tendon repair using shape memory alloy suture: a biomechanical evaluation. Clin Orthop 2002;402:251–9.
[151] Zhao C, Amadio PC, Momose T, Couvreur P, Zobitz ME, An KN. The effect of suture technique on adhesion formation after flexor tendon repair for partial lacerations in a canine model. J Trauma 2001;51(5):917–21.
[152] Elliot D, Moiemen NS, Flemming AF, Harris SB, Foster AJ. The rupture rate of acute flexor tendon repairs mobilized by the controlled active motion regimen. J Hand Surg [Br] 1994;19(5): 607–12.
[153] Tang JB, Shi D, Gu YQ, Chen JC, Zhou B. Double and multiple looped suture tendon repair. J Hand Surg [Br] 1994;19(6):699–703.
[154] McLarney E, Hoffman H, Wolfe SW. Biomechanical analysis of the cruciate four-strand flexor tendon repair. J Hand Surg [Am] 1999;24(2): 295–301.
[155] Singer M, Maloon S. Flexor tendon injuries: the results of primary repair. J Hand Surg [Br] 1988; 13(3):269–72.
[156] Singer G, Ebramzadeh E, Jones NF, Meals R. Use of the Taguchi method for biomechanical comparison of flexor-tendon-repair techniques to allow immediate active flexion. A new method of analysis and optimization of technique to improve the quality of the repair. J Bone Joint Surg [Am] 1998; 80(10):1498–506.
[157] Savage R, Risitano G. Flexor tendon repair using a "six strand" method of repair and early active mobilisation. J Hand Surg [Br] 1989;14(4): 396–9.
[158] Lister GD, Kleinert HE, Kutz JE, Atasoy E. Primary flexor tendon repair followed by immediate controlled mobilization. J Hand Surg [Am] 1977; 2(6):441–51.
[159] Ejeskar A. Flexor tendon repair in no-man's-land: results of primary repair with controlled mobilization. J Hand Surg [Am] 1984;9(2):171–7.
[160] Edinburg M, Widgerow AD, Biddulph SL. Early postoperative mobilization of flexor tendon injuries using a modification of the Kleinert technique. J Hand Surg [Am] 1987;12(1):34–8.
[161] Saldana MJ, Ho PK, Lichtman DM, Chow JA, Dovelle S, Thomes LJ. Flexor tendon repair and rehabilitation in zone II open sheath technique versus closed sheath technique. J Hand Surg [Am] 1987; 12(6):1110–4.
[162] Saldana MJ, Chow JA, Gerbino P Jr, Westerbeck P, Schacherer TG. Further experience in rehabilita-

tion of zone II flexor tendon repair with dynamic traction splinting. Plast Reconstr Surg 1991;87(3): 543–6.

[163] Cullen KW, Tolhurst P, Lang D, Page RE. Flexor tendon repair in zone 2 followed by controlled active mobilisation. J Hand Surg [Br] 1989;14(4): 392–5.

[164] May EJ, Silfverskiold KL, Sollerman CJ. The correlation between controlled range of motion with dynamic traction and results after flexor tendon repair in zone II. J Hand Surg [Am] 1992;17(6): 1133–9.

[165] Adolfsson L, Soderberg G, Larsson M, Karlander LE. The effects of a shortened postoperative mobilization programme after flexor tendon repair in zone 2. J Hand Surg [Br] 1996;21(1): 67–71.

[166] Baktir A, Turk CY, Kabak S, Sahin V, Kardas Y. Flexor tendon repair in zone 2 followed by early active mobilization. J Hand Surg [Br] 1996;21(5): 624–8.

[167] Choueka J, Heminger H, Mass DP. Flexor tendon forces during simulated active and active resisted motion: an in-vitro biomechanical study in a curvilinear model. Presented at the Third Triennial International Hand and Wrist Biomechanics Symposium; Minneapolis, Minnesota; September 1, 1998.

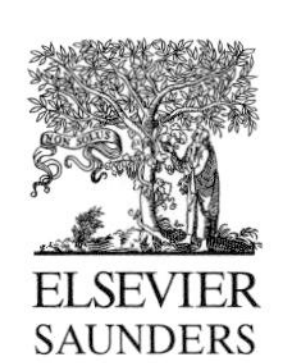
ELSEVIER
SAUNDERS

Hand Clin 21 (2005) 151–157

HAND
CLINICS

Flexor Tendons: Anatomy and Surgical Approaches

Christopher H. Allan, MD

Orthopaedics and Sports Medicine, Harborview Medical Center, University of Washington School of Medicine, Department of Orthopaedics, Box 359798, 325 Ninth Avenue, Seattle, WA 98104, USA

The extrinsic flexor tendons of the hand represent the terminal functional units of the forearm motors to the digits and are named based on the location of those forearm muscles. The flexor digitorum profundus (FDP; profound = deep) tendons arise from the deeper layer of flexor muscles, whereas the flexor digitorum superficialis (FDS) tendons are the continuation of the more superficial muscle layer. The flexor pollicis longus (FPL) tendon also arises from the deeper muscle layer and is the only thumb flexor with a tendon occupying a sheath.

As these tendons enter the hand they traverse the carpal tunnel. The finger flexors are arranged with the profundus tendons deepest in the carpal tunnel. Above them are located the index and small finger superficialis tendons, and finally the superficialis tendons of the middle and ring fingers. At this level the median nerve, closely apposed to the undersurface of the superficialis musculature in the forearm, has become the most palmar structure (Fig. 1).

In the hand, the flexor tendons are enclosed in synovial sheaths that lubricate them and minimize friction as they pass beneath the transverse carpal ligament and within the digits (Fig. 2).

These synovial sheaths demarcate different zones along the course of the tendons (Fig. 3). Zone I represents the region distal to the synovial sheath, occupied by the profundus tendon only. Zone II extends the length of the fibro-osseous sheath of the digit, where (in the nonthumb digits) FDP and FDS glide within the sheath's narrow confines (Figs. 4 and 5). Zone III extends from the proximal aspect of the digital synovial sheath (approximately the level of the metacarpal neck) to the distal aspect of the transverse carpal ligament. Occasionally the small finger flexor sheath is continuous throughout the digit and palm and so zone II is considered to begin with the A1 pulley (discussed later). Zone IV comprises the carpal tunnel, and zone V is proximal to it (Fig. 3).

Zone II receives a great deal of attention because of its anatomic complexity and because of resulting difficulties in obtaining good clinical results after flexor tendon injury and repair in this location. In zone II the synovial sheath is organized into thickenings or segments of transverse or oblique fibers comprising annular or cruciate pulleys, respectively (Figs. 4 and 5). The entirety of the sheath, pulleys and all, serves to retain the flexor tendons close to the phalanges throughout a complete range of motion. Bowstringing of tendons, which would be an obstacle to grasp, is thereby prevented. The cruciate pulleys are located at or near the interphalangeal joints, and their configuration allows them to collapse with flexion of those joints, allowing for shortening of the flexor sheath without bunching of tissue.

In the case of the thumb, an abbreviated sheath with one oblique and two annular pulleys is found (Fig. 6).

These anatomic facts form the basis for approaches to injured flexor tendons; in the nonthumb digits the cruciate pulleys can be sacrificed readily to gain access without compromising the sheath's retaining function. Although all pulleys should be preserved as much as possible, even if only those overlying the proximal and middle phalanges (A2 and A4, respectively) are preserved, then full flexion sufficient to allow for digit tip to distal palmar crease contact should still be possible [1].

E-mail address: callan@u.washington.edu

0749-0712/05/$ - see front matter
doi:10.1016/j.hcl.2004.11.003

hand.theclinics.com

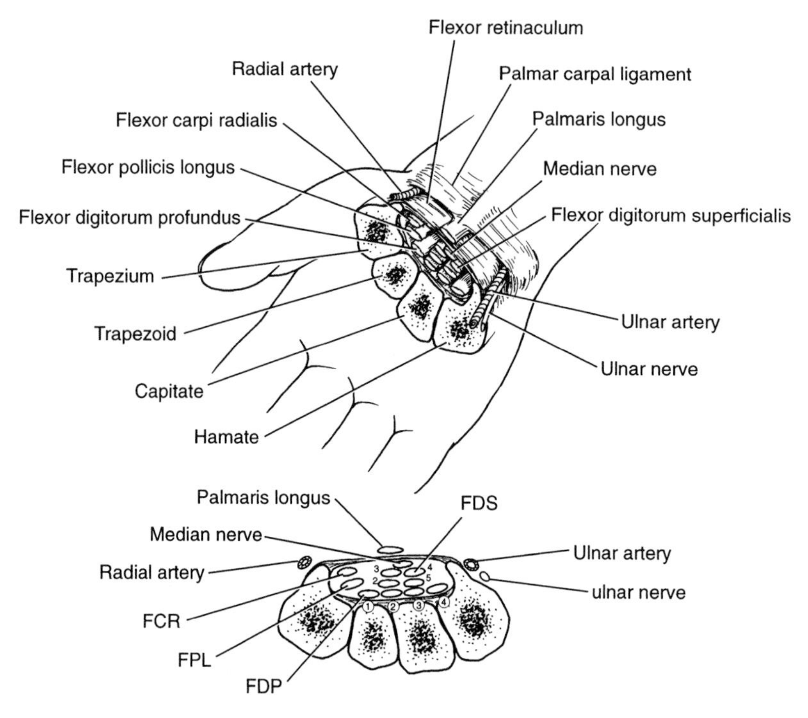

Fig. 1. Flexor tendon anatomy at the wrist.

The flexor tendons in zone II are nourished by synovial fluid within the sheath and through direct vascular inflow by way of the vincula (from the Latin *vincire* and *vinctum*, to bind) [2]. Each flexor receives a vinculum longus and a vinculum brevis (Fig. 7), conveying vessels that ramify along the dorsal course of the tendons. Repairs often are planned to avoid the dorsal aspect of the flexors to preserve this blood supply [3].

Surgical approaches

Flexor tendon injuries occur most commonly in association with lacerations or other open

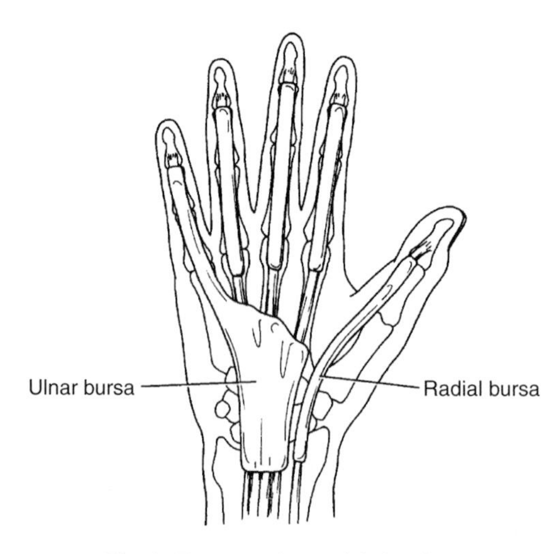

Fig. 2. Bursae and synovial sheaths.

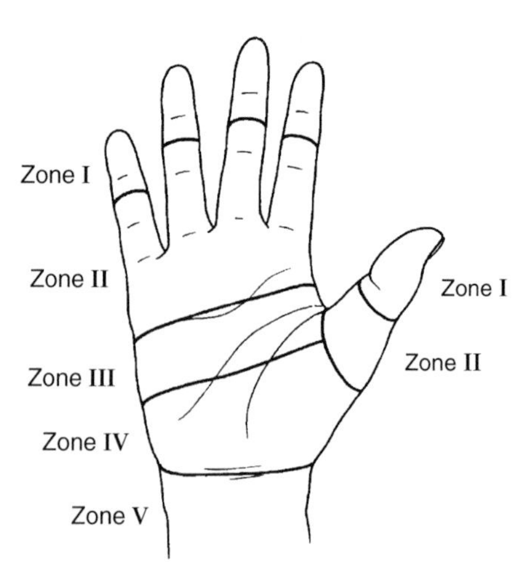

Fig. 3. Flexor tendon zones.

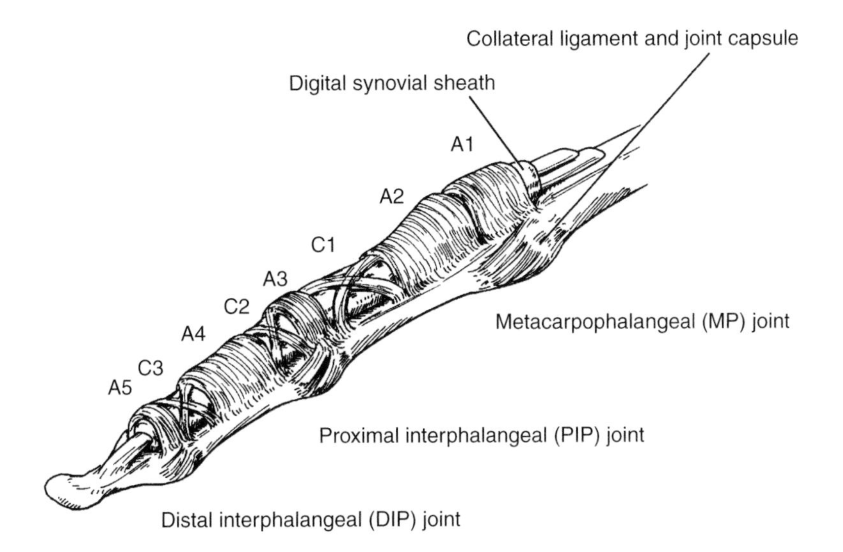

Fig. 4. Digital flexor sheath: annular (A1–A5) and cruciate (C1–C3) pulleys.

wounds of digits, and in such situations the surgical approach therefore is dictated to some extent by the nature of the wound. The chief principles guiding the choice of incision are to avoid crossing flexion creases at right angles (to prevent later flexion contracture caused by scar) and to protect the underlying neurovascular bundles from harm.

Oblique Bruner incisions or straight midlateral incisions should allow for safe exposure of the flexor sheath in zones I or II, and these may be combined as needed [4]. In the palm, incisions along the course of or perpendicular to flexion creases may be used. In any case, it is important to avoid creating narrow skin flaps, because the tip of such a flap may not survive (Fig. 8).

Flexor tendon injuries in the palm, wrist, or forearm tend to be simpler to expose and repair, in part because of the absence of the constricting fibro-osseous sheath. In zone III the lumbrical (which originates from the FDP at this level) may be intact, preventing retraction of the cut ends of a profundus tendon. In zone IV an open release of the carpal tunnel generally exposes both ends of

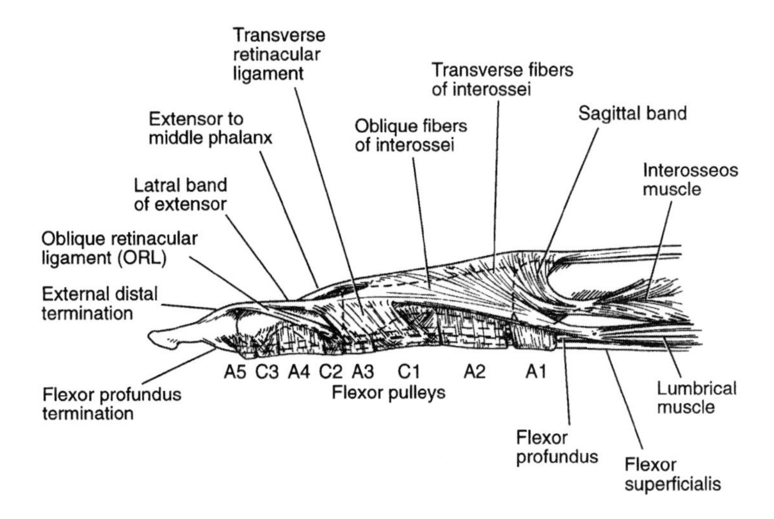

Fig. 5. Relationship of flexor sheath and pulleys to intrinsic and extensor apparatus.

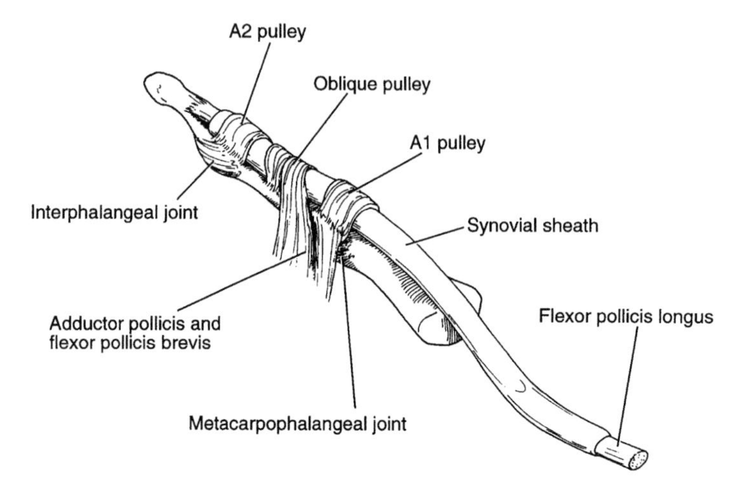

Fig. 6. Thumb flexor sheath and pulleys.

a lacerated tendon, although keeping some part of the transverse carpal ligament intact to prevent bowstringing is preferred if at all possible. Zone V injuries occur so close to the muscle belly that significant retraction does not occur, but injuries at this level often involve multiple structures and so substantial extension of lacerations distally and proximally may be necessary to allow identification and repair of multiple tendons, nerves, and vessels. In this situation extending one end of the incision distally and the other proximally minimizes the risk for flap necrosis.

Another factor dictating the planning of an incision should be the location of the laceration along the course of the tendon sheath. If the digit was held in flexion at the time of the injury, the distal tendon end (or ends, if both FDS and FDP have been cut) likely require a greater distal exposure for retrieval and repair than is true for tendon injuries to an extended digit (Fig. 9). Often this can be determined through direct inspection of the wound in the operating room after irrigation and with tourniquet control. Passive flexion of the digit may bring the distal cut ends readily

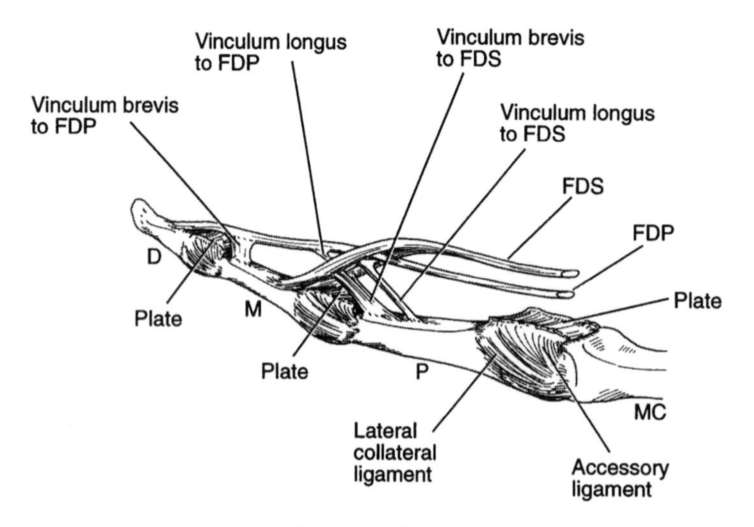

Fig. 7. The vincula.

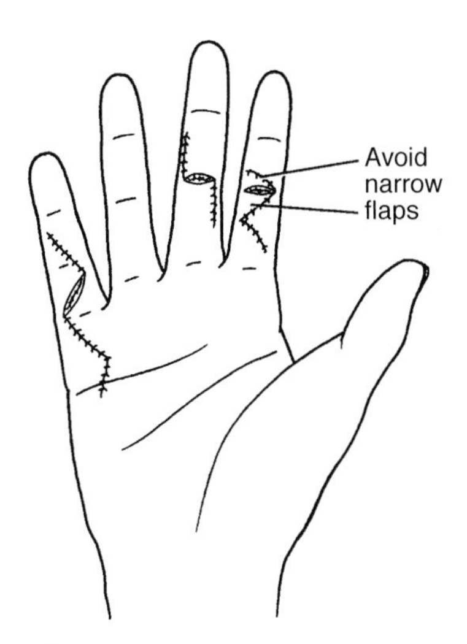

Fig. 8. Incisions for exposure and repair of flexor tendon lacerations.

into view, minimizing the extent of distal exposure required. When this is not the case, a more extensive distal incision—sometimes surprisingly so—must be used. With identification and protection of the neurovascular bundles, the entire volar surface of the flexor sheath can be exposed.

After exposure of the distal cut ends, the proximal ends must be retrieved. As stated, this tends not to be difficult in the case of injuries proximal to zone II. For injuries within the digit, flexion of the wrist and fingers and kneading of the volar forearm musculature from proximal to distal to "milk" the cut ends into the wound may be successful, though this seems to be true only rarely. As a next step, a curved tendon passer, hemostat, small hooked skin retractor, or other device then may be inserted into the sheath and directed proximally to attempt to grasp the proximal cut ends. Care must be taken to avoid harm to nerves and vessels, which are immediately adjacent to the course of the flexor tendons at most locations in the hand.

If this fails to retrieve the cut ends after more than a few gentle attempts have been made, it is probably safest and quickest to proceed with exposure of the tendons in the palm. A transverse incision is made at the level of the A1 pulley and the tendons are exposed. The cut tendons occasionally can be advanced gently distally, using a nontoothed forceps, into the wound in the digit. If this does not succeed, a small pediatric feeding tube (5 French is commonly used) is inserted in the proximal wound, into the sheath, and out the distal wound [5]. A suture is used to tie the cut tendons to the feeding tube, and the tube is gently pulled distally, usually bringing the tendons into the distal wound (Fig. 10). A 25-gauge needle can be placed transversely through the retrieved tendon ends, proximal and distal, to retain them at the proposed site of repair.

A final issue in exposure of injured flexor tendons has to do with the overlying flexor sheath. The generally transverse orientation of the fibers making up the sheath leads to pullout of sutures parallel to these fibers, as would be used to repair a longitudinal incision. It is often necessary, though, to open the sheath at some location other

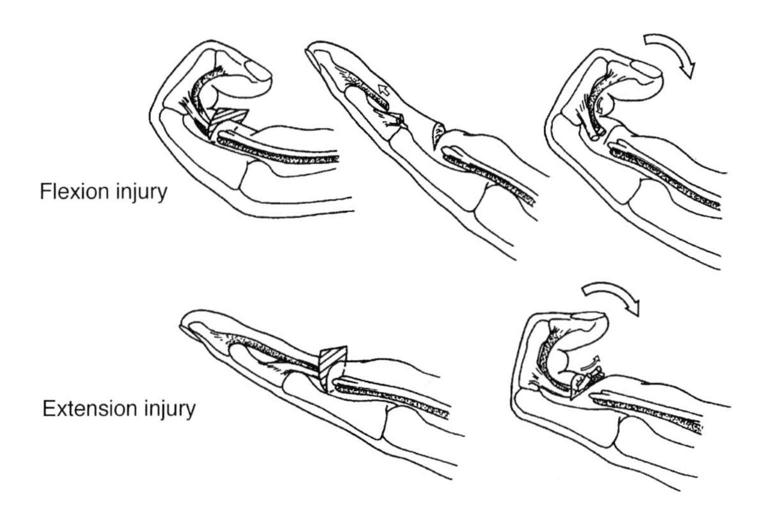

Fig. 9. Effect of digit posture at time of injury on location of distal cut tendon ends in zone II injuries.

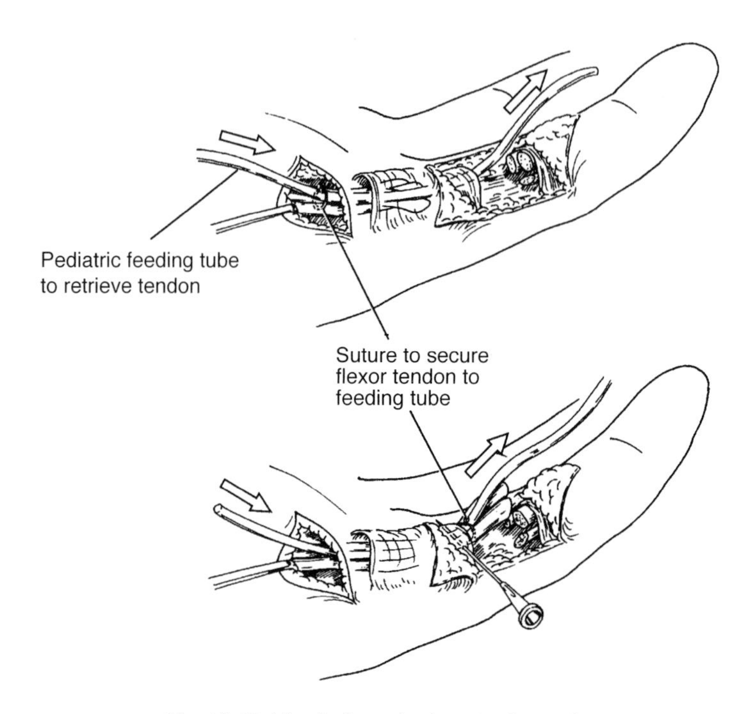

Fig. 10. Retrieval of proximal cut tendon ends.

than the original wound—or to extend the original wound—to perform an adequate repair. One compromise is to use L-shaped or funnel incisions where needed, the transverse limbs of which may be repaired reliably, and which give greater exposure than straight longitudinal incisions [6]. Such funnel-shaped flaps also can be helpful when passing the proximal tendon end into a more distal part of the sheath to allow for repair (Fig. 11).

Summary

The nature of the original injury is the chief determinant of outcome and is out of the control of the surgeon. Every step thereafter can be

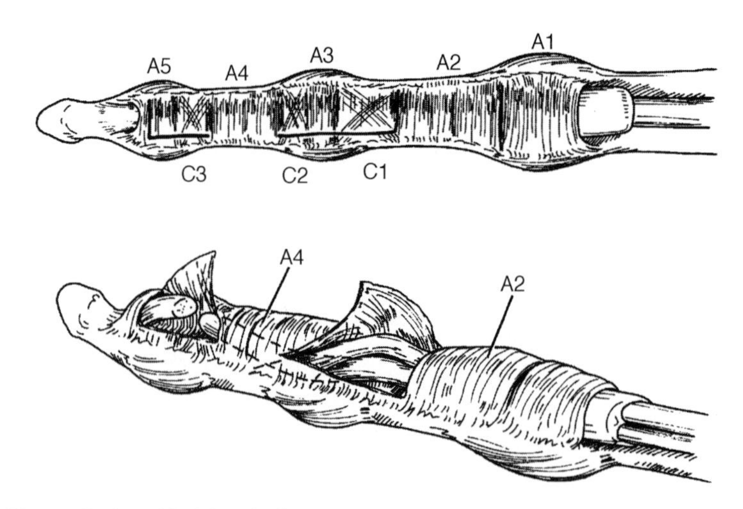

Fig. 11. L-shaped incisions in flexor sheath for greater exposure and ease of repair.

influenced by him or her, though, and a thorough knowledge of anatomy and surgical approaches allows for the best possible repair under any set of circumstances.

References

[1] Trumble T. Principles of hand surgery and therapy. Philadelphia: WB Saunders Co.; 2000.
[2] Strickland JW. Flexor tendon injuries: I. Foundations of treatment. J Am Acad Orthop Surg 1995;3(1): 44–54.
[3] Amadio PC, Hunter JM, Jaeger SH, Wehbe MA, Schneider LH. The effect of vincular injury on the results of flexor tendon surgery in zone 2. J Hand Surg [Am] 1985;10(5):626–32.
[4] Strickland JW. Flexor tendon injuries: II. Operative technique. J Am Acad Orthop Surg 1995;3(1): 55–62.
[5] Sourmelis SG, McGrouther DA. Retrieval of the retracted flexor tendon. J Hand Surg [Br] 1987; 12(1):109–11.
[6] Lister G. Indications and techniques for repair of the flexor tendon sheath. Hand Clin 1985;1(1):85–95.

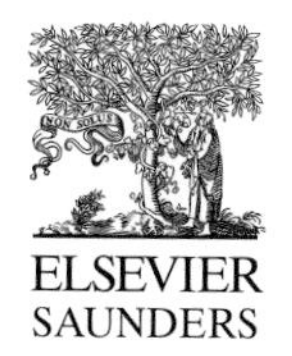

ELSEVIER
SAUNDERS

Hand Clin 21 (2005) 159–166

HAND
CLINICS

Flexor Tendon Biology

Martin I. Boyer, MD, MSc, FRCS(C)

Department of Orthopaedic Surgery, Washington University at Barnes-Jewish Hospital, One Barnes Hospital Plaza, Saint Louis, MO 63110, USA

Significant advances in the understanding of intrasynovial flexor tendon repair and rehabilitation have been made since the early 1970s [1,2], when reports first demonstrated that flexor tendon lacerations within the fibro-osseous digital sheath could be repaired primarily and rehabilitated successfully without early tendon excision and delayed intrasynovial grafting [3]. The concept of adhesion-free, or primary tendon healing (that tendons could heal intrinsically without the ingrowth of fibrous adhesions from the surrounding sheath), has been validated experimentally and clinically in studies over the past 25 years [4–13]. Recent attempts to understand and improve the results of intrasynovial flexor tendon repair have focused on restoration of the gliding surface [13–22], augmentation of early postoperative repair site biomechanic strength [23–36], and on the elucidation of the molecular biology of early postoperative tendon healing [2,23,37,38–40]. The goals of the surgical treatment of patients with intrasynovial flexor tendon lacerations remain unchanged: to achieve a primary tendon repair of sufficient tensile strength to allow application of a postoperative mobilization rehabilitation protocol. This program should inhibit the formation of intrasynovial adhesions and restore the gliding surface while facilitating the healing of the repair site [41].

Tendon structure and nutrition

The intrasynovial portion of the digital flexor tendon consists of longitudinally oriented collagen fascicles separated spatially into equal radial and ulnar halves and functionally into volar and dorsal sections. The dorsal part of the tendon contains most of the direct vascular supply of the tendon, which originates from the two vinculae supplied directly by ladder branches of the radial and ulnar digital arteries. By contrast, the volar portion of the intrasynovial flexor tendon, which in absolute terms constitutes less than half of the thickness of the tendon itself, contains little or no direct blood supply [42]. Cells within this avascular portion of the tendon obtain nutrient supply and eliminate waste products primarily by passive diffusion of the relevant solutes and gases [43].

The dorsal and volar surfaces of the flexor tendons are covered by a thin visceral gliding layer of epitenon. The flexor tendons course through a synovial lined fibro-osseous tunnel that provides a biomechanic advantage (on the basis of the pulley system) and the synovial source of nutrition from the internal parietal layer of sheath [44]. Although studies of intrasynovial flexor tendon physiology have demonstrated the importance of intrinsic and extrinsic sources of nutrition [45–52], tendon nutrition by passive diffusion is likely of greater importance overall.

A recent investigation of tendon ultrastructure by Ritty [53] has shed new light on the organization of fibroblasts within the interior aspect of the flexor digitorum profundus (FDP) tendon. It has been shown that internal tendon fibroblasts are organized into longitudinally oriented linear arrays surrounded by their own unique extracellular matrix. Identification of the components of this matrix demonstrated substantial contributions of fibrillin-2, type VI collagen, and versican. In addition, a new fibrillin-2 containing macromolecular assembly has been shown to run axially

E-mail address: boyerm@msnotes.wustl.edu (M.I. Boyer).

doi:10.1016/j.hcl.2004.11.009

along the tendon arrays. These assemblies contain the internal tendon fibroblasts, have a constant diameter, and often are greater than 1 mm long. Investigation of the interplay between the tendon fibroblasts within these microenvironments and externally applied forces or biologic factors during early rehabilitation following repair may increase the quantity or quality of endotenon fibroblast participation during early tendon repair.

Biomechanics

Attempts to improve the time-zero early postoperative strength of the repair construct have focused on biomechanic and biologic attempts to modify the early postoperative repair site. Attempts to vary the configuration of the core suture [14,30,31,54–61], to alter the number of suture strands passing across the repair site [29,33–36,54–57,62–71], to investigate the use of core sutures of different caliber and materials [72–74], and to investigate variation in the pattern and depth of placement of the circumferential epitenon suture [65,75–77] have all been evaluated as to their beneficial effects on time-zero and in vivo postoperative tendon healing. Although clinical application of repair site augmentations, such as onlay tendon grafts, patches, or synthetic materials, has been disappointing because of increased repair site bulk and poor ability to restore the gliding surface, recent ex vivo results suggest that these techniques may warrant further investigation [78]. In addition, investigation of the feasibility of the direct application, within carrier media, to the repair site of growth factors or compounds beneficial to the healing of dense regular connective tissue holds promise (R.H. Gelberman, personal communication, 2004).

Ex vivo and in vivo investigations in linear, in situ, and other models have suggested that core suture configurations with the greatest tensile strength are those in which there are multiple sites of tendon suture interaction [23,59,79–84]. Although the Kessler or modified Kessler techniques still enjoy widespread acceptance [1], newer techniques such as Tajima [85,86], Strickland [25,34,41,86], Cruciate [54,57], Becker [25,30,34,79,80], and Savage [31,36,58,59,68,86] configurations all offer greater suture hold on the tendon that is independent of the suture knot. These modern methods of core suture technique have been shown not only to offer greater time-zero repair site tensile strength, but also improved strength up to and including 6 weeks postoperatively [23,36,82]. A significant relationship between tendon cross-sectional dimension and suture hold on the tendon stump, however, has not been proven [24]. The nature of the tendon–suture interaction from an ultrastructural point of view remains unevaluated.

It is well accepted that core suture techniques using a greater number of suture strands crossing the repair site between proximal and distal tendon demonstrate higher tensile strength stumps than core suture techniques of similar pattern with less sutures across the repair site [26,35,36,71]. This fact holds true in ex vivo time-zero studies and in in vivo studies for up to 6 weeks postoperatively. The results of numerous studies using commonly used core suture techniques have demonstrated the superiority of the four-strand core suture over the two-strand core suture and the greater strengths achieved with six- and eight-strand core suture techniques. The limiting factor to more widespread use of modern multistrand suture techniques remains the surgeon's ability to perform the repair using atraumatic technique such that trauma to the tendon stumps and the circumferential visceral epitenon is minimized.

Other variables relevant to core suture placement shown to have a positive effect on time-zero core suture tensile strength include the dorsovolar location of the core suture, the cross-sectional area of tendon grasped or locked by the redirecting loop of suture, and the total number of times that the tendon has been grasped by the suture. Studies in an ex vivo in situ human model have shown that greater time-zero strength is achieved with a more dorsal placement of the core suture within the tendon stumps [29,34,87]. This has a negative theoretic effect on intrasynovial flexor tendon vascularity, because the more dorsal suture placement interferes with internal tendon vascularity to a greater extent, especially in the areas in which the long and short vincula enter the FDP tendon. Ex vivo studies have suggested that the redirecting loop of the core suture that is positioned to lock rather than grasp the tendon stumps show greater time-zero strength, and in addition, increasing the number of locks or grasps increases the time-zero tensile strength of the flexor tendon repair site [88–90]. The placement of the suture knot either within or away from the repair site has not been shown conclusively to have an effect on core suture tensile strength [72,91,92]. Greater quantity of suture within the repair site may increase repair site bulk and decrease tendon glide, whereas knot placement away from the repair site may affect tendon gliding detrimentally because of increased friction between tendon and sheath proximal or distal to the repair site. Techniques of intrasynovial core suture placement that do not require the tying of sutures have not gained widespread acceptance [93].

An additional technique by which hand surgeons have attempted to augment repair site strength is by alteration of the configuration of circumferential epitendinous suture. Several studies have suggested that a clinically and statistically significant component of time-zero repair site strength is provided by a circumferential epitendinous suture passed multiple times across the repair site [65,75]. Most investigations suggest that although the epitendinous suture does increase time-zero and early postoperative strength of the repair site, it cannot be relied on to provide the most repair site tensile strength. It has been shown, however, that the role of the epitendinous suture, regardless of its configuration, is twofold: first, to decrease repair site bulk by smoothing out the tendon stump surface, and second, to increase tensile strength of the repair site to decrease early postoperative repair site gap formation. Based on recent studies of core suture biomechanics and in vivo clinical and experimental studies of tendon force in canines and humans, a four-strand core suture technique supplemented by a running epitendinous suture is recommended to achieve sufficient repair site tensile strength to allow for postoperative passive motion rehabilitation to proceed without significant risk for gap formation at the repair site. Increased depth and frequency of epitendinous suture passes do not seem to exert negative effects on the epitenon cell layer's contribution to the intrinsically healing tendon.

The repair site gap

Although greater degrees of strength have been achieved with modern core and epitendinous suture techniques, the effect of small degrees of early repair site dehiscence or repair site gap formation on tendon healing and accrual of repair site strength has been appreciated only recently [27]. Previous investigators have hypothesized that the presence of repair site gaps was accompanied uniformly by the presence of intrasynovial flexor tendon adhesions, decreased tendon glide, and digital stiffness [66,94–96]. A recent in vivo canine study has refuted this assumption and has demonstrated that the presence of a repair site gap, even greater than 3 mm, is not correlated with the presence of intrasynovial adhesions or with decreased digital arc of motion [27]. Although large gaps did not seem to affect tendon function (ie, excursion), large repair site gaps that occurred during the first 21 days postoperatively were observed to have a significant negative effect on tendon structure (ie, the accrual of tendon repair site tensile strength). In tendons without gaps or with gaps less than 3 mm in length, a significant increase in repair site tensile strength was seen between 3 and 6 weeks postoperatively, whereas in tendons with a repair site gap greater than 3mm, significant accrual of repair site strength did not occur. Although the biologic processes at work within the larger repair site gaps remain open to further investigation, large repair site gaps seen early in the postoperative period pose a greater risk for rupture as motion rehabilitation progresses after 3 weeks. Evaluation of imaging modalities such as ultrasound, MRI, and plain radiographs to determine precisely the extent of repair site gap has yielded inconsistent results that are not yet applicable to the clinical situation.

Repair site biochemistry

Important strides have been made recently in the investigation of specific biologic processes active at the repair site during the early postoperative period. Increased levels of local cellular division as demonstrated histologically and measured by increased levels of histone H4 mRNA and increased synthesis of type I collagen mRNA and protein has been demonstrated within repair site cells and cells within the adjacent epitenon early in the postoperative period [38,97,98]. Goldfarb has shown, however, that neither the total amount nor the maturity of the collagen at the repair site increased significantly during the first 6 weeks postoperatively [99]. The accrual of repair site tensile strength demonstrated between 3 and 6 weeks postoperatively in tendons with repair site gap of less than 3 mm therefore must be caused by mechanisms other than increased synthesis or more rapid maturation of collagen at the repair site. The precise biochemical processes deficient in those tendons not accruing strength after 3 weeks postoperatively are unknown at present.

Fibroblasts grown in culture have demonstrated responsiveness to externally applied stress on cellular and molecular levels [37]; however, the exact relationship between synthesis of collagen and integrins and the accrual of tensile strength at tendon repair site remains unknown. Fibronectin, an abundant extracellular matrix protein involved in cell–matrix communication, and $\alpha_5\beta_1$, $\alpha_v\beta_3$ integrins, cell-surface compounds involved in the binding of fibroblasts to extracellular matrix, are likewise upregulated during the early postoperative period in tendons undergoing early passive motion mobilization following repair [100–104]. The clinical relevance of the observed increase in local synthesis and accumulation of compounds that enable communication between the extracellular matrix and the interior of the fibroblast during the early postoperative period is important insofar as locally applied rehabilitation stresses might be mimicked by application of these factors administered exogenously or by genetic engineering of the repair site. Tendons immobilized following repair demonstrated significantly decreased fibronectin concentration when compared with mobilized tendons [100].

Upregulation in the synthesis of mRNA angiogenic mediators such as basic fibroblast growth factor (bFGF) and vascular endothelial growth factor (VEGF) has been demonstrated within the flexor tendon repair site and in surrounding epitenon and has been shown to precede temporally and be distinct spatially from longitudinal blood vessel growth on the tendon surface and within the flexor tendon substance [38,39,47,105]. The cellular origin of these angiogenic mediators and their role in blood vessel ingrowth through the avascular region of the flexor tendon remains unknown. Although the ingrowth of new blood vessels through the avascular zone of the FDP tendon following repair and early motion rehabilitation has been shown to be independent of the formation of restrictive intrasynovial adhesions, the benefit of increasing the levels of local angiogenic mediators remains theoretical. Although Lineaweaver has shown that exogenous application of VEGF can increase the tensile strength achieved following repair of Achilles tendons in a rat model [106], the potential risks for overproduction or over-accumulation of angiogenic mediators at the surgical site may result in earlier or more extensive formation of restrictive adhesions. This concern is underscored by the increased expression of transforming growth factor beta (TGF-beta) [37,40,107], known to be associated with the local formation of scar tissue, in these in vivo models.

The identification of fibroblast responsiveness in culture to insulin-like growth factor (IGF) [45] and its expression by flexor tendon cells in vitro [108] has been demonstrated. The beneficial effects of increasing IGF levels locally to improve early tendon structure following repair remains untested, however. Similarly, local application of epidermal-derived growth factor (EDGF) has been shown to have a positive effect on fibroblast migration in vitro. Its beneficial effects in vivo in earlier population of the repair site with cells involved in matrix production, however, are untested also [109].

The future of intrasynovial tendon repair and rehabilitation

Future attempts to improve the pace and the extent of flexor tendon repair site healing probably lie within the biologic realm, because the benefits of modern multiple strand core suture techniques combined with early postoperative motion rehabilitation likely have been maximized (J.W. Strickland, personal communication, 2002). The next phase of fruitful investigation will attempt the optimization of dosage, delivery, tempo, and timing of the beneficial genes or compounds, alone or in combination, to the postoperative repair site at the time of surgical treatment.

References

[1] Kessler I, Nissim F. Primary repair without immobilization of flexor tendon division within the digital sheath. An experimental and clinical study. Acta Orthop Scand 1969;40(5):587–601.

[2] Verdan CE. Half a century of flexor-tendon surgery. Current status and changing philosophies. J Bone Joint Surg [Am] 1972;54(3):472–91.

[3] Bunnell S. Surgery of the hand. Philadelphia: Lippincott; 1948. p. 381–466.

[4] Gelberman RH, Amiel D, Gonsalves M, Woo S, Akeson WH. The influence of protected passive mobilization on the healing of flexor tendons: a biochemical and microangiographic study. Hand 1981;13(2):120–8.

[5] Gelberman RH, Manske PR, Akeson WH, Woo SL, Lundborg G, Amiel D. Flexor tendon repair. J Orthop Res 1986;4(1):119–28.

[6] Gelberman RH, Manske PR, Vande Berg JS, Lesker PA, Akeson WH. Flexor tendon repair in vitro: a comparative histologic study of the rabbit, chicken, dog, and monkey. J Orthop Res 1984;2(1): 39–48.

[7] Gelberman RH, Vandeberg JS, Manske PR, Akeson WH. The early stages of flexor tendon healing: a morphologic study of the first fourteen days. J Hand Surg [Am] 1985;10(6 Pt 1):776–84.
[8] Gelberman RH, Woo SL, Lothringer K, Akeson WH, Amiel D. Effects of early intermittent passive mobilization on healing canine flexor tendons. J Hand Surg [Am] 1982;7(2):170–5.
[9] Manske PR, Gelberman RH, Lesker PA. Flexor tendon healing. Hand Clin 1985;1(1):25–34.
[10] Manske PR, Gelberman RH, Vande Berg JS, Lesker PA. Intrinsic flexor-tendon repair. A morphological study in vitro. J Bone Joint Surg [Am] 1984;66(3):385–96.
[11] Manske PR, Lesker PA. Biochemical evidence of flexor tendon participation in the repair process—an in vitro study. J Hand Surg [Br] 1984; 9(2):117–20.
[12] Manske PR, Lesker PA. Histologic evidence of intrinsic flexor tendon repair in various experimental animals. An in vitro study. Clin Orthop 1984;182: 297–304.
[13] Manske PR, Lesker PA, Gelberman RH, Rucinsky TE. Intrinsic restoration of the flexor tendon surface in the nonhuman primate. J Hand Surg [Am] 1985;10(5):632–7.
[14] Aoki M, Kubota H, Pruitt DL, Manske PR. Biomechanical and histologic characteristics of canine flexor tendon repair using early postoperative mobilization. J Hand Surg [Am] 1997;22(1):107–14.
[15] Boardman ND III, Morifusa S, Saw SS, McCarthy DM, Sotereanos DG, Woo SL. Effects of tenorrhaphy on the gliding function and tensile properties of partially lacerated canine digital flexor tendons. J Hand Surg [Am] 1999;24(2):302–9.
[16] Gelberman RH, Vande Berg JS, Lundborg GN, Akeson WH. Flexor tendon healing and restoration of the gliding surface. An ultrastructural study in dogs. J Bone Joint Surg [Am] 1983;65(1):70–80.
[17] Nyska M, Porat S, Nyska A, Rousso M, Shoshan S. Decreased adhesion formation in flexor tendons by topical application of enriched collagen solution—a histological study. Arch Orthop Trauma Surg 1987;106(3):192–4.
[18] Peterson WW, Manske PR, Kain CC, Lesker PA. Effect of flexor sheath integrity on tendon gliding: a biomechanical and histologic study. J Orthop Res 1986;4(4):458–65.
[19] Porat S, Rousso M, Shoshan S. Improvement of gliding function of flexor tendons by topically applied enriched collagen solution. J Bone Joint Surg [Br] 1980;62B(2):208–13.
[20] Zhao C, Amadio PC, An KN, Zobitz ME. Gliding characteristics of tendon repair in partially lacerated canine flexor digitorum profundus tendons. Anaheim: 45th Ann Orthop Res Soc; 1999. p. 120.
[21] Zhao C, Amadio PC, Zobitz ME, An KN. Gliding characteristics of tendon repair in canine flexor digitorum profundus tendons. J Orthop Res 2001; 19(4):580–6.
[22] Zhao C, Amadio PC, Zobitz ME, Momose T, Couvreur P, An K. Gliding resistance after repair of partially lacerated human flexor digitorum profundus tendon in vitro. Clin Biomech (Bristol, Avon) 2001;16(8):696–701.
[23] Boyer MI, Gelberman RH, Burns ME, Dinopoulos H, Hofem R, Silva MJ. Intrasynovial flexor tendon repair. An experimental study comparing low and high levels of in vivo force during rehabilitation in canines. J Bone Joint Surg [Am] 2001;83A(6): 891–9.
[24] Boyer MI, Meunier MJ, Lescheid J, Burns ME, Gelberman RH, Silva MJ. The influence of cross-sectional area on the tensile properties of flexor tendons. J Hand Surg [Am] 2001;26(5):828–32.
[25] Choueka J, Heminger H, Mass DP. Cyclical testing of zone II flexor tendon repairs. J Hand Surg [Am] 2000;25(6):1127–34.
[26] Dinopoulos HT, Boyer MI, Burns ME, Gelberman RH, Silva MJ. The resistance of a four- and eight-strand suture technique to gap formation during tensile testing: an experimental study of repaired canine flexor tendons after 10 days of in vivo healing. J Hand Surg [Am] 2000;25(3):489–98.
[27] Gelberman RH, Boyer MI, Brodt MD, Winters SC, Silva MJ. The effect of gap formation at the repair site on the strength and excursion of intrasynovial flexor tendons. An experimental study on the early stages of tendon-healing in dogs. J Bone Joint Surg [Am] 1999;81(7):975–82.
[28] Hamman J, Ali A, Phillips C, Cunningham B, Mass DP. A biomechanical study of the flexor digitorum superficialis: effects of digital pulley excision and loss of the flexor digitorum profundus. J Hand Surg [Am] 1997;22(2):328–35.
[29] Komanduri M, Phillips CS, Mass DP. Tensile strength of flexor tendon repairs in a dynamic cadaver model. J Hand Surg [Am] 1996;21(4):605–11.
[30] Miller L, Mass DP. A comparison of four repair techniques for Camper's chiasma flexor digitorum superficialis lacerations: tested in an in vitro model. J Hand Surg [Am] 2000;25(6):1122–6.
[31] Noguchi M, Seiler JG III, Gelberman RH, Sofranko RA, Woo SL. In vitro biomechanical analysis of suture methods for flexor tendon repair. J Orthop Res 1993;11(4):603–11.
[32] Silva MJ, Hollstien SB, Fayazi AH, Adler P, Gelberman RH, Boyer MI. The effects of multiple strand techniques on the tensile properties of flexor digitorum profundus to bone repair. J Bone Joint Surg [Am] 1998;80(10):1507–14.
[33] Silva MJ, Hollstien SB, Fayazi AH, Adler P, Gelberman RH, Boyer MI. The effects of multiple-strand suture techniques on the tensile properties of repair of the flexor digitorum profundus tendon to bone. J Bone Joint Surg [Am] 1998;80(10): 1507–14.

[34] Stein T, Ali A, Hamman J, Mass DP. A randomized biomechanical study of zone II human flexor tendon repairs analyzed in an in vitro model. J Hand Surg [Am] 1998;23(6):1046–51.
[35] Winters SC, Gelberman RH, Woo SL-Y, Chan SS, Grewal R, Seiler JG. The effects of multiple-strand suture methods on the strength and excursion of repaired intrasynovial flexor tendon: a biomechanical study in dogs. J Hand Surg [Am] 1998;23(1): 97–104.
[36] Winters SC, Seiler JG III, Woo SL, Gelberman RH. Suture methods for flexor tendon repair. A biomechanical analysis during the first six weeks following repair. Ann Chir Main Memb Super 1997;16(3):229–34.
[37] Banes AJ, Horesovsky G, Larson C, et al. Mechanical load stimulates expression of novel genes in vivo and in vitro in avian flexor tendon cells. Osteoarthritis Cartilage 1999;7(1):141–53.
[38] Bidder M, Towler DA, Gelberman RH, Boyer MI. Expression of mRNA for vascular endothelial growth factor at the repair site of healing canine flexor tendon. J Orthop Res 2000;18(2): 247–52.
[39] Chang J, Most D, Thunder R, Mehrara B, Longaker MT, Lineaweaver WC. Molecular studies in flexor tendon wound healing: the role of basic fibroblast growth factor gene expression. J Hand Surg [Am] 1998;23(6):1052–8.
[40] Chang J, Thunder R, Most D, Longaker MT, Lineaweaver WC. Studies in flexor tendon wound healing: neutralizing antibody to TGF-beta1 increases postoperative range of motion. Plast Reconstr Surg 2000;105(1):148–55.
[41] Strickland JW. Development of flexor tendon surgery: twenty-five years of progress. J Hand Surg [Am] 2000;25(2):214–35.
[42] Lundborg G, Myrhage R, Rydevik B. The vascularization of human flexor tendons within the digital synovial sheath region—structural and functional aspects. J Hand Surg [Am] 1977;2(6): 417–27.
[43] Lundborg G, Holm S, Myrhage R. The role of the synovial fluid and tendon sheath for flexor tendon nutrition. An experimental tracer study on diffusional pathways in dogs. Scand J Plast Reconstr Surg 1980;14(1):99–107.
[44] Doyle JR, Blythe WF. Anatomy of the flexor tendon sheath and pulleys of the thumb. J Hand Surg [Am] 1977;2(2):149–51.
[45] Abrahamsson SO, Lundborg G, Lohmander LS. Tendon healing in vivo. An experimental model. Scand J Plast Reconstr Surg Hand Surg 1989; 23(3):199–205.
[46] Gelberman RH. Flexor tendon physiology: tendon nutrition and cellular activity in injury and repair. Instr Course Lect 1985;34:351–60.
[47] Gelberman RH, Khabie V, Cahill CJ. The revascularization of healing flexor tendons in the digital sheath. A vascular injection study in dogs. J Bone Joint Surg [Am] 1991;73(6):868–81.
[48] Lundborg G, Rank F. Experimental intrinsic healing of flexor tendons based upon synovial fluid nutrition. J Hand Surg [Am] 1978;3(1):21–31.
[49] Manske PR, Bridwell K, Whiteside LA, Lesker PA. Nutrition of flexor tendons in monkeys. Clin Orthop 1978;136:294–8.
[50] Manske PR, Lesker PA. Flexor tendon nutrition. Hand Clin 1985;1(1):13–24.
[51] Manske PR, Lesker PA. Nutrient pathways of flexor tendons in primates. J Hand Surg [Am] 1982;7(5):436–44.
[52] Manske PR, Lesker PA, Bridwell K. Experimental studies in chickens on the initial nutrition of tendon grafts. J Hand Surg [Am] 1979;4(6):565–75.
[53] Ritty TM, Roth R, Heuser JE. Tendon cell array isolation reveals a previously unknown fibrillin-2-containing macromolecular assembly. Structure (Camb) 2003;11(9):1179–88.
[54] Barrie KA, Wolfe SW, Shean C, Shenbagamurthi D, Slade JF III, Panjabi MM. A biomechanical comparison of multistrand flexor tendon repairs using an in situ testing model. J Hand Surg [Am] 2000;25(3):499–506.
[55] Howard RF, Ondrovic L, Greenwald DP. Biomechanical analysis of four-strand extensor tendon repair techniques. J Hand Surg [Am] 1997;22(5): 838–42.
[56] Labana N, Messer T, Lautenschlager E, Nagda S, Nagle D. A biomechanical analysis of the modified Tsuge suture technique for repair of flexor tendon lacerations. J Hand Surg [Br] 2001;26(4):297–300.
[57] McLarney E, Hoffman H, Wolfe SW. Biomechanical analysis of the cruciate four-strand flexor tendon repair. J Hand Surg [Am] 1999;24(2):295–301.
[58] Sanders DW, Bain GI, Johnson JA, Milne AD, Roth JH, King GJ. In-vitro strength of flexor-tendon repairs. Can J Surg 1995;38(6):528–32.
[59] Savage R, Risitano G. Flexor tendon repair using a "six strand" method of repair and early active mobilisation. J Hand Surg [Br] 1989;14(4):396–9.
[60] Strickland JW. Flexor tendons—acute injuries. In: Green DP, Hotchkiss RN, Pederson WC, editors. Green's operative hand surgery. New York: Churchill Livingstone; 1999. p. 1851–97.
[61] Tang JB, Pan CZ, Xie RG, Chen F. A biomechanical study of Tang's multiple locking techniques for flexor tendon repair. Chir Main 1999;18(4):254–60.
[62] Barrie KA, Tomak SL, Cholewicki J, Wolfe SW. The role of multiple strands and locking sutures on gap formation of flexor tendon repairs during cyclical loading. J Hand Surg [Am] 2000;25(4): 714–20.
[63] Bhatia D, Tanner KE, Bonfield W, Citron ND. Factors affecting the strength of flexor tendon repair. J Hand Surg [Br] 1992;17(5):550–2.
[64] Gill RS, Lim BH, Shatford RA, Toth E, Voor MJ, Tsai TM. A comparative analysis of the six-strand

double-loop flexor tendon repair and three other techniques: a human cadaveric study. J Hand Surg [Am] 1999;24(6):1315–22.

[65] Lotz JC, Hariharan JS, Diao E. Analytic model to predict the strength of tendon repairs. J Orthop Res 1998;16(4):399–405.

[66] Pruitt DL, Manske PR, Fink B. Cyclic stress analysis of flexor tendon repair. J Hand Surg [Am] 1991; 16(4):701–7.

[67] Raposio E, Cella A, Barabino P, Santi P. Two modified techniques for flexor tendon repair. Plast Reconstr Surg 1999;103(6):1691–5.

[68] Shaieb MD, Singer DI. Tensile strengths of various suture techniques. J Hand Surg [Br] 1997;22(6): 764–7.

[69] Smith AM, Evans DM. Biomechanical assessment of a new type of flexor tendon repair. J Hand Surg [Br] 2001;26(3):217–9.

[70] Tang JB, Wang B, Chen F, Pan CZ, Xie RG. Biomechanical evaluation of flexor tendon repair techniques. Clin Orthop 2001;386:252–9.

[71] Thurman RT, Trumble TE, Hanel DP, Tencer AF, Kiser PK. Two-, four-, and six-strand zone II flexor tendon repairs: an in situ biomechanical comparison using a cadaver model. J Hand Surg [Am] 1998;23(2):261–5.

[72] Momose T, Amadio PC, Zhao C, Zobitz ME, An KN. The effect of knot location, suture material, and suture size on the gliding resistance of flexor tendons. J Biomed Mater Res 2000;53(6): 806–11.

[73] Norris SR, Ellis FD, Chen MI, Seiler JG III. Flexor tendon suture methods: a quantitative analysis of suture material within the repair site. Orthopedics 1999;22(4):413–6.

[74] Wada A, Kubota H, Miyanishi K, Hatanaka H, Miura H, Iwamoto Y. Comparison of postoperative early active mobilization and immobilization in vivo utilising a four-strand flexor tendon repair. J Hand Surg [Br] 2001;26(4):301–6.

[75] Diao E, Hariharan JS, Soejima O, Lotz JC. Effect of peripheral suture depth on strength of tendon repairs. J Hand Surg [Am] 1996;21(2):234–9.

[76] Mashadi ZB, Amis AA. Strength of the suture in the epitenon and within the tendon fibres: development of stronger peripheral suture technique. J Hand Surg [Br] 1992;17(2):172–5.

[77] Papandrea R, Seitz WH Jr, Shapiro P, Borden B. Biomechanical and clinical evaluation of the epitenon-first technique of flexor tendon repair. J Hand Surg [Am] 1995;20(2):261–6.

[78] Slade JF, Bhargava M, Barrie KA, Shenbagamurthi D, Wolfe SW. Zone II tendon repairs augmented with autogenous dorsal tendon graft: a biomechanical analysis. J Hand Surg [Am] 2001; 26(5):813–20.

[79] Becker H. Primary repair of flexor tendons in the hand without immobilisation—preliminary report. Hand 1978;10(1):37–47.

[80] Becker H, Davidoff M. Eliminating the gap in flexor tendon surgery. A new method of suture. Hand 1977;9(3):306–11.

[81] Ikuta Y, Tsuge K. Postoperative results of looped nylon suture used in injuries of the digital flexor tendons. J Hand Surg [Br] 1985;10(1):67–72.

[82] Silva MJ, Brodt MD, Boyer MI, et al. Effects of increased in vivo excursion on digital range of motion and tendon strength following flexor tendon repair. J Orthop Res 1999;17(5):777–83.

[83] Tsuge K, Ikuta Y, Matsuishi Y. Intra-tendinous tendon suture in the hand—a new technique. Hand 1975;7(3):250–5.

[84] Tsuge K, Yoshikazu I, Matsuishi Y. Repair of flexor tendons by intratendinous tendon suture. J Hand Surg [Am] 1977;2(6):436–40.

[85] Tajima T. History, current status, and aspects of hand surgery in Japan. Clin Orthop 1984;184:41–9.

[86] Wagner WF Jr, Carroll CT, Strickland JW, Heck DA, Toombs JP. A biomechanical comparison of techniques of flexor tendon repair. J Hand Surg [Am] 1994;19(6):979–83.

[87] Soejima O, Diao E, Lotz JC, Hariharan JS. Comparative mechanical analysis of dorsal versus palmar placement of core suture for flexor tendon repairs. J Hand Surg [Am] 1995;20(5):801–7.

[88] Hatanaka H, Manske PR. Effect of suture size on locking and grasping flexor tendon repair techniques. Clin Orthop 2000;375:267–74.

[89] Hatanaka H, Manske PR. Effect of the cross-sectional area of locking loops in flexor tendon repair. J Hand Surg [Am] 1999;24(4):751–60.

[90] Hatanaka H, Zhang J, Manske PR. An in vivo study of locking and grasping techniques using a passive mobilization protocol in experimental animals. J Hand Surg [Am] 2000;25(2):260–9.

[91] Aoki M, Pruitt DL, Kubota H, Manske PR. Effect of suture knots on tensile strength of repaired canine flexor tendons. J Hand Surg [Br] 1995;20(1): 72–5.

[92] Pruitt DL, Aoki M, Manske PR. Effect of suture knot location on tensile strength after flexor tendon repair. J Hand Surg [Am] 1996;21(6):969–73.

[93] Seradge H, Tian W, Kashef GH, Seradge A, Owen W. The Oklahoma repair technique: a biomechanical study of a new suture repair technique. J OK State Med Assoc 2000;93(12):551–6.

[94] Barmakian JT, Lin H, Green SM, Posner MA, Casar RS. Comparison of a suture technique with the modified Kessler method: resistance to gap formation. J Hand Surg [Am] 1994;19(5):777–81.

[95] Silfverskiöld KL, May EJ. Gap formation after flexor tendon repair in zone II. Results with a new controlled motion programme. Scand J Plast Reconstr Surg Hand Surg 1993;27(4):263–8.

[96] Silfverskiöld KL, May EJ, Tornvall AH. Gap formation during controlled motion after flexor tendon repair in zone II: a prospective clinical study. J Hand Surg [Am] 1992;17(3):539–46.

[97] Garner WL, McDonald JA, Koo M, Kuhn C III, Weeks PM. Identification of the collagen-producing cells in healing flexor tendons. Plast Reconstr Surg 1989;83(5):875–9.

[98] Gelberman RH, Amiel D, Harwood F. Genetic expression for type I procollagen in the early stages of flexor tendon healing. J Hand Surg [Am] 1992; 17(3):551–8.

[99] Goldfarb CA, Harwood F, Silva MJ, Gelberman RH, Amiel D, Boyer MI. The effect of variations in applied rehabilitation force on collagen concentration and maturation at the intrasynovial flexor tendon repair site. J Hand Surg [Am] 2001;26(5): 841–6.

[100] Amiel D, Gelberman R, Harwood F, Siegel D. Fibronectin in healing flexor tendons subjected to immobilization or early controlled passive motion. Matrix 1991;11(3):184–9.

[101] Banes AJ, Link GW, Bevin AG, et al. Tendon synovial cells secrete fibronectin in vivo and in vitro. J Orthop Res 1988;6(1):73–82.

[102] Gelberman RH, Steinberg D, Amiel D, Akeson W. Fibroblast chemotaxis after tendon repair. J Hand Surg [Am] 1991;16(4):686–93.

[103] Harwood FL, Goomer RS, Gelberman RH, Silva MJ, Amiel D. Regulation of alpha(v)beta3 and alpha5beta1 integrin receptors by basic fibroblast growth factor and platelet-derived growth factor-BB in intrasynovial flexor tendon cells. Wound Repair Regen 1999;7(5):381–8.

[104] Harwood FL, Monosov AZ, Goomer RS, et al. Integrin expression is upregulated during early healing in a canine intrasynovial flexor tendon repair and controlled passive motion model. Connect Tissue Res 1998;39(4):309–16.

[105] Boyer MI, Watson JT, Lou J, Manske PR, Gelberman RH, Cai SR. Quantitative variation in vascular endothelial growth factor mRNA expression during early flexor tendon healing: an investigation in a canine model. J Orthop Res 2001;19(5):869–72.

[106] Zhang F, Liu H, Stile F, et al. Effect of vascular endothelial growth factor on rat Achilles tendon healing. Plast Reconstr Surg 2003;112(6):1613–9.

[107] Robbins JR, Evanko SP, Vogel KG. Mechanical loading and TGF-beta regulate proteoglycan synthesis in tendon. Arch Biochem Biophys 1997; 342(2):203–11.

[108] Tsuzaki M, et al. Insulin-like growth factor-I is expressed by avian flexor tendon cells. J Orthop Res 2000;18(4):546–56.

[109] Jann HW, Stein LE, Slater DA. In vitro effects of epidermal growth factor or insulin-like growth factor on tenoblast migration on absorbable suture material. Vet Surg 1999;28(4):268–78.

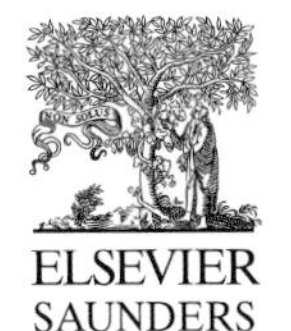

ELSEVIER
SAUNDERS

Hand Clin 21 (2005) 167–171

HAND
CLINICS

Zone I Flexor Tendon Injuries

Brian A. Murphy, MD*, Daniel P. Mass, MD

University of Chicago, Section of Orthopaedic Surgery and Rehabilitation Medicine, Department of Surgery, 5841 South Maryland Avenue, MC 3079, Chicago, IL 60637-1470, USA

Zone I flexor tendon injuries include injuries to the flexor digitorum profundus (FDP) tendon. These injuries occur distal to the superficialis insertion over the middle phalanx or proximal distal phalanx, and as such are isolated injuries to the FDP. The mechanism most commonly is closed avulsion from the distal phalanx or a laceration, but other mechanisms such as open avulsion or crush injury can occur. On physical examination, the cascade of the fingers is disrupted, and distal interphalangeal (DIP) joint flexion must be isolated to determine if the FDP tendon is continuous, because other mechanisms are present to enable finger flexion at the other joints.

FDP avulsion injuries have been labeled "jersey" fingers because of their mechanism of injury, which typically involves hyperextension of the DIP joint against a maximally contracted flexion force, occurring often in tackling sports [1]. The flexed finger is caught in the jersey of the player being tackled, and a forceful extension moment occurs as the player attempts to escape the tackle. These injuries occur as tendinous avulsions with or without a bony fragment involved from the base of the distal phalanx. These injuries occur most often in the ring finger [2], although avulsions in all of the fingers and the thumb have been reported. Various theories exist to explain the prevalence of ring finger injuries. Manske reported an experimental study in which the insertion of the profundus to the ring finger was weaker than that of the long finger [2], and Bynum and Gilbert have shown that the ring finger becomes the most prominent finger with the fingers in a partially flexed position [3]. The factors influencing the prognosis include the level to which the tendon retracts, the delay between injury and treatment, the presence and size of bony fragments, and the blood supply to the tendon in this location [1,4].

Avulsion injuries are classified by Leddy and Packer into three types [1]. Type I injuries represent avulsions in which the proximal tendon stump has retracted into the palm. These must be treated in an urgent fashion to avoid degeneration of the tendon and myostatic contracture. This occurs because of the severe damage to the vascularity of the tendon with this injury, as both vincula are ruptured when the tendon retracts to the level of the palm. The resulting hematoma in the flexor sheath also contributes to the risk for scar formation and contracture; hence the need for urgent repair. The diagnosis often is delayed because the finger still can flex at the metacarpal phalangeal (MCP) and proximal interphalangeal (PIP) joints because of the action of the intact intrinsic and flexor digitorum superficialis (FDS) tendons, respectively. Treatment options after a delay in diagnosis include DIP fusion, reconstruction of the FDP, no treatment (just leaving the finger alone), or excision of the profundus if it becomes a painful nodule after retracting into the palm. The FDP can be reconstructed in a one-stage procedure with the graft placed around rather than through the FDS decussation [5]. The loss of DIP flexion is not severely disabling; however, the loss of strength from the deficient FDP can be troublesome. Stiffness of the PIP joint can occur, often with some degree of fixed flexion contracture [6]. Fortunately these injuries are rare [7].

* Corresponding author.

E-mail address: bmurphy@surgery.bsd.uchicago.edu (B.A. Murphy).

doi:10.1016/j.hcl.2004.12.004

Type II injuries occur as the avulsed tendon retracts to the level of the FDS decussation at the PIP joint. These are the most common form of avulsions [7]. A small piece of bone may be attached to the tendon stump, aiding in the radiographic diagnosis. The short vinculum is ruptured, but the long vinculum remains intact, and the tendon length is preserved. These injuries therefore can be addressed up to 3 months after the injury with good results [7], as long as the tendon has not further retracted. Silva et al [8] have shown in a canine model that the FDP tendon hypertrophies after it is divided from its insertion site, and at 21 days the tendon still is able to hold a suture well. This reinforces the notion that delayed repair is still possible. If retraction occurs, the injury is converted to a type I injury, with the commensurate prognosis. Type II injuries generally have a better prognosis than type I.

Type III injuries involve a larger piece of bone that gets caught at the level of the A4 pulley. Both vincula remain intact, and a small measure of DIP flexion can occur through the vincula. The bony injuries can be treated by open reduction and internal fixation of the fracture fragment, which indirectly repairs the tendon. Kang et al reported on a series of five cases in which miniplates and cortical screws were used for avulsed fragments of sufficient size [9], and the use of lag screws also has been advocated [10]. If the fracture fragment is too small for fixation or if a pure tendon avulsion has occurred, the tendon should be reattached directly to the distal phalanx. The type III injuries also can involve a fracture with subsequent avulsion of the tendon from the bony fragment and retraction of the tendon into the palm. This has been classified as a type IIIA injury, and fortunately is exceedingly rare.

Treatment varies according to the type of injury. When the tendinous avulsion needs to be repaired, a periosteal flap can be raised, under which the tendon can be inserted. For a type I injury, the injury site is exposed using a Bruner incision and the flexor sheath distal to the A4 pulley is opened. A separate incision can be made in the palm to find the proximal stump. A pediatric gastrostomy tube then can be threaded through the flexor sheath to bring the proximal end into the injury site. The proximal end of the tendon traditionally has been secured with a Kessler or Bunnell repair, and then the suture ends tied over a button on the dorsum of the distal phalanx (Fig. 1).

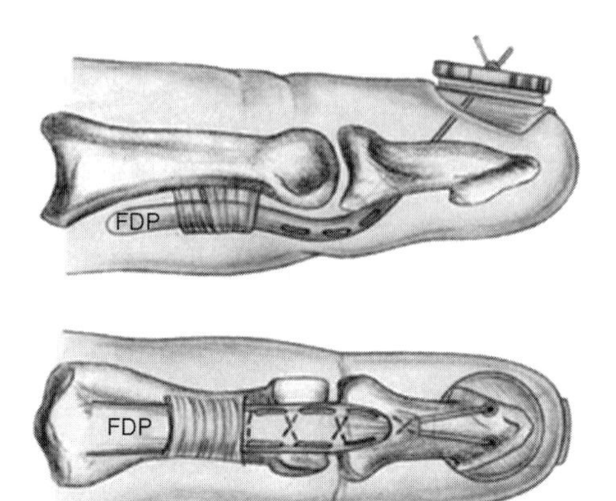

Fig. 1. Sketch of flexor digitorum profundus (FDP) avulsion repaired over a button. (*From* Berger RA, Weiss AC. Hand surgery. Philadelphia, PA: Lippincott Williams & Wilkins; 2004. p. 679–98; with permission.)

A weaker unlocked repair must be done with this technique to allow for subsequent suture removal. Early motion could not be initiated because of the risk for re-rupture, and the risk for infection from the sutures lying outside the skin did exist. The nail bed also could be injured by improper placement of the sutures on the dorsal aspect of the distal phalanx. The authors' preferred technique involves suture anchors, which are tolerated much better by patients than is a button (Fig. 2).

Two Mitek microsuture anchors with 4-0 Ethibond anchored in the distal phalanx with modified

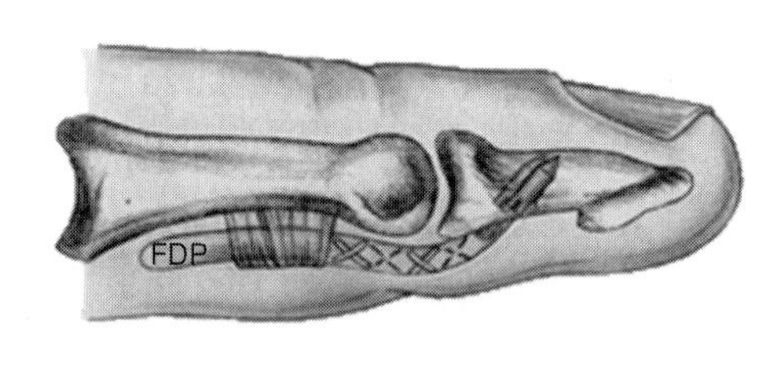

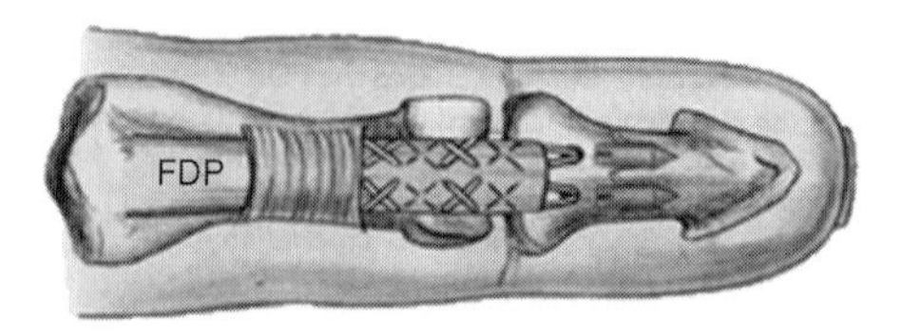

Fig. 2. Sketch of flexor digitorum profundus (FDP) avulsion repair with micro Mitek. (*From* Berger RA, Weiss AC. Hand surgery. Philadelphia, PA: Lippincott Williams & Wilkins; 2004. p. 679–98; with permission.)

Becker repairs on the radial and ulnar sides of the tendon demonstrate a pull-out strength of 70 N, which is strong enough to begin early active motion. Two micro anchors have been shown to be stronger than the pull-out suture or one mini-suture anchor by itself [11]. Type II injuries do not require dissection into the palm to retrieve the proximal end of the tendon, because the tendon is at the level of the PIP joint or proximal phalanx. The repair is the same as for the type I injuries. In bony type III injuries, Kirschner wires can be used in a dorsal to volar fashion. Alternatively if the fragment is large enough, mini-fragment screws can be used to secure the fracture [10]. The fragment needs to be 2.5 times the diameter of the screw to allow for proper fixation without splitting the fragment. A mini-plate also has been advocated in a case series [9].

The FDP tendon also can be injured in zone I through a laceration. The proximal end usually retracts to the level of the PIP joint or distal proximal phalanx [12]. The flexor sheath is exposed using Bruner incisions over the level to which the tendon has retracted. The length of the distal stump depends on the position of the finger at the time of the laceration. If the finger was flexed, the distal stump may be short when the finger is extended. Enough distal stump may or may not exist to perform a formal tendon repair. If enough tendon is present, the authors prefer to perform a locked cruciate with 3-0 Ethibond and an epitendinous volar 6-0 nylon repair under the A4 pulley. This requires roughly 0.75 cm of distal tendon for the locking sutures. To repair the tendon under the A4 pulley, one must advance the proximal end of the tendon enough to perform the repair distal to the pulley, or the pulley can be released partially to allow for the repair. The flexor sheath can be opened in the spaces between the pulleys to allow for retrieval and advancement of the tendon. The proximal end can be retrieved with a pediatric gastrostomy tube and be held in place either with the tube or with a 25-gauge needle placed horizontally through the tendon and pulley. If the distal stump is too small for a formal repair, the tendon can be advanced and anchored to the distal phalanx as one would repair an avulsion, or a repair maintaining the original length can be performed. It has been demonstrated that advancement of up to 1 cm was not detrimental to the function of the tendon, but most surgeons prefer to maintain length of the tendon and avoid potential weakness of the other profundus tendons from the quadriga effect and possible flexion contractures [13]. Performing a formal repair in the proximal stump and bringing the suture through the distal stump without a formal repair maintains length. A 4-0 nylon Kessler repair is placed in the proximal stump, and the sutures are attached to two Keith needles. The Keith needles then are brought out through the distal stump and out the tip of the finger, instead of the bone (Fig. 3).

The sutures then are tied over a button at the proper tension to avoid shortening of the tendon. An injury to the A4 pulley often occurs concomitantly. If more than 50% of the pulley has been damaged, it should be reconstructed with a strip of dorsal wrist retinaculum (Fig. 4) or a synovial-lined donor tendon.

Otherwise the damaged portion should be débrided. Postoperatively, if a formal repair of the tendon can be accomplished, an early motion protocol can be used for postoperative treatment. This typically involves short arc motion and place and hold exercises. If the repair used a button, it must be protected.

The results of this injury traditionally have not been as good as those of other flexor tendon injuries. Full motion usually is not regained, whereas good and excellent results were reported only in up to 67% in one series. The percentage dropped to less than 50% with DIP flexion as the determining factor [14]. Silva et al have shown in

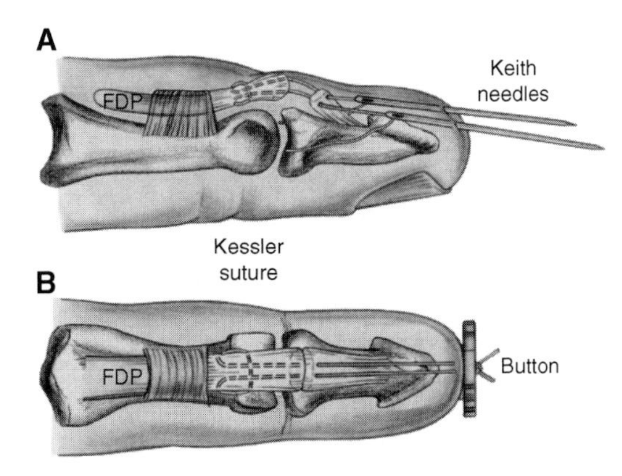

Fig. 3. Profundus pullout through fingertip. (*A*) Kessler repair to proximal profundus end attached to two Keith needles that are pushed through the distal profundus and out the distal tip of the finger. (*B*) Suture tied over a button at the tip. FDP, flexor digitorum profundus. (*From* Berger RA, Weiss AC. Hand surgery. Philadelphia, PA: Lippincott Williams & Wilkins; 2004. p. 679–98; with permission.)

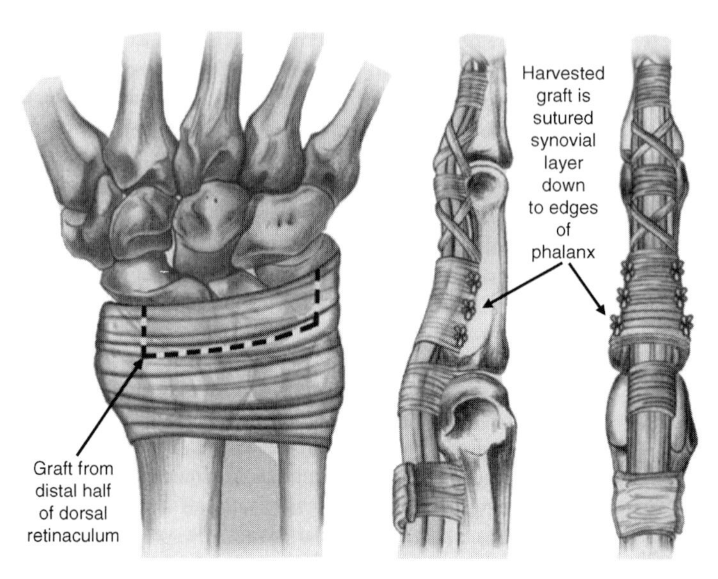

Fig. 4. Dorsal retinacular reconstruction. Half of the dorsal retinaculum is harvested and sutured synovial layer down to the edges of the proximal or middle phalanx, because there is usually a scar rim of the original pulley. (*From* Berger RA, Weiss AC. Hand surgery. Philadelphia, PA: Lippincott Williams & Wilkins; 2004. p. 679–98; with permission.)

a canine model that the ultimate force of the insertion site did not increase 6 weeks after injury and suture repair [15]. This longer healing course differs from the healing properties of midsubstance tendon repairs and may account for the poor outcomes. Leversedge et al performed a vascular study demonstrating a hypovascular watershed area between the vascular supply from the vincula and the vascular supply that comes from the distal phalanx itself, which occurs 1 cm proximal to the insertion of the FDP tendon [16]. This hypovascularity may play a role in the slower healing response, but the difference in healing mechanisms between midsubstance and insertional tendon injuries of the flexor tendons has not been fully elucidated. The surgeon and the patient should be prepared for the possibility of less than optimal outcomes with these injuries.

References

[1] Leddy JP, Packer JW. Avulsion of the profundus tendon insertion in athletes. J Hand Surg 1977;2A: 66–9.

[2] Manske PR, Lesker PA. Avulsion of the ring finger flexor digitorum profundus tendon: an experimental study. Hand 1978;10:52–5.

[3] Bynum DK, Gilbert JA. Avulsion of the flexor digitorum profundus: anatomic and biomechanical considerations. J Hand Surg 1988;13A:222–7.

[4] Leddy JP. Avulsions of the flexor digitorum profundus. Hand Clin 1985;1:77–83.

[5] McClinton MA, Curtis RM, Wilgis EF. One hundred tendon grafts for isolated flexor digitorum profundus injuries. J Hand Surg 1982;7A: 224–9.

[6] Thayer DT. Distal interphalangeal joint injuries. Hand Clin 1988;4:1–4.

[7] Lubahn JD, Hood JM. Fractures of the distal interphalangeal joint. Clin Orth and Related Res 1996; 327:12–20.

[8] Silva MJ, Ritty TM, Ditsios K, Burns ME, Boyer MI, Gelberman RH. Tendon injury response: assessment of biomechanical properties, tissue morphology and viability following flexor digitorum profundus tendon transection. J Orthop Res 2004; 22:990–7.

[9] Kang N, Pratt A, Burr N. Miniplate fixation for avulsion injuries of the flexor digitorum profundus insertion. J Hand Surg [Br] 2003;28:363–8.

[10] Shabat S, Sagiv P, Stern A, Nyska M. Avulsion fracture of the flexor digitorum profundus tendon ("Jersey finger") type III. Arch Orthop Trauma Surg 2002;122:182–3.

[11] Brustein M, Pellegrini J, Choueka J, et al. Bone suture anchors versus the pullout button for repair of distal profundus tendon injuries: a comparison of strength in human cadaveric hands. J Hand Surg 2001;26A:489–96.

[12] Evans RB. A study of the zone I flexor tendon injury and its implications for treatment. J Hand Ther 1990;3:133–48.

[13] Malerich MM, Baird RA, McMaster W, Erickson JM. Permissible limits of flexor digitorum profundus

tendon advancement—an anatomic study. J Hand Surg 1987;12A:30–3.
[14] Moiemen NS, Elliot D. Primary flexor tendon repair in zone 1. J Hand Surg [Br] 2000;25:78–84.
[15] Silva MJ, Boyer MI, Ditsios K, et al. The insertion site of the canine flexor digitorum profundus tendon heals slowly following injury and suture repair. J Orthop Res 2002;20:447–53.
[16] Leversedge FJ, Ditsios K, Goldfarb CA, Silva MJ, Gelberman RH, Boyer MI. Vascular anatomy of the human flexor digitorum profundus tendon insertion. J Hand Surg 2002;27A:806–12.

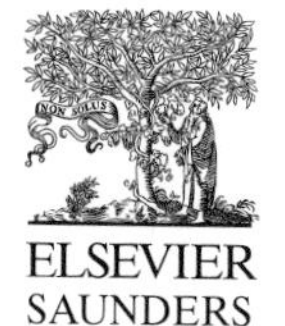
ELSEVIER
SAUNDERS

Hand Clin 21 (2005) 173–179

HAND
CLINICS

Acute Flexor Tendon Repairs in Zone II

Robert W. Coats II, MD[a], Julio C. Echevarría-Oré, MD[b], Daniel P. Mass, MD[a,*]

[a]*Section of Orthopaedic Surgery and Rehabilitation Medicine, Department of Surgery, University of Chicago Pritzker School of Medicine, University of Chicago Hospital, 5841 South Maryland Avenue, MC 3079, Chicago, IL 60637, USA*

[b]*Department of Orthopaedics and Traumatology, Hospital Nacional Edgardo Rebagliati Martins, Lima, Perú*

Early repair of flexor tendon injuries has become the standard of care, even when the tendon injury lies between the A1 pulley on the volar aspect of the metacarpophalangeal (MCP) joint to the insertion of the flexor digitorum superficialis (FDS) tendon insertion on the middle phalanx or zone II, as described by Verdan. Bunnell, in 1918, admonished surgeons that "it is better to remove the tendons entirely from the finger and graft in new tendons throughout its length." Although this concept has been abandoned, Bunnell's second admonishment, strict adherence to meticulous atraumatic technique, cannot be overemphasized [1,2]. Flexor tendon repairs in "no man's land" have improved with advances in understanding of flexor tendon anatomy, biomechanics, nutrition, and healing [3]. Improvements in repair techniques have reduced clinically significant repair gap formation, allowing rapid postoperative active and passive mobilization therapy protocols. Increased repair strength, decreased gap formation, and rapid tendon mobilization encourages intrinsic tendon healing, while avoiding extrinsic adhesion formation. We can now go from this (Fig. 1) to this (Fig. 2) in 6 weeks.

To obtain adequate strength and gliding in this region, the following anatomic factors must be taken into consideration: (1) two tendons are encased in a narrow fibro-osseous pulley system compartment, (2) the vascular supply of flexor tendons is mainly dorsal, and (3) the superficialis and profundus tendons have unique spatial relationships (Fig. 3).

The repair technique must provide enough tensile strength to start early active motion without compromising the vascular supply through the vincula or significantly increasing the work of flexion. The goal of gliding implies providing a smooth tendon surface that decreases friction within the pulley system, therefore preventing extrinsic scarring and rigid adhesions. This enhances tendon nutrition through diffusion, intrinsic healing, and collagen remodeling.

Clinical history and physical examination

Almost all zone II tendon injuries, whether partial or complete, are caused by a laceration from a sharp object, such as a knife or broken glass. For presurgical planning it is helpful to know if the fingers were in extension rather than flexion when the injury occurred. If both tendons are cut at the same level, it is easier to find the tendon ends through a smaller incision. Both repairs will be at the same level, however, increasing the risk for extrinsic healing between the two tendons, possibly creating one scar unit [4]. Tendon injuries can be tested by tenodesis rather than active flexion, which does not hurt the patient (Fig. 4). A thorough neurovascular evaluation of the digits must be performed, and if injured, the digital nerves and arteries should be repaired during the same operative setting. Fracture must be ruled out, and if present, rigid osteosynthesis is performed at the same time as tendon repair (Fig. 5).

* Corresponding author.

E-mail address: dmass@surgery.bsd.uchicago.edu (D.P. Mass).

0749-0712/05/$ - see front matter
doi:10.1016/j.hcl.2004.11.001

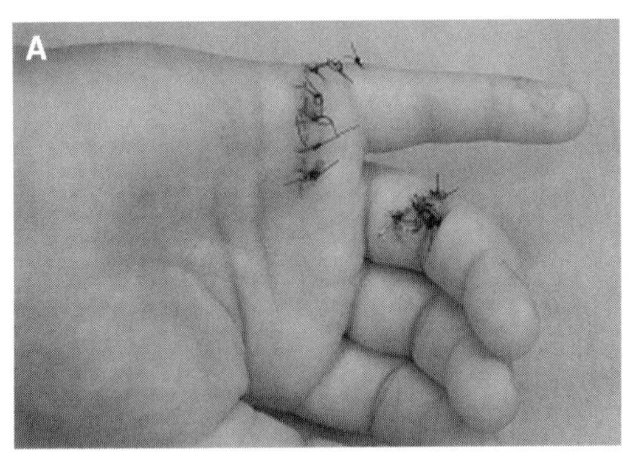

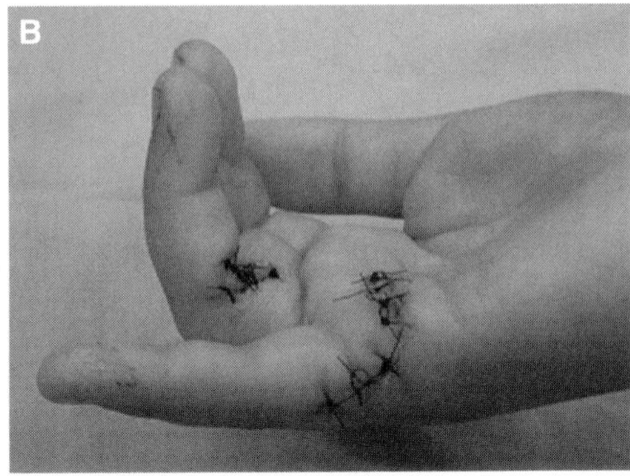

Fig. 1. (*A*) AP of little finger with sublimus and profundus laceration. (*B*) Lateral of little finger with sublimus and profundus laceration.

Indications for surgery

Because of the considerations mentioned previously, the only way to achieve adequate function of the injured tendons is by surgical repair. Isolated injury to the superficialis or profundus can be left unrepaired but only after explaining the potential compromised function of that digit. The patient's ability to participate in a postoperative rehabilitation protocol is an equally important consideration. Poor rehabilitation of a good zone II flexor tendon repair is potentially more debilitating than an untreated injury.

When dealing with partial tendon lacerations, it is important to consider that in a clinical setting most wounds create a volar laceration of the

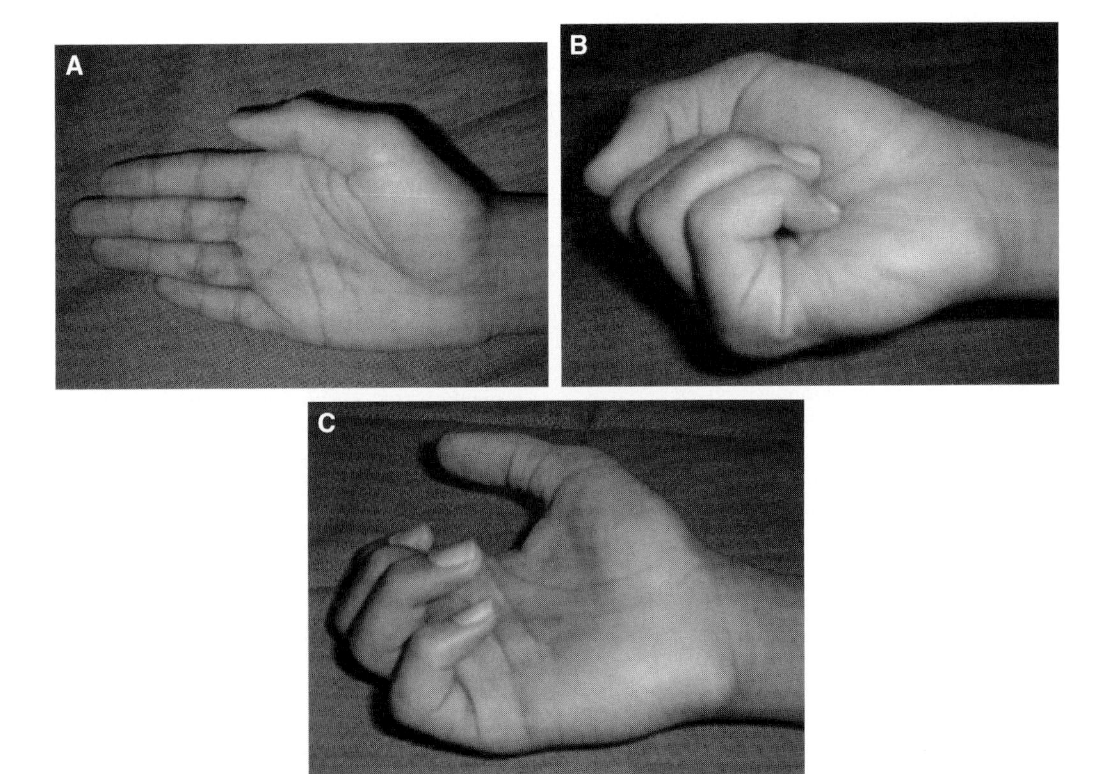

Fig. 2. (*A*) Active extension at 6 weeks. (*B*) Active flexion at 6 weeks. (*C*) Active claw at 6 weeks.

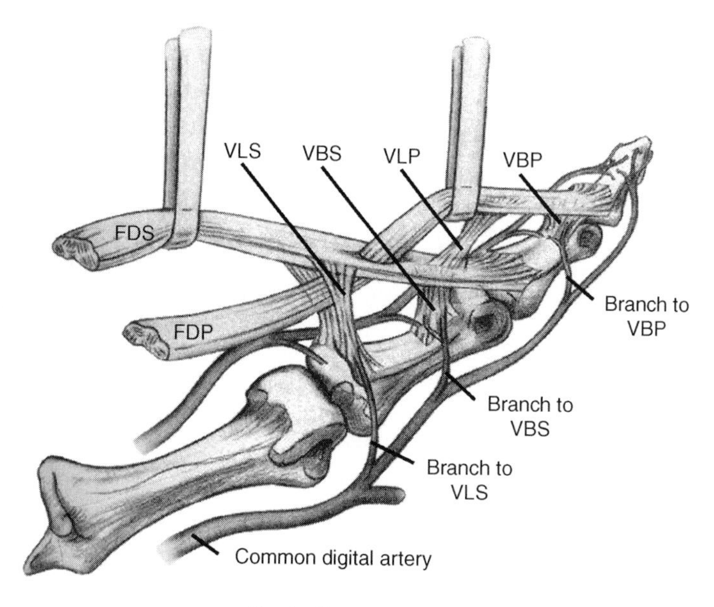

Fig. 3. Camper's chiasm.

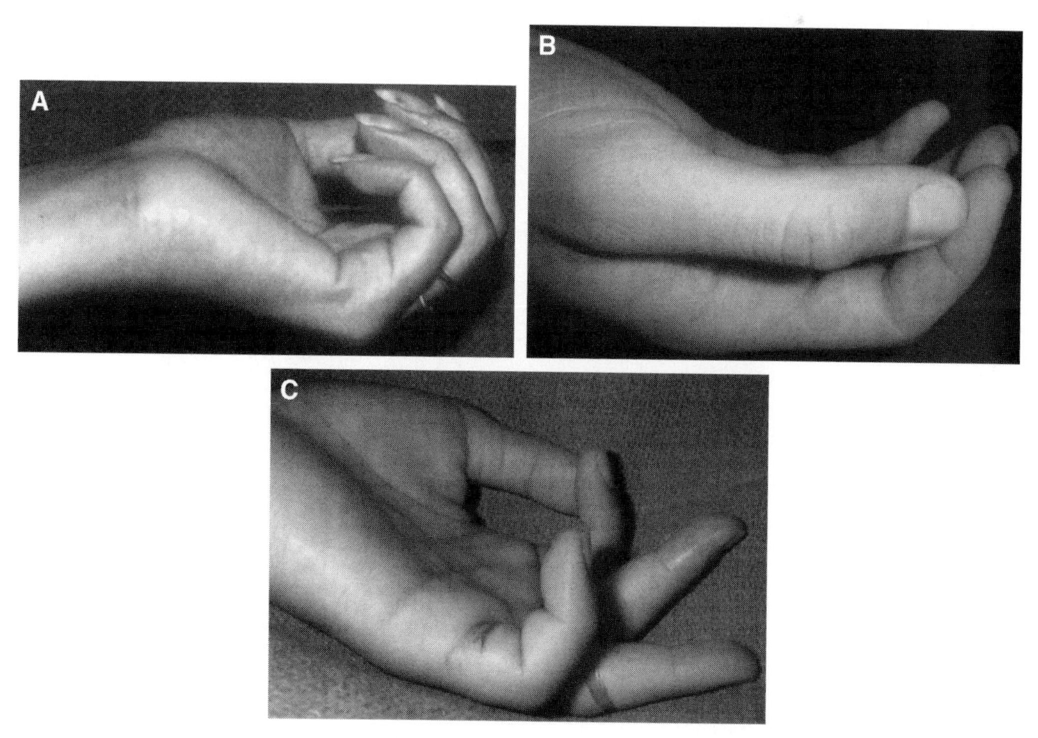

Fig. 4. (*A*) Normal tenodesis cascade of the fingers. (*B*) Break of ring finger cascade—profundus avulsion. (*C*) Break of long and ring finger cascade—long finger has superficialis laceration, ring has both tendons cut.

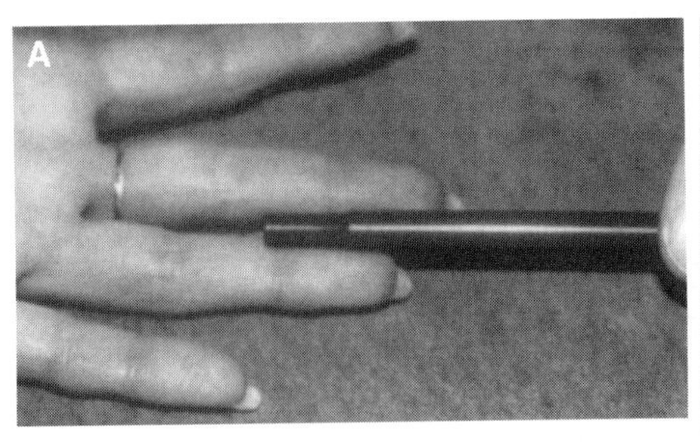

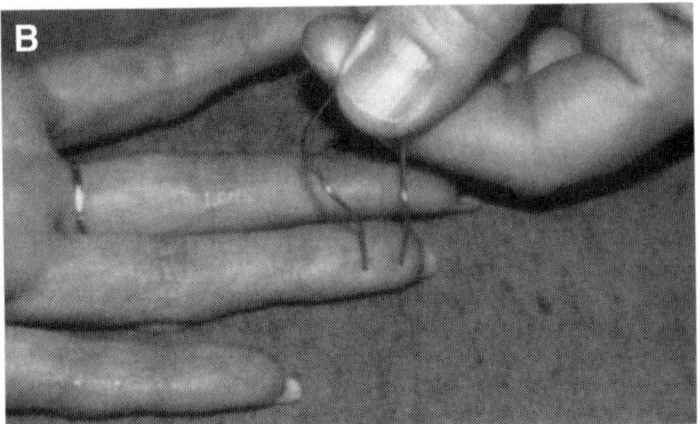

Fig. 5. Sensory tests. (*A*) Testing for sweat. (*B*) Testing for 2 point discrimination.

tendon. In such cases, it is necessary to determine if the laceration is total or partial, how much is involved, and whether there is triggering or trapping with active motion. Partial lacerations involving up to 90% of the tendon cross-section may be amenable to trimming if there is triggering during active motion. Sheath closure then is followed by protected motion [5,6].

The primary repair of flexor tendons is contraindicated when there have been severe multiple tissue injuries to the fingers, when the wounds are dirty or contaminated, or when there has been skin loss overlying the flexor system [3].

Surgical technique

These injuries may be operable on an elective basis within 2 or 3 days as long as one of the digital arteries is intact. All flexor tendon repairs must be performed in a formal operating room with at least an axillary block and preferably under loupe magnification. A tourniquet is placed before the limb is prepared and draped. Incisions are marked before limb exsanguination and tourniquet inflation.

Either Bruner zigzag or midaxial incisions are used (Fig. 6), depending on the geometry of the laceration and the anticipated neurovascular involvement. Opening of a transverse incision with extension through a midaxial incision is particularly useful in the event of an FDS and FDP injury with a nerve injury on one side. Bruner incisions are preferred for isolated tendon injuries or those with multiple structure involvement on both sides of the digit. If tendon retraction into the palm is anticipated, appropriate skin incisions must be planned, allowing them to be connected to the digital incisions if necessary.

Once the tendon sheath has been exposed, the laceration site can be identified. At this point it is crucial to assess the status of the A2 and A4 pulley, because these are of paramount importance in the biomechanics of tendon excursion. If the laceration has not involved either of these pulleys, it is possible to open one side of the tendon sheath for wider exposure without injuring these structures. When the laceration is within the midsubstance of an otherwise intact A2 or A4 pulley, unilateral opening of the pulley system proximally or distally creates a triangular shaped flap and allows exposure of the tendon ends (Fig. 7). Partial pulley injuries require debridement of the ends, preserving as much pulley as possible. Because the A2 pulley is functionally more important than the others, when its

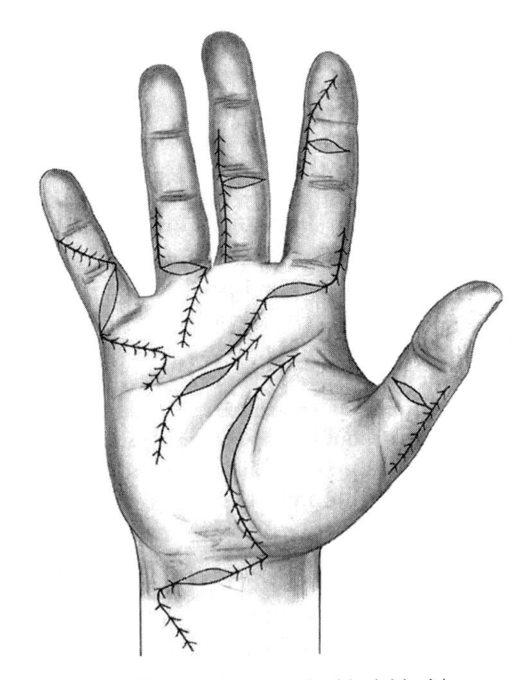

Fig. 6. Bruner zig-zag and midaxial incision.

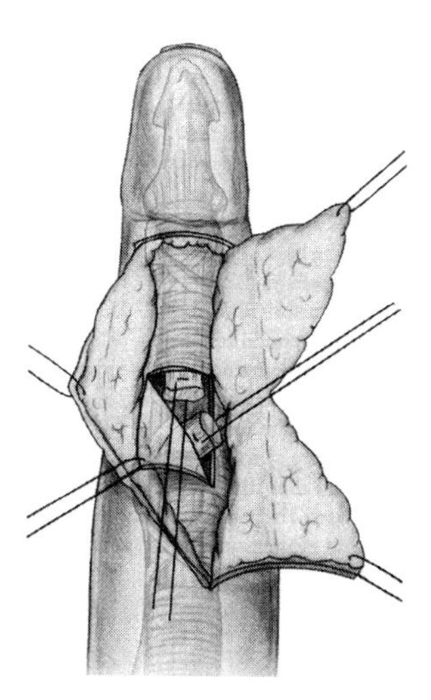

Fig. 7. Opening of the pulley sheath for exposure.

proximal or distal one half is injured, partial pulley reconstruction may be considered [7]. If the entire A2 or A4 pulley is destroyed, pulley reconstruction is indicated (see article on pulleys by Mehta and Phillips elsewhere in this issue).

After adequate exposure of the tendon sheath, the proximal and distal tendon stumps must be delivered to the operating field [8]. In case the proximal stumps are not in the sheath nor are they able to be "milked in" by flexing the wrist and

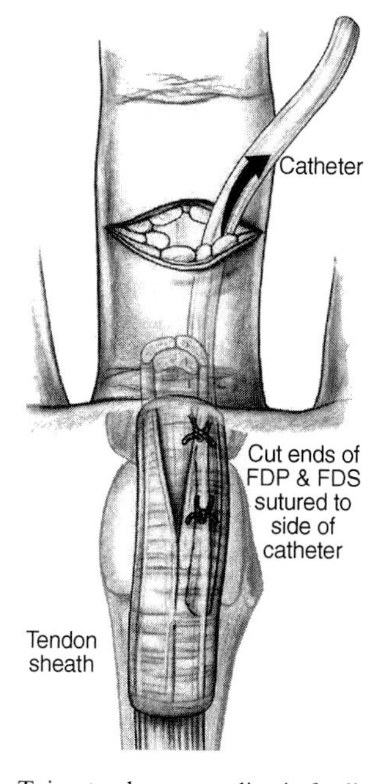

Fig. 8. Tying tendons to pediatric feeding tube.

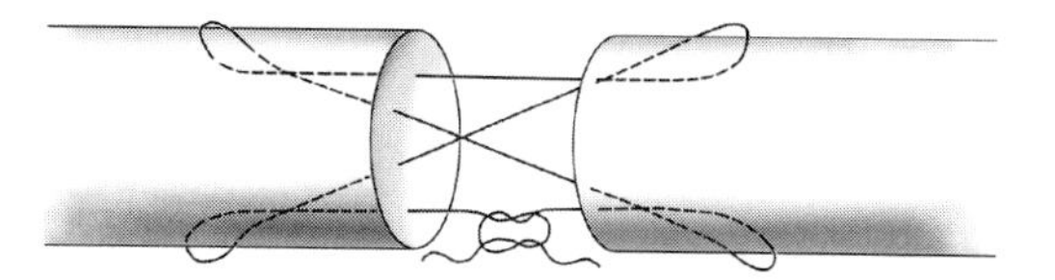

Fig. 9. Cruciate repair.

MCP joints, it is necessary to explore the palm. Once the proximal stumps are found, they must be brought into the digital incision. This is accomplished by placing sutures to be grasped by a small mosquito hemostat placed distally, or by advancing proximally a #5 pediatric feeding catheter through the tendon sheath and then tying the tendons to its side to pull them to the site of repair (Fig. 8). The distal stumps usually are found by flexing the distal joints. If this proves unsuccessful, distal sheath opening and subsequent repair is necessary. Hypodermic (25-gauge) needles may be placed through both stumps and a pulley to prevent retraction while the repair is performed.

In most zone II injuries, the FDS is divided into two slips that fan out and twist around the profundus tendon until remerging to insert on the middle third of the middle phalanx. A modified cruciate repair (Fig. 9) or other 4-strand repair is performed on one slip, thus allowing adequate strength and maintaining slip approximation to prevent narrowing of the superficialis opening (Camper's chiasm) around the profundus [9,10]. The other slip is resected. If only one slip of the FDS is lacerated, that side is excised to open the chiasm. The profundus tendon is repaired with a modified cruciate tendon suture using 3-0 or 4-0 (depending on the size of the tendon) Ethibond (Excel Ethicon, Inc.; Somerville, New Jersey) or Tycron that has adequate strength for

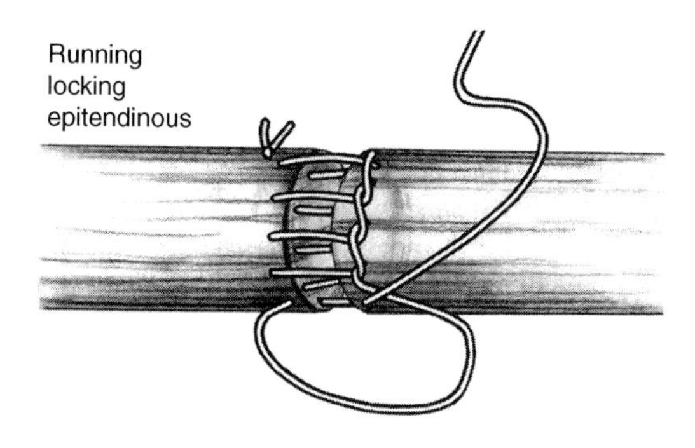

Fig. 10. Epitendinous repair.

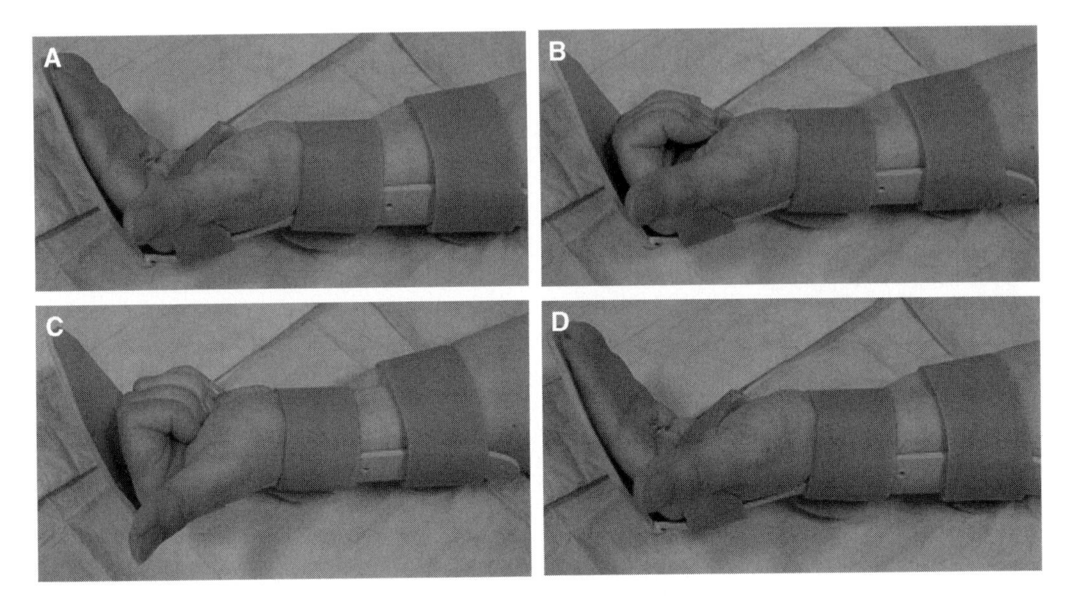

Fig. 11. Active motion protocol without resistance in a splint. (*A*) Resting position. (*B*) Flexion to proximal palm. (*C*) Flexion to distal palm. (*D*) Return to extension.

an active motion protocol [9,10], favorable gliding characteristics, and minimal repair site gapping. This is followed by a locking circumferential repair with 6-0 nylon [10], though it is preferable to perform the back wall epitendinous repair first to set the position of the core suture (Fig. 10).

After verifying the tendon repair, the sheath opening must be addressed. Closure of the sheath with 6-0 dissolving suture is the goal, but the sheath may be left open if tendon strangulation is an issue. It is necessary to preserve as much of the A2 and A4 pulleys as possible, to have an effective pulley system that allows full finger flexion. The other pulleys can be opened and even excised, depending on their involvement. If the distal part of the A2 and A3 pulley is missing, severe bowstringing across the proximal interphalangeal (PIP) joint causes a flexion contracture and loss of full finger flexion unless the distal A2 pulley is reconstructed. If less than one half of the A2 and A4 pulley remains, these are reconstructed using the dorsal retinaculum [11] or the palmaris longus.

Postoperative rehabilitation

In the immediate postoperative period, the patients are put in clam digger splints, but with the wrist in 30° of extension, the MCP joints in 60° of flexion, and both interphalangeal joints in full extension. After 2 or 3 days they are put in a Kleinert rubber band splint for home exercises. During sleep hours, patients have their fingers immobilized with the DIP and PIP joints in full extension to prevent flexion contractures. If possible, arrangements must be made for daily hand therapy for protected active range of motion (ROM) (Fig. 11). The authors start active flexion and extension in the splint without resistance. We use Strickland's place and hold technique [12], with the wrist in 30° of extension, active interphalangeal joint flexion with the MCP joints in 60° of flexion, if there are reliability problems with active motion.

The postoperative protocol is modified for children. Young children are placed in a clam digger long arm cast to the finger tips and older children in a clam digger short arm cast. The wrist is left in 30° of extension, with the MCP joints in 60° of flexion and the interphalangeal joints fully extended. In all cases a thick dressing is placed volarly under the fingers, from the MCP joint distally. This dressing is removed once the cast has hardened, providing space for the fingers to move actively in a protective shell. The authors have had no ruptures with this technique (Fig. 12).

Pitfalls

A common pitfall that occurs when repairing the FDS slips at Camper's chiasm is suturing the

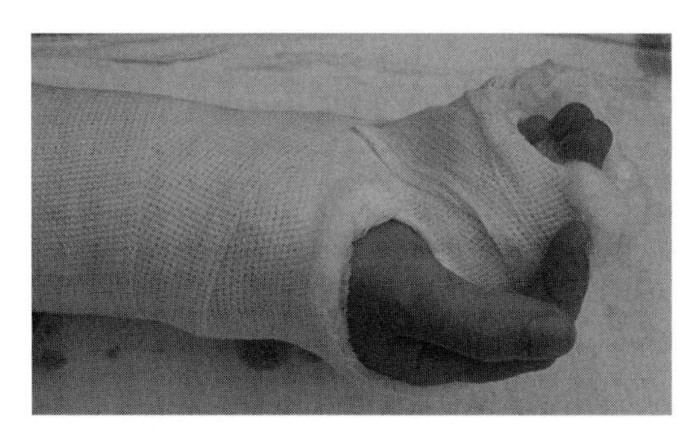

Fig. 12. Pediatric cast for tendon repair/active motion space.

tendon in an incorrect rotational alignment. Once lacerated, the proximal stumps rotate 90° in an outward fashion, whereas the distal stumps rotate inward. In this situation, occasionally the stumps of each slip are sutured as found, decreasing the effective size of the opening of the FDP. Careful attention must be made to the orientation of the FDS slips in this zone.

When performing zone II flexor tendon repairs, it is essential to have the tendon ends well approximated. If the back wall of the epitendinous repair is completed first, the tendon ends line up well and can be abutted during placement of the core sutures. The epitendinous repair allows for easy manipulation of the tendon during repair, adds strength to the repair, and helps tendon gliding by smoothing the repair site.

Summary

Flexor tendon repair in zone II is still a technically demanding procedure, but the outcomes have become more predictable and satisfying. Of keystone importance for obtaining the goals of normal strength and gliding of repaired flexor tendons are an atraumatic surgical technique, an appropriate suture material, a competent pulley system, and the use of early motion rehabilitation protocols. The overall goal of hand and finger function also implies timely addressing of neurovascular injuries. New devices such as the Teno-Fix (Ortheon Medical; Winter Park, Florida) have shown adequate strength in the laboratory but are bulky and untested for work of flexion. Insufficient clinical data and high cost may prevent widespread use.

References

[1] Bunnell S. Repair of tendons in the fingers and description of two new instruments. Surg Gynecol Obstet 1918;26:103–10.

[2] Bunnell S. Repair of tendons in the fingers. Surg Gynecol Obstet 1922;35:88–97.

[3] Strickland J. Flexor tendon repair. Hand Clin 1985; 1:55–68.

[4] Mass D. Early repairs of flexor tendon injuries. In: Berger R, Weiss A, editors. Hand surgery. Philadelphia: Lippincott, Williams and Wilkins; 2004. p. 679–98.

[5] Al-Qattan MM. Conservative management of zone II partial flexor tendon lacerations greater than half the width of the tendon. J Hand Surg 2000; 25A:1118–21.

[6] Erhard L, Zobitz ME, Zhao C, Amadio PC, An KA. Treatment of partial lacerations in flexor tendons by trimming—a biomechanical in vitro study. J Bone Joint Surg [Am] 2002;84(6):1006–12.

[7] Hamman J, Ali A, Phillips C, Cunningham B, Mass DP. A biomechanical study of the flexor digitorum superficialis: effects of digital pulley excision and loss of the flexor digitorum profundus. J Hand Surg 1997;22A:328–35.

[8] Sourmelis SG, McGrouther DA. Retrieval of the retracted flexor tendon. J Hand Surg 1997;12B: 109–11.

[9] McLarney E, Hoffman H, Wolfe SW. Biomechanical analysis of the cruciate four-strand flexor tendon repair. J Hand Surg 1999;24A:295–301.

[10] Miller L, Mass DP. A comparison of four repair techniques for Camper's chiasm flexor digitorum superficialis lacerations: tested in an in vitro model. J Hand Surg 2000;25A:1122–6.

[11] Lister G. Reconstruction of pulleys employing extensor retinaculum. J Hand Surg 1979;4:461–4.

[12] Strickland JW. The Indiana method of flexor tendon repair. Atlas Hand Clin 1996;1:77–103.

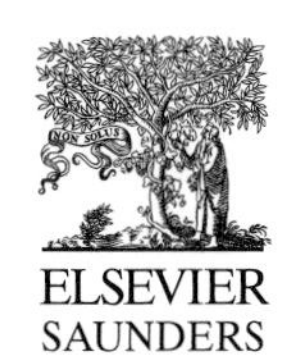

ELSEVIER
SAUNDERS

Hand Clin 21 (2005) 181–186

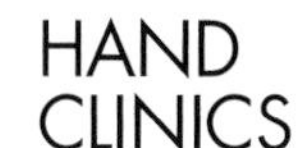

HAND
CLINICS

Treatment of Acute Flexor Tendon Injury: Zones III–V

George S. Athwal, MD, FRCSC, Scott W. Wolfe, MD*

Hospital for Special Surgery, 535 East 70th Street, New York, NY 10021, USA

The mass of literature on flexor tendon injury centers on the treatment of zone II lacerations. Recent advancements in tendon repair and rehabilitation have been directed toward improving results of zone II injury [1]. It is often stated that lessons learned from the treatment of these injuries can be transferred to the other zones. Although this may be true in general, several key differences exist between zones. Surgeons must be familiar with these differences when evaluating, treating, and rehabilitating patients with zone III–V tendon injuries.

The classification of the zone of injury is by way of the following standard parameters: zone III is the area proximal to the origin of the flexor tendon sheath to the distal aspect of the transverse carpal ligament, zone IV is within the carpal tunnel, and zone V is proximal to the carpal tunnel to the musculotendinous junction [2]. Tendons, nerves, and blood vessels are located in close proximity in the hand and forearm; therefore, combined injuries are the norm. Innocuous skin wounds may mask the extent of deep structural injury (Fig. 1). As many as nine digital flexors, three wrist flexors, two major nerves, and two major arteries may be involved. Extensive volar lacerations in zone V have been termed "spaghetti wrist" or "full house" injuries [3–7].

Anatomy

The anatomy of the palm and volar surface of the forearm is complex. Important nerves and vessels are in close proximity to the flexor tendons. Knowledge of these anatomic structures and their interrelations is paramount in the treatment of flexor tendon injuries of the palm and forearm.

In the forearm, the flexor muscles are grouped in three layers: the superficial layer, containing the pronator teres, palmaris longus, flexor carpi radialis (FCR), and flexor carpi ulnaris (FCU); the middle layer, composed exclusively of the flexor digitorum superficialis (FDS); and the deep layer, comprised of the flexor digitorum profundus (FDP), flexor pollicis longus (FPL), and pronator quadratus. As the pronator teres inserts along the midshaft of the radius, it is not involved with flexor tendon injuries in zones III–V. The pronator quadratus arises from the distal one quarter of the anteromedial ulna and projects laterally to insert on the distal one quarter of the anterior radius. It may be concomitantly injured in flexor tendon injuries; however, it does not have a discrete tendon that can be repaired easily.

The palmaris longus arises from the common flexor origin and inserts into the flexor retinaculum and palmar aponeurosis. It has a short muscle belly and a long tendon that is used commonly as a donor for tendon grafting. It is unilaterally absent in approximately 16% of the population and bilaterally absent in approximately 9% [8]. The FCR also originates from the common flexor origin and inserts on the palmar bases of the second and third metacarpals. In zone V, the FCR tendon travels ulnar to the radial artery. The FCU has a humeral and an ulnar head. The ulnar nerve travels between these two heads in the proximal forearm and exits to lie anterior to the muscle belly until the distal forearm. As they cross the wrist, the artery and nerve are deep to the FCU tendon, which inserts on the pisiform.

* Corresponding author.
E-mail address: wolfes@hss.edu (S.W. Wolfe).

0749-0712/05/$ - see front matter
doi:10.1016/j.hcl.2004.11.007

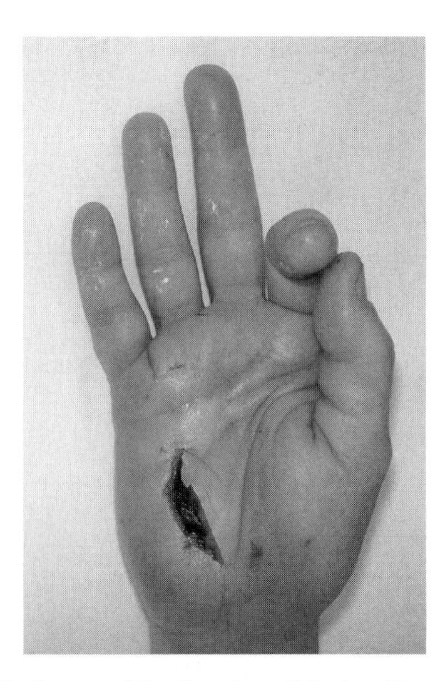

Fig. 1. Posture of the ulnar three digits in a 50-year-old woman who fell forward onto a 16-oz bottle of juice, sustaining a deep glass wound to the hypothenar eminence. Exploration revealed complete transection to deep and superficial tendons of the ulnar three digits, transection of the superficial palmar arch, and the deep motor branch of the ulnar nerve.

The FDS arises from a long curved oblique line that begins at the medial epicondyle and extends to the volar middle third of the radius. These two origins connect in the proximal forearm to create a fibrous aponeurotic band that overlies but can surround the median nerve and the ulnar artery [1]. The muscle divides into four muscle bellies, and at the wrist crease, the tendons are aligned into two rows. The FDS to the middle and ring digits are more superficial than those to the index and little finger. In some individuals the FDS tendon slip to the little finger may be absent or hypoplastic [9].

The FDP resides in the deep compartment and arises from the anterior ulna and interosseous membrane. The portion of the muscle to the index finger separates from the main muscle belly more proximally, contributing to a variable degree of index independence [1,10]. The tendons of the FDP lie in a single row, deep to the FDS, as they cross the wrist. The FPL arises from the anterior surface of the mid-radius and the interosseous membrane and passes through the carpal canal to insert on the distal phalanx of the thumb. An accessory head of the FPL exists in approximately 50% of people [11] and originates from the coronoid or medial epicondyle.

The median nerve enters the forearm between the two heads of pronator teres and travels distally between the FDS and FDP. At the level of the wrist, the nerve is located between and just dorsal to the tendons of the palmaris longus and FCR. The nerve has also become superficial to the tendons of FDS and FDP. The ulnar nerve approaches the wrist deep to the FCU and medial to the ulnar artery. It enters the palm through Guyon's canal and then divides into motor and sensory branches.

The radial artery travels beneath the brachioradialis in the mid-forearm; as it approaches the wrist it wraps around the scaphotrapezial joint and enters the deep palm through the dorsal first web space. The artery ends in the deep palmar arch. The ulnar artery passes under the fibrous arch of the FDS with the median nerve and then travels medial to the FDS and FDP and deep to the FCU. The artery enters the palm through Guyon's canal and terminates in the superficial palmar arch.

Etiology

Injury to the flexor tendons in zones III–V is commonly caused by lacerations (Fig. 2). These injuries occur predominantly in males and the most common means is by broken glass [3,5–7, 12–14]. Mechanisms such as deliberately punching a plate glass window and falling with glass or other sharp objects held within the hand are common. Suicide attempts and self-mutilation, although frequent, seem to be a much less common cause of deep injury [3,6,14]. Crush injuries cause significant damage to the soft tissues and bone; however, tendons are remarkably resistant and only rarely rupture [15]. Farmyard injuries and traumatic amputations also cause flexor tendon injuries; however, they are categorically different because of their high energy and polytraumatic nature.

Diagnosis

The diagnosis of isolated flexor tendon injuries is usually straightforward; however, isolated injuries rarely occur in zones III–V. It is important to determine the mechanism of injury, degree of possible contamination, and time delay to presentation. The treating surgeon must examine fully the injured extremity to determine the degree of injury. Innocuous skin lacerations may hide extensive injuries, because the size and mechanism of the injury does not correlate with the number of anatomic structures injured [16].

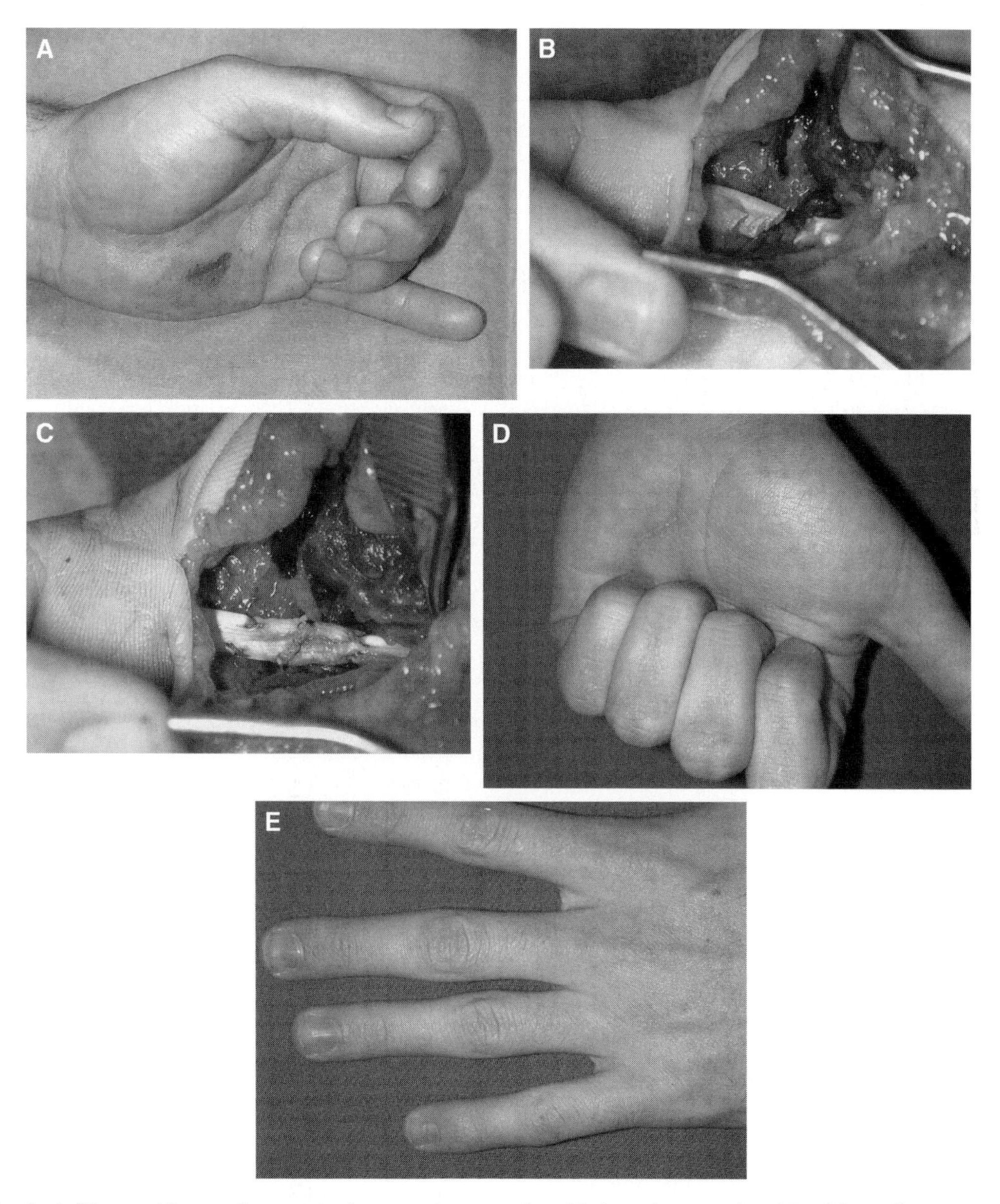

Fig. 2. A 24-year-old executive sustained penetrating wound to his hypothenar region (*A*) while peeling a potato. Exploration revealed complete disruption of the FDS and FDP tendons to the little finger (*B*). Each tendon was repaired with a 3-0 braided polyester locked cruciate repair augmented with a back-wall first epitenon technique of 6-0 nylon (*C*). Follow-up at 5 months showed full digital flexion (*D*) and extension (*E*).

Observation of the digital cascade may be a clue to the extent of injury (see Figs 1 and 2A). Active functional testing of the flexor tendons at the distal interphalangeal and proximal interphalangeal joints more definitively assesses FDS and FDP function. In the uncooperative adult or the frightened child a squeeze test, analogous to the Thompson test for Achilles tendon ruptures, may be useful. It is based on the passive excursion of the flexor tendons with pressure applied to the muscle belly. The tenodesis effect, which is observed with normal wrist flexion and extension, may also aid in diagnosis. The diagnosis of partial tendon laceration is particularly difficult because of intact motor function that is usually weakened, and pain that may be thought to arise from concomitant injuries.

Detailed examination of the peripheral nerves and vessels around the zone of injury and distally in the hand is vital. Vascular injuries may be missed if the Allen test is not preformed, as pulses distal to the lacerated radial or ulnar arteries may be palpable secondary to good backflow through the palmar arches [16]. Gibson et al [16], in a prospective study to determine the accuracy of preoperative examination in zone V injuries, found that approximately 50% of all examinations had three or more errors and approximately 20% had five or more errors. The most commonly missed injury was laceration to the ulnar artery. Injuries to the FCU and FDS to the index finger were the most commonly missed tendon injuries. Injuries to the median and ulnar nerves were the least commonly missed; however, they were still missed 15% and 14% of the time, respectively. Of interest, they found that examinations by more experienced surgeons were only slightly more accurate than those preformed by second and third year residents. They postulated that other factors contributed to the high error rate, such as patient anxiety, pain, intoxication, or psychologic issues. In many cases, accurate diagnosis cannot be obtained with clinical examination, and exploration is required.

Treatment

A viable hand with few injured structures and small clean wounds may be cleansed in the emergency department for planned definitive exploration and treatment in a delayed fashion. With higher severity wounds, traumatic wound protocols should be initiated with antibiotics, tetanus status, irrigation, and debridement. The treating surgeon should have a low threshold for surgical exploration with loupe magnification, particularly in children, in whom the examination is fraught with missed injuries.

A systematic approach to injuries in zones III–V simplifies the problem and decreases complications. General or upper extremity regional anesthesia and tourniquet control are preferred. Wounds are extended proximally and distally, avoiding perpendicular crossing of flexion creases, to allow adequate exposure of injured structures. Injuries sustained in zone IV require carpal tunnel release for exposure, and release of the transverse carpal ligament for injuries in zones III and distal V may be prudent for exposure and prophylaxis from postoperative swelling. Proximal tendon ends in zone III injuries may be retrieved by a milking maneuver with the wrist in flexion [17].

Injured and uninjured structures are identified and tagged from deep to superficial. If the deep motor branch of the ulnar nerve has been lacerated in zone III, it is repaired first, with or without a repair of the deep palmar arch as necessary. The digital flexor tendons are repaired next, in a deep to superficial sequence. A 3-0 or 4-0 nonabsorbable suture is used in a locking fashion to provide at least a four-strand repair. The authors prefer the use of the locked cruciate repair [18] because of its favorable mechanical profile and gap resistance [18–22]. Gap formation is further reduced by use of a nonabsorbable monofilament 6-0 epitendinous suture (see Fig. 2C).

Partial and complete lacerations to the median or ulnar nerves are repaired with 8-0 or 9-0 nylon using an epineural technique under microscopic magnification. Magnification allows the identification of nerve orientation by way of hints from epineural vessels and fascicular anatomy.

Vascular repair in the viable hand is controversial. Carroll [23] noted that in wrist lacerations, the radial and ulnar arteries may be ligated without consequence. Gelberman et al [24] found few signs of ischemia or symptoms of cold intolerance in unrepaired single artery injuries and also demonstrated increased flow in the remaining intact artery. They did, however, report that combined nerve and artery injuries had the most disabling symptoms. Potenza [25], however, noted cold insensitivity, intrinsic muscle atrophy, and trophic skin changes after ligation of a single artery. Others have found cold intolerance to be common although not associated with any injury pattern [5]. The authors routinely repair single artery lacerations using microsurgical technique.

Postoperative considerations

After surgery, patients are placed in a dorsal extension-blocking splint with the wrist in 20°–40° of flexion, the metacarpophalangeal joints in 40°–60° of flexion, and the interphalangeal joints in full extension [1,4]. Several rehabilitation programs exist for flexor tendon repair and most involve some form of early motion and differential tendon gliding maneuvers [1]. In the senior author's experience, early motion flexion protocols may be used in zone III–V injuries, though adhesions are not as frequent outside of zone II, and repairs in these zones generally result in satisfactory outcomes regardless of rehabilitation technique. It should be noted that early active motion has not been demonstrated to improve the results of flexor tendon repair in any zone when compared with more conservative passive motion and place/hold protocols. Unrestricted active motion also may increase the risk for repair site rupture [1].

Outcomes

Despite their frequent occurrence, there is a paucity of literature on the outcomes of flexor tendon injuries in zones III–V. Tendons, nerves, and vessels are found in close proximity and are located superficially in the palm, wrist, and forearm. These factors account for the common occurrence of combined injuries. Outcomes of tendon injuries therefore also depend on the degree of nerve and vascular damage.

Yii et al [14] analyzed flexor tendon repairs in zone V mobilized with an early active motion regimen. They found independent FDS action in 66% of patients with one or both flexor tendons lacerated. In FDS only lacerations, independent function was present in 96%, whereas in hands with combined FDS and FDP lacerations, independent FDS function was only present in 61%. This difference in independent FDS action was statistically significant, indicating that more extensive injuries resulted in a greater degree of adhesions. Analysis of range of motion, using the American Society for Surgery of the Hand criteria, demonstrated 90% good and excellent results. Digits with FDS only injuries had 100% good and excellent results, whereas combined FDS and FDP injuries had 89% good and excellent results. Yii et al also examined, by multivariant analysis, the impact of spaghetti wrist injuries on hand function. A statistically significant difference was observed in patients in independent FDS function between spaghetti and non-spaghetti injuries. A non-spaghetti injury was defined as division of fewer than 10 longitudinal structures [14]. The difference in digital range of motion between spaghetti and non-spaghetti injuries, however, was not statistically significant.

Stefanich et al [12] also examined outcomes after zone V tendon lacerations in 23 patients mobilized with the Kleinert protocol. Subjective hand function was normal in only 8 of 23 patients. Independent FDS action was present in only 7 of 23 patients (30%). Eight patients recovered 100% of total active digital motion; the average total active motion per digit was thumb, 90%; index, 88%; middle, 93%; ring, 91%; and small finger, 89%. When comparing the injured to the uninjured side, pinch strengths and grip strengths recovered to 85% and 79%, respectively.

Rogers et al [6] retrospectively reviewed 26 cases of simultaneous lacerations of the median and ulnar nerves with flexor tendons at the wrist. Eight of 26 were available for final review and most had gained a good range of motion in the affected hand. Almost half of the digits examined had full active range of motion; however, a number had significant fixed deformities occurring most commonly in patients who had not complied with postoperative rehabilitation.

Puckett and Meyer [3] reported results of extensive volar wrist lacerations in 37 patients also mobilized with the Kleinert protocol. The average number of structures injured per patient was eight and the average number of tendons lacerated was six. Thirty-three wrists had good or excellent range of motion, which represented 97% of the patients with complete follow-up. No patients required tenolysis and there were no tendon ruptures.

Results of nerve repairs are more difficult to assess. Most patients regain protective sensation and approximately half regain some degree of two-point discrimination [4–6]. In general, patients with better two-point discrimination have more normal hand use and sensory function [3]. Return of ulnar motor function is generally poor, whereas median nerve function is generally more satisfactory [5,7]. Most studies would agree that combined median and ulnar nerve injuries showed the poorest outcome [4,7,26].

Age is also an important determinant in nerve injuries [4,5,13]. Inconomou et al [13] reviewed major penetrating glass injuries to the upper extremities in seven children. In nerve injuries below the elbow, they reported that five patients regained normal sensory function and two fair. Similarly, the motor recovery was full in five and good in two.

The significance of arterial injury in a viable hand is unknown. Complications caused by the repair or ligation of arteries are difficult to grade and therefore are lacking in studies. Repair of single artery lacerations is controversial; however, most investigators performed repairs when feasible [3,4,7,13].

Tendon related complications in zones III–V are not as common as in zone II. Tenolysis infrequently is required and tendon ruptures are similarly rare [4,12,14]. Poor compliance and motivation, however, is common among the patient population that tends to sustain flexor tendon injuries in zones III–V [4,5]. Several investigators have cited difficulty in locating and motivating patients to return for follow-up evaluation, leading to the possibility of a significant bias in reported outcomes and complications [4–7].

Summary

Many of the principles of flexor tendon repair and rehabilitation can be applied to zones III–V. Injuries in zones III–V are rarely isolated and neurovascular involvement is common. Because of the often extensive and unknown degree of injury, there should be a low threshold for surgical wound exploration. Primary repair of injured tendons and neurovascular structures is recommended by way of a systematic approach. Good to excellent outcomes in range of motion and tendon function can be expected; however, functional outcomes of associated nerve injuries are varied, with younger patients generally demonstrating the best results (Fig. 2E).

References

[1] Boyer MI, Strickland JW, Engles D, Sachar K, Leversedge FJ. Flexor tendon repair and rehabilitation: state of the art in 2002. Instr Course Lect 2003;52:137–61.

[2] Kleinert HE, Verdan C. Report of the Committee on Tendon Injuries (International Federation of Societies for Surgery of the Hand). J Hand Surg [Am] 1983;8:794–8.

[3] Puckett CL, Meyer VH. Results of treatment of extensive volar wrist lacerations: the spaghetti wrist. Plast Reconstr Surg 1985;75(5):714–21.

[4] Chin G, Weinzweig N, Mead M, Gonzalez M. Spaghetti wrist: management and results. Plast Reconstr Surg 1998;102(1):96–102.

[5] Hudson DA, de Jager LT. The spaghetti wrist. Simultaneous laceration of the median and ulnar nerves with flexor tendons at the wrist. J Hand Surg [Br] 1993;18(2):171–3.

[6] Rogers GD, Henshall AL, Sach RP, Wallis KA. Simultaneous laceration of the median and ulnar nerves with flexor tendons at the wrist. J Hand Surg [Am] 1990;15(6):990–5.

[7] Kabak S, Halici M, Baktir A, Turk CY, Avsarogullari L. Results of treatment of the extensive volar wrist lacerations: 'the spaghetti wrist.' Eur J Emerg Med 2002;9(1):71–6.

[8] Thompson NW, Mockford BJ, Cran GW. Absence of the palmaris longus muscle: a population study. Ulster Med J 2001;70(1):22–4.

[9] Idler RS. Anatomy and biomechanics of the digital flexor tendons. Hand Clin 1985;1:3–11.

[10] Bogumill GP. Functional anatomy of the flexor tendon system of the hand. Hand Surg 2002;7(1):33–46.

[11] Al-Qattan MM. Gantzer's muscle. An anatomical study of the accessory head of the flexor pollicis longus muscle. J Hand Surg [Br] 1996;21(2):269–70.

[12] Stefanich RJ, Putnam MD, Peimer CA, Sherwin FS. Flexor tendon lacerations in zone V. J Hand Surg [Am] 1992;17(2):284–91.

[13] Iconomou TG, Zuker RM, Michelow BJ. Management of major penetrating glass injuries to the upper extremities in children and adolescents. Microsurgery 1993;14(2):91–6.

[14] Yii NW, Urban M, Elliot D. A prospective study of flexor tendon repair in zone 5. J Hand Surg [Br] 1998;23(5):642–8.

[15] Buchler U, Hastings H Jr. Combined injuries. In: Green DP, Hotchkiss RN, Pederson WC, editors. Operative hand surgery. 4th edition. Philadelphia: Churchill Livingstone; 1998. p. 1631–50.

[16] Gibson TW, Schnall SB, Ashley EM, Stevanovic M. Accuracy of the preoperative examination in zone 5 wrist lacerations. Clin Orthop 1999;365:104–10.

[17] Pennington DG. Atraumatic retrieval of the proximal end of a severed digital flexor tendon. Plast Reconstr Surg 1977;60(3):468–9.

[18] McLarney E, Hoffman H, Wolfe SW. Biomechanical analysis of the cruciate four-strand flexor tendon repair. J Hand Surg [Am] 1999;24:295–301.

[19] Barrie KA, Wolfe SW. The relationship of suture design to biomechanical strength of flexor tendon repairs. Hand Surg 2001;6(1):89–97.

[20] Barrie KA, Tomak SL, Cholewicki J, Merrell GA, Wolfe SW. Effect of suture locking and suture caliber on fatigue strength of flexor tendon repairs. J Hand Surg [Am] 2001;26(2):340–6.

[21] Barrie KA, Tomak SL, Cholewicki J, Wolfe SW. The role of multiple strands and locking sutures on gap formation of flexor tendon repairs during cyclical loading. J Hand Surg [Am] 2000;25(4):714–20.

[22] Barrie KA, Wolfe SW, Shean C, Shenbagamurthi D, Slade JF III, Panjabi MM. A biomechanical comparison of multistrand flexor tendon repairs using an in situ testing model. J Hand Surg [Am] 2000; 25(3):499–506.

[23] Carroll RE, Match RM. Common errors in the management of wrist lacerations. J Trauma 1974;14(7): 553–62.

[24] Gelberman RH, Blasingame JP, Fronek A, Dimick MP. Forearm arterial injuries. J Hand Surg [Am] 1979;4(5):401–8.

[25] Potenza AD. Flexor tendon injuries. Orthop Clin N Am 1970;1(2):355–73.

[26] Widgerow AD. Full house/spaghetti wrist injuries. S Afr J Surg 1990;28:6–10.

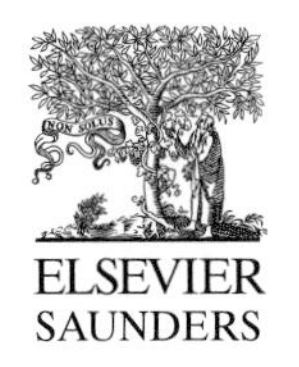

ELSEVIER
SAUNDERS

Hand Clin 21 (2005) 187–197

HAND
CLINICS

Complex Injuries Including Flexor Tendon Disruption

Jon D. Hernandez, MD, PhD[a], Peter J. Stern, MD[b,*]

[a]*Mary S. Stern Hand Surgery, Hand Surgery Specialists, 528 Oak Street, Suite 200, Cincinnati, OH 45206, USA*
[b]*Orthopaedic Surgery, University of Cincinnati, College of Medicine, 528 Oak Street, Suite 200, Cincinnati, OH 45206, USA*

Complex injuries to the hand account for 60% of emergency and 20% of post-traumatic secondary reconstructive cases at university-based centers performing hand surgery [1]. When compared with isolated injuries, the number of procedures necessary to treat complex hand injuries is doubled, work incapacity is increased almost fivefold, and permanent disability is more likely.

Complex injuries to the hand result in damage to a combination of its tissue components: bone, joints, tendon, nerves, vessels, and skin. Although these components are defined as distinct anatomic structures, it is the combined integrated function of these structures that allows the hand to serve as a primary mechanism by which one performs the multitude of tasks within our environment. Trauma to the hand involving combined tissue injury can result in severe functional deficits if left untreated or treated inappropriately.

Flexor tendon injuries are a common part of complex injuries to the hand and can present in a wide spectrum of severity and location. When tendon injuries are being assessed, it is important to evaluate the neighboring soft tissue and bony structures. Treatment options depend on associated injuries and may include primary repair (including replantation), delayed primary or secondary repair, or amputation. Regardless of treatment, these injuries have long- and short-term consequences that are best managed by a physician–therapist team approach.

This article deals with flexor tendon disruption associated with combined injuries to the hand. The mechanisms by which these injuries occur include high-energy trauma, crush injuries, and industrial accidents. Although these injuries have been associated with a higher complication rate than isolated injuries, a better understanding of the treatment principles has resulted in a reduction in the rate of complications [1]. The ensuing discussion relates to flexor tendon repair and healing in the presence of associated soft tissue and bony injuries.

Types of complex flexor tendon injuries

In general, complex injuries involving the flexor tendons include volar combined injuries and dorsal and volar combined injuries [1]. Volar combined injuries include damage to the skin, neurovascular bundle, extrinsic flexor tendon, intrinsic apparatus (lumbricals, in the hand), and skeletal structures. The dorsal skin, venous system, extrinsic extensors, and intrinsic system (in the digits) are spared. The most common cause of volar combined injuries is a laceration from a sharp piece of glass or knife blade usually presenting with minimal crush or contamination.

Dorsal and volar combined injuries include variable degrees of damage to the dorsal and palmar aspects of the digit with complete amputation representing the extreme. Crushing injuries typically seen in industrial accidents are the most common cause. Local segmental devascularization is often present and can result in distal vascular compromise.

Tendon healing

Tendons heal by intrinsic and extrinsic mechanisms. Extrinsic healing requires the proliferation

* Corresponding author.
E-mail address: pjstern@hss.com (P.J. Stern).

0749-0712/05/$ - see front matter
doi:10.1016/j.hcl.2004.12.001

and migration of macrophages and fibroblasts from the surrounding soft tissue as shown by Potenza [2,3] and Peacock [4,5]. Intrinsic healing takes place when cells within the tendon participate in the healing process as has been observed by several investigators [6–9].

Flexor tendons rarely are injured in isolation and thus rarely undergo healing in isolation. Functional healing is the combined healing of multiply injured tissues. According to Buchler [1], "The ultimate functional outcome in combined injuries relates not only to the sum of the various lesional components but more significantly to the multiple *interactions* among the involved structures as they undergo healing." Following tenorrhaphy, intrinsic healing predominates over extrinsic healing when early motion is begun postoperatively [10–12] and allows for less adhesion formation and better strength. When repairs are performed within zone II of the flexor tendon fibro-osseous sheath, allowing early motion is critical [13–15] and results in improved final motion.

Treatment

General concepts

Most complex injuries are open, and thus, treatment always begins with a thorough irrigation and debridement. Foreign material and debris must be removed from the wound and can be accomplished with saline irrigation and sharp debridement. Occasionally detergents can be added to the solution for removal of oil-based materials. Necrotic tissue likewise should be débrided, because this can serve as a medium for bacterial growth. Cultures need not be taken at the time of initial debridement.

In sharp lacerations, all injured structures are repaired primarily by direct suture. Untidy lacerations with limited defects require a thorough assessment of the associated injuries, particularly with respect to the neurovascular elements, because structural damage may be concealed and extend beyond the site of injury.

Tendon

Information on tendon repair and biomechanics is discussed in detail elsewhere in this issue. The focus of this section is on the concepts of tendon healing in the presence of associated injuries. Tendon healing in complex injuries is vital to restoration of hand function. Bony and soft tissue integrity plays an important part in tendon repair. To function and heal best, tendons need to lie in a well vascularized bed. Tendons that are exposed or that run through poorly vascularized soft tissue become adherent, resulting in poor range of motion. Bony integrity is paramount to the initiation of early motion. Stable fixation of associated fractures is necessary for early motion protocols, whereas delayed motion caused by unstable fractures results in contractures and adhesions. The tendon sheath and pulleys play an important role in allowing fine motor movements. When disrupted, bowstringing and contractures can result, hindering final function and limiting range of motion. Every attempt should be made to preserve the A2 and A4 pulleys when repairing flexor tendons in zone II (Fig. 1). When these pulleys are injured, they can be repaired primarily with a graft [16] or reconstructed in a staged manner over a silicone rod to allow healing before tendon motion through

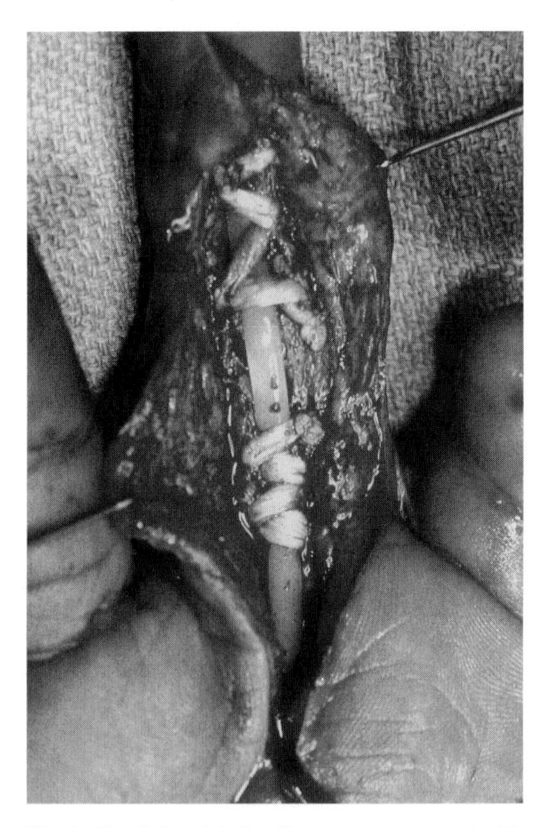

Fig. 1. The A-2 and A-4 pulleys are reconstructed with a free palmaris longus graft over a silicone rod. (*From* Hunter JM, Mackin EJ, Callahan AD. Rehabilitation of the hand and upper extremity. 5th edition. St. Louis: CV Mosby; 2002; with permission.)

the pulley [17]. Wehbe et al [18] recommended two-stage flexor tendon reconstruction for severely injured digits in which major reconstruction was necessary at the initial operative setting.

Bone and joint

In a study by Duncan et al [19] evaluating severe open fractures of the hand, metacarpal fractures had significantly better outcomes than phalangeal fractures. Fractures involving the proximal phalanx or the proximal interphalangeal joint had the poorest prognosis, especially when they were associated with tendon injury.

When there are concomitant fractures in a combined injury, stable internal fixation is desirable to provide a biomechanic environment that allows early tendon mobilization, fewer adhesions, and thus better motion and function. This can be accomplished by a variety of methods. Plate and screw fixation are ideal for fractures, because length can be restored and stable fixation achieved to allow for dynamic rehabilitation protocols. Although biomechanic stability is best achieved by plating dorsally, the authors prefer lateral plate placement to avoid bulk beneath the dorsal apparatus. Plate placement can be through a midaxial incision such that tendon repair and osseous fixation can be accomplished through the same incision. With complex injuries, lacerations are usually present. In these cases the incision should be planned around the laceration in a manner that prevents further damage to the soft tissue envelope.

Many fractures in complex injuries are not suited for plate fixation, because periosteal stripping during the injury itself and that required for plate fixation could further jeopardize soft tissue integrity and bone healing and possibly result in avascular necrosis. In these events, intraosseous wires or Kirschner pins may be useful, because both limit the amount of further dissection and permit easier soft tissue closure. When there has been extensive soft tissue loss or comminution, an external fixator may be ideal to allow access to the injury and avoid the need for implant coverage. Intramedullary fixation is also a reasonable alternative, particularly for short oblique and transverse fractures [20].

Segmental bone loss is common in high-energy injuries. Failure to preserve length may disrupt the delicate balance between flexor and extensor forces. At least 5 mm of bone loss generally can be tolerated by the flexor system; however, shortening is poorly tolerated by the extensor system, particularly in phalangeal fractures. In volar combined injuries in which the extensor system remains intact, excessive skeletal shortening leads to relative extensor lengthening and results in proximal interphalangeal (PIP) extension deficits and possibly subsequent contracture. Vahey et al demonstrated that for every millimeter of bone–tendon discrepancy there was a 12° extension lag at the PIP joint [21]. When there is extensive soft tissue injury and bone loss, delayed reconstruction is preferred. Length and alignment are maintained with the use of an external fixator (Fig. 2). Placement of a spacer (silicone or polymethylmethacrylate with or without antibiotic impregnation) helps maintain stability and length and also maintains a soft tissue cavity for later graft placement. Ultimately a corticocancellous graft is used to reconstitute osseous integrity. Length should be determined by radiographs of the contralateral digit.

In combined volar and dorsal injuries in which the extensor and flexor mechanisms are divided, limited skeletal shortening is permissible to gain adequate soft tissue length for extensor and flexor tendon repair. This concept is used in replantation of amputated digits. The method of fixation depends on the level of postoperative rehabilitation. Stable osteosynthesis is required if tendon repair is achieved that would allow for active or passive range of motion. If early motion is not anticipated, then less rigid methods of fixation may be used. When early motion is not possible, however, and thus immobilization is necessary, a tenolysis should be anticipated.

When an associated joint injury is present, the surgeon should decide during the initial presentation whether reconstruction is attainable. Simple intra-articular fractures often require screw or Kirschner pin fixation only. More complex fractures, however, in which articular fragments are completely separated from the shaft (eg, bicondylar fracture), may require more stable fixation, such as a blade plate (Fig. 3). When articular reconstruction is not feasible because of intra-articular comminution or bone loss, treatment options include skeletal traction [22], arthrodesis [23,24], or silicone replacement [25]. Arthrodesis may result in excessive shortening and may be complicated by delayed consolidation.

Vascular

Combined hand injuries often involve the arterial system as a result of its superficial

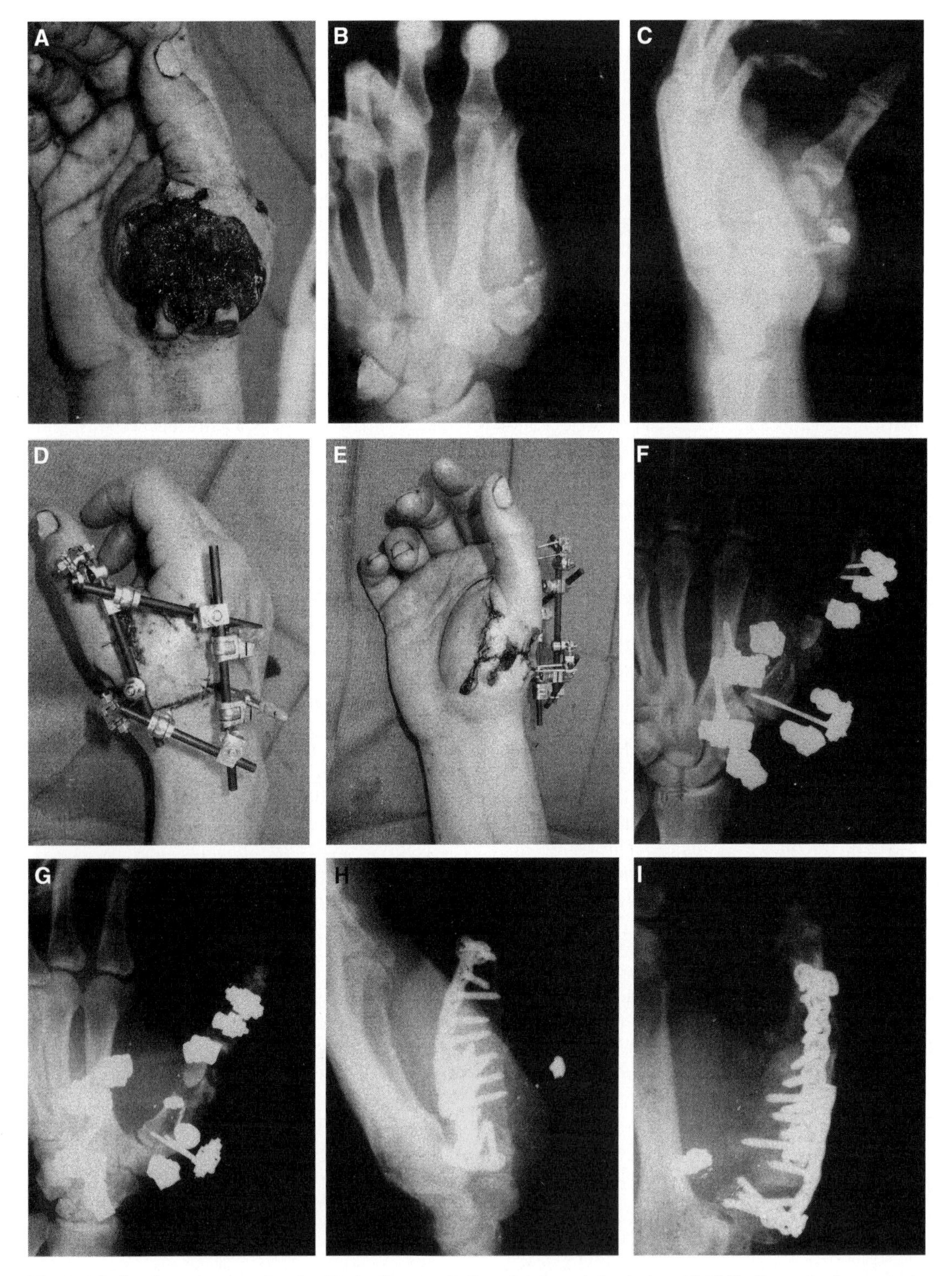

Fig. 2. (*A*) Gunshot wound to thumb with significant soft tissue injury and shortening. (*B,C*) Radiographs demonstrate a metacarpal defect in which only the proximal base and distal articular fragment remain. (*D,E*) Thumb length is restored and maintained with an external fixator. (*F,G*) The radiographic results are shown. (*H,I*) Later, reconstruction was achieved with a corticocancellous autogenous graft stabilized with plates and screws.

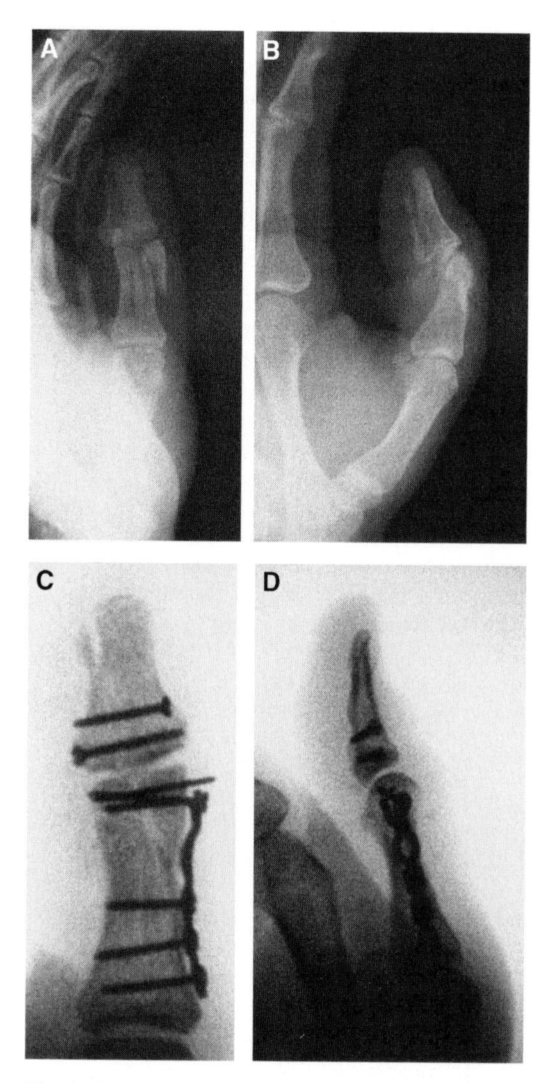

Fig. 3. (*A,B*) A crushing injury to the thumb results in a complex intra-articular fracture of the thumb interphalangeal joint. (*C,D*) Fixation and stabilization was achieved using screw fixation for the distal phalanx, whereas a mini-condylar blade plate was used for the bicondylar proximal phalangeal fracture.

location. Injury may be caused by direct laceration, avulsion, or endothelial damage without loss of vessel continuity. In volar combined injury, associated arterial lesions not only endanger survival of its tributary parts, but also are commonly associated with nerve injury. Because of the association between adequacy of perfusion and the quality of nerve regeneration, it is important to restore blood flow. This can be accomplished by direct suture or by interpositional vein grafting [26].

Isolated arterial injuries are unlikely to cause ischemia because of the rich collateral network. Combined complex injuries, however, are more likely to result in tissue ischemia and necrosis, because multiple vascular insults often are encountered. Several factors related to the severity of the injury can influence the extent of ischemia, including the level of sympathetic tone, systemic factors such as pre-existing vascular disease, smoking, the hemodynamic state of the patient, and the postinjury management. Increased sympathetic tone (vascular spasm) or systemic hypotension (shock) can result in a larger area of necrosis unless the arterial flow is reestablished.

Once an arterial insufficiency is identified, arterial reconstruction is indicated if salvage of the digit is appropriate. In those injuries with associated fractures, the bone must be stabilized before vascular repair. If the anastomosis can be accomplished without tension, then direct end-to-end repair is appropriate. If tension is present direct repair is likely to result in thrombosis, and, therefore, other methods are used. The stump ends can be mobilized or the bone can be shortened to provide a tension-free direct end-to-end repair. If these methods fail or cannot be performed, however, then reconstruction with a reversed interpositional vein graft is appropriate.

Soft tissue injury can result in venous congestion, particularly with dorsal and volar–dorsal combined injuries (including complete amputation). Venous distension, increased turgor, and bluish color suggest venous congestion, and, when present, venous repair should be considered. Vein repair should follow the reestablishment of arterial flow.

Nerves

Nerve injury is often a component of severe volar combined or crushing injuries. When nerve injury is present function is compromised, because there is a loss of sensibility in the involved digits. Sensibility also may be compromised with tendon injury alone, because object recognition in the absence of vision requires finger movement. The combination of nerve and tendon injuries thus can markedly affect hand function [27].

Nerve damage can occur in the form of avulsion, laceration, or crush, resulting in disruption or internal damage to the nerve. In the event that a nerve has undergone sharp laceration in a well vascularized clean wound with adequate soft tissue coverage and skeletal stability, the nerve ends should undergo immediate primary repair. In combined injuries the conditions mentioned previously often are not met. Although most nerve injuries in the forearm and arm are amenable to secondary repair, lesions of the proper digital nerves, the common digital nerves of the palm, and the motor nerves of the ulnar, median and radial nerves should not be left for secondary reconstruction. This would later require a difficult dissection into a scarred area with only minimal improvement in the chances for nerve regeneration. Every effort thus should be made to achieve primary repair.

Neurorrhaphy (primary or secondary) performed under tension results in fibrosis. Nerve gaps often occur in combined injuries, caused by the initial trauma or from excision of damaged tissue during debridement. The temptation to pull small defects together by direct suture repair should be resisted. Mobilization of the nerve ends provides some excursion of the nerve to allow a tension-free repair; however, the amount of possible nerve mobilization is controversial, because it has been shown that over-mobilization can be detrimental to nerve recovery [28].

Nerve grafting allows for unlimited excision of damaged nerve for adequate debridement, decreased scar formation, and repair with maintenance of coaptation throughout full range of motion to allow early rehabilitation. Nerve autografts and allografts can be used for nerve defects [29]. Autogenous donor nerves include the sural, lateral antebrachial cutaneous, medial antebrachial cutaneous, and distal posterior interosseous nerves. Although studies have shown that nerves can regenerate across short nerve gaps through various conduits, such as veins [30,31], pseudosheaths [32], and bioabsorbable tubes [33], their functional results remain unclear. Risitano et al [34] reported very good to good clinical results when using a simple vein graft to bridge sensory nerve gaps in acute hand injuries in cases in which primary repair was not feasible. For large nerve gaps, end-to-side nerve repair has been suggested [35], but whether this is reliable in hand injuries has yet to be demonstrated.

Skin

Complex injuries to the hand, from simple lacerations to major defects, involve the skin and subcutaneous tissue to varying degrees. Protecting flexor tendon repair with soft tissue coverage is vital in restoring function. Additional goals of soft tissue coverage include restoring sensibility, achieving cosmesis, and sometimes filling defects. Buchler [36] described three adjacent zones of injury. The central zone is characterized by loss or destruction of tissue with a variable degree of contamination. Extensive devascularization is present at the adjacent zone, and the peripheral zone demonstrates normal-appearing tissue. Soft tissue coverage can be performed immediately [37] or in a delayed fashion after an initial irrigation and debridement and fracture stabilization allowing time to plan definitive procedures. When flexor tendons are exposed, desiccation is of concern and definitive coverage should be secured as early as possible.

The simplest soft tissue coverage that meets the reconstructive requirements (Box 1) is recommended and is usually the safest procedure. Options include skin grafts, local or rotational flaps, pedicle flaps, and free flaps. The nature of the injury and the experience of the surgeon dictate which is used.

The preferred coverage of defects with a well vascularized bed are skin grafts that are of two main types: split-thickness skin grafts (STSGs) and full-thickness skin grafts (FTSGs). Although STSGs are associated with a high degree of take (success), contraction and durable durability are of concern particularly on the volar surface. For this reason, the authors prefer FTSGs, particularly on the flexor (contact) surface of a finger. FTSGs, however, have a slightly lower rate of take. Factors contributing to decreased take include failure to ensure that the graft is in good contact with the recipient tissue (eg, hematoma), a poorly vascularized bed, and motion beneath the graft.

Box 1. Soft tissue reconstructive ladder

High complexity	Distant pedicle flap
	Free flap
	Regional flap
	Local flap
	Skin graft
	Delayed primary closure
Low complexity	Primary closure

From Hunter JM, Mackin EJ, Callahan AD. Rehabilitation of the hand and upper extremity. 5th edition. St. Louis: CV Mosby; 2002; with permission.

Areas of poorly vascularized beds such as exposed nerves, cartilage, metal implants, tendon without paratenon, cortical bone denuded of periosteum, or a failed reconstruction require vascularized soft tissue support, ie, flaps. Types of flaps used in the hand include local, regional, and distant (pedicle or free) that may be random, in which there is no named blood supply, or axial, in which a named vessel is contained within the flap.

Local random flaps are limited by the size of the defect and have little applicability to the coverage of flexor tendons. They are designed such that one border of the flap is adjacent to the defect to be covered and include transposition, rotation, and advancement flaps (eg, V-Y and Moberg advancement flaps) and are well described by Lister [38].

Regional flaps are soft tissue flaps taken from the same extremity. The cross-finger flap can be used to cover exposed flexor tendons of the thumb and fingers (Fig. 4). Other examples include the first dorsal metacarpal artery flap that often is used to cover small dorsal or volar thumb defects, and the radial forearm flap, an axial pattern flap based on the radial artery, which is used commonly for larger coverage, such as over the dorsal or palmar surface of the carpus and metacarpals. Disadvantages of the radial forearm flap include sacrifice of the radial artery and an unsightly donor defect, which usually (if greater than 4 cm in width) must be covered with a skin graft. The reverse radial forearm fascial flap relies on distally-based perforating vessels [39], thus avoiding the pitfalls mentioned previously, because it maintains radial artery integrity and does not involve the transfer of skin and subcutaneous tissue. The flap must be covered by an STSG, however.

The groin flap is the most common distant axial-pattern flap used for coverage in the upper

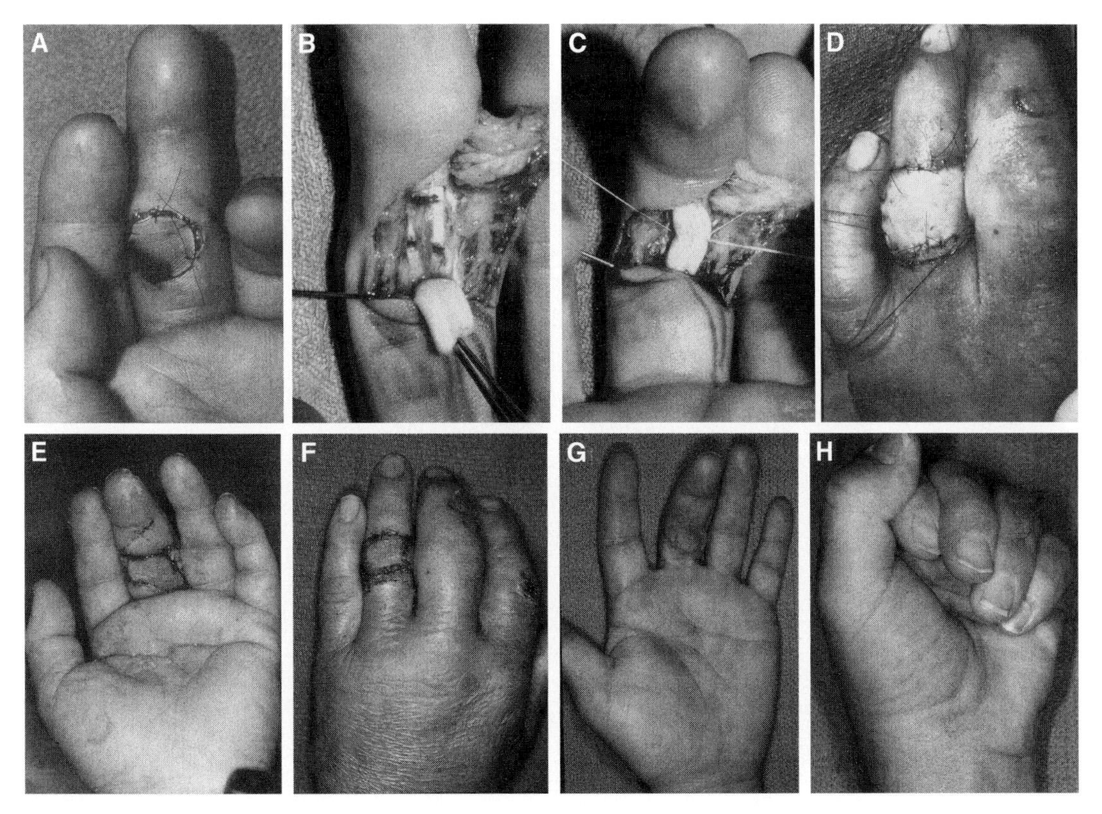

Fig. 4. Cross-finger flap. (*A*) A necrotic island of skin is the result of a knife laceration. Removal of the necrotic tissue exposes the lacerated (*B*) FDP and FDS tendons, which underwent (*C*) four-stranded tendon repairs. (*D*) A cross-finger flap was raised from the dorsum of the adjacent digit and the resulting defect was covered with a full thickness skin graft. (*E*) The raised flap then was used to cover the exposed tendon repair. Several weeks postoperatively the (*F*) donor and (*G*) recipient sites are well healed. The final functional results of (*G*) extension and (*H*) flexion are shown.

extremity. It has become the standard of wound coverage in the hand, especially for large areas of injured tissue and exposed vital structures [40]. The groin flap can cover dorsal, volar, or combined hand defects. Advantages include its size (up to 30 cm^2) [41], durable coverage, constant anatomy (supplied by the superficial circumflex iliac artery), inconspicuous donor site, and ease of application (Fig. 5). Disadvantages include two to three stages for application and take-down and maintenance of the hand in a dependent position for 3–4 weeks, which may produce edema and interfere with rehabilitation.

Free flaps are of virtually unlimited size, may be closely matched to the missing tissue, and may incorporate vascularized elements of all or most of the essential structural elements for segmental reconstruction [36]. Free flaps therefore offer advantages in the treatment of severe hand injuries. Commonly used free flaps in upper extremity coverage include fasciocutaneous (lateral arm and periscapular) and muscle flaps (latissimus, rectus abdominis, and gracilis). Transferred muscle flaps must be covered by an STSG if not transferred as a myocutaneous flap. Because free flaps are transferred in a single setting, aggressive rehabilitation can be initiated sooner. An additional advantage includes the use of the transferred muscle as a functioning free muscle transplantation [42].

Replantation, revascularization, and amputation

Although microsurgical techniques have made possible the salvage of devascularized upper extremity parts, the surgeon must determine whether replantation, revascularization, or amputation should be considered. Trauma can result in complete amputation or devascularization of any portion of the upper extremity. Revascularization refers to restoration of arterial inflow or venous outflow or both, whereas replantation refers to the reattachment of a completely amputated part using bony fixation, tendon repair, and revascularization techniques previously described. Successful replantation or revascularization may

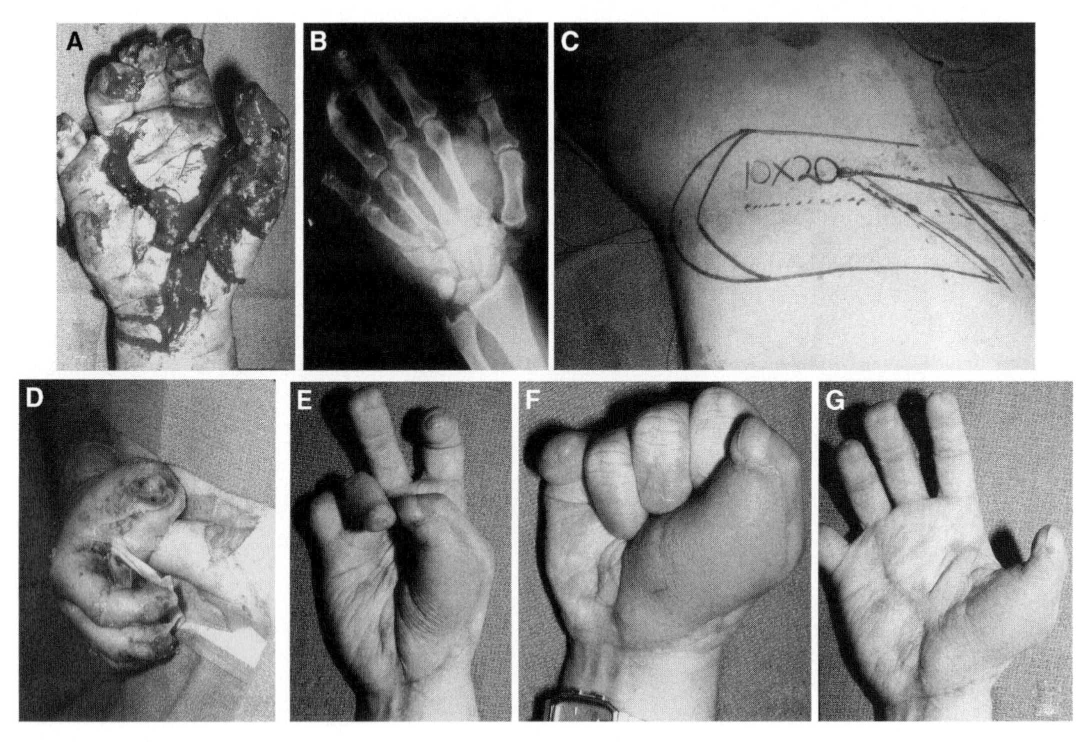

Fig. 5. Groin flap. (*A*) A crushing injury to the right hand results in multiple injuries, including a soft tissue defect exposing the FPL tendon. (*B*) A thumb carpometacarpal dislocation is present on radiographs. In addition to reconstructive procedures of the thumb motor intrinsics, the patient also underwent a groin flap to cover the soft tissue defect and exposed FPL. The groin flap is outlined (*C*) and once mobilized it provides coverage of the defect (*D*). The final outcome reveals that the patient is able to oppose the thumb (*E*), make a fist (*F*) and open the hand (*G*).

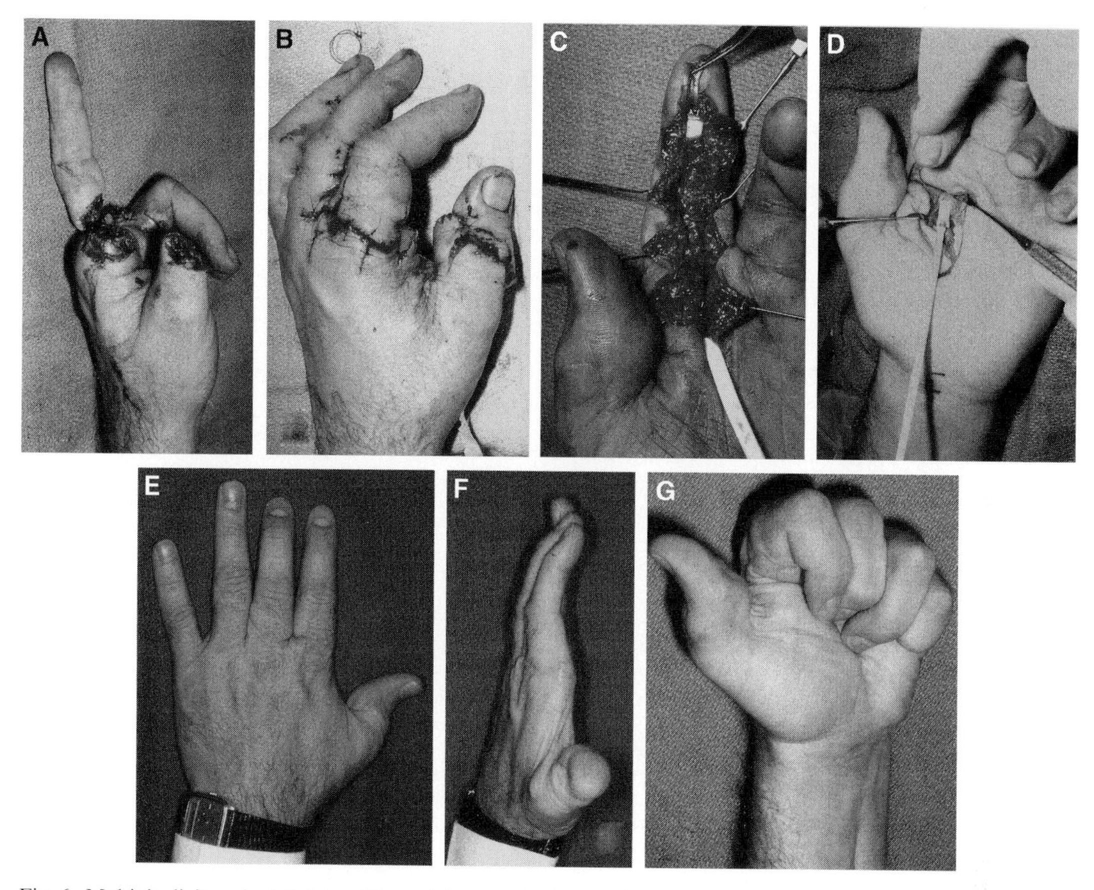

Fig. 6. Multiple digit replant. (*A*) A skill saw injury results in complete amputation of the thumb and index finger and near complete amputation of the long finger. (*B*) Immediate clinical result following replantation and revascularization is shown. (*C,D*) Failure of the FDP tendon repair to the index finger is treated with a two-stage reconstruction. (*C*) In the first stage a silicone rod is placed through the tendon sheath. (*D*) In the second stage the silicone rod is removed and a palmaris longus autograft then is used to reconstruct the FDP. (*E–G*) The final functional results are shown.

necessitate additional surgery (Fig. 6) or lead to stiffness, insensibility, or pain resulting in a more dysfunctional hand than might immediate revision amputation. The decision to replant or revascularize an injured part versus revision amputation therefore should be made with respect to optimizing overall hand function in regard to the individual patient needs.

Ideal candidates have sustained sharp, guillotine-type injuries of the thumb, multiple digits, hand, wrist, or forearm with wounds that are only minimally contaminated. Those patients not meeting these criteria should be considered for amputation.

Summary

The treatment of tendon injury in combined complex injuries to the hand is dictated by the presence of concomitant injuries. Early range of motion is desirable. To achieve this, fractures must be stabilized and the soft tissue envelope and vascular integrity maintained or reconstituted. In those instances in which these conditions cannot be met, the surgeon and patient should be prepared for secondary surgeries, including reconstruction or tenolysis. Although nerve integrity is not necessary for early functional success following tenorrhaphy, nerve injuries should be repaired or grafted primarily as the injury permits. In cases in which vascular compromise is encountered, the options of revascularization versus primary amputation should be discussed with the patient. With an understanding of the treatment principles, the complications associated with complex tendon injuries can be minimized. It is important to stress that optimal functional outcome is multifactorial and includes a physician–therapist team-oriented approach.

References

[1] Buchler U, Hastings H Jr. Combined Injuries. In: Green DP, Hotchkiss RN, Pederson WC, editors. Green's operative hand surgery. 4th edition. Philadelphia: Churchill Livingstone; 1999. p. 1631–50.
[2] Potenza AD. Tendon healing within the flexor digital sheath in the dog. Am J Orthop 1962;44:49–64.
[3] Potenza AD. Critical evaluation of flexor-tendon healing and adhesion formation within artificial digital sheaths. J Bone Joint Surg [Am] 1963;45: 1217–33.
[4] Peacock EE Jr. Fundamental aspects of wound healing relating to the restoration of gliding function after tendon repair. Surg Gynecol Obstet 1964;119: 241–50.
[5] Peacock EE Jr. Biological principles in the healing of long tendons. Surg Clin N Am 1965;45:461–76.
[6] Becker H, Graham MF, Cohen IK, Diegelmann RF. Intrinsic tendon cell proliferation in tissue culture. J Hand Surg [Am] 1981;6(6):616–9.
[7] Lundborg G, Hansson HA, Rank F, Rydevik B. Superficial repair of severed flexor tendons in synovial environment. An experimental, ultrastructural study on cellular mechanisms. J Hand Surg [Am] 1980; 5(5):451–61.
[8] Lundborg G, Rank F. Experimental studies on cellular mechanisms involved in healing of animal and human flexor tendon in synovial environment. Hand 1980;12(1):3–11.
[9] Lundborg G, Rank F, Heinau B. Intrinsic tendon healing. A new experimental model. Scand J Plast Reconstr Surg 1985;19(2):113–7.
[10] Gelberman RH, Woo SL, Lothringer K, Akeson WH, Amiel D. Effects of early intermittent passive mobilization on healing canine flexor tendons. J Hand Surg [Am] 1982;7(2):170–5.
[11] Gelberman RH, Vande Berg JS, Lundborg GN, Akeson WH. Flexor tendon healing and restoration of the gliding surface. An ultrastructural study in dogs. J Bone Joint Surg [Am] 1983;65(1):70–80.
[12] Manske PR, Gelberman RH, Vande Berg JS, Lesker PA. Intrinsic flexor-tendon repair. A morphological study in vitro. J Bone Joint Surg [Am] 1984;66(3): 385–96.
[13] Chow JA, Thomes LJ, Dovelle S, Milnor WH, Seyfer AE, Smith AC. A combined regimen of controlled motion following flexor tendon repair in "no man's land." Plast Reconstr Surg 1987;79(3):447–55.
[14] Lister GD, Kleinert HE, Kutz JE, Atasoy E. Primary flexor tendon repair followed by immediate controlled mobilization. J Hand Surg [Am] 1977; 2(6):441–51.
[15] Strickland JW, Glogovac SV. Digital function following flexor tendon repair in zone II: a comparison of immobilization and controlled passive motion techniques. J Hand Surg [Am] 1980;5(6):537–43.
[16] Boyes JH, Stark HH. Flexor-tendon grafts in the fingers and thumb. A study of factors influencing results in 1000 cases. J Bone Joint Surg [Am] 1971; 53(7):1332–42.
[17] Lister GD. Reconstruction of pulleys employing extensor retinaculum. J Hand Surg [Am] 1979;4(5): 461–4.
[18] Wehbe MA, Mawr B, Hunter JM, Schneider LH, Goodwyn BL. Two-stage flexor-tendon reconstruction. Ten-year experience. J Bone Joint Surg [Am] 1986;68(5):752–63.
[19] Duncan RW, Freeland AE, Jabaley ME, Meydrech EF. Open hand fractures: an analysis of the recovery of active motion and of complications. J Hand Surg [Am] 1993;18(3):387–94.
[20] Gonzalez MH, Igram CM, Hall RF. Intramedullary nailing of proximal phalangeal fractures. J Hand Surg [Am] 1995;20(5):808–12.
[21] Vahey JW, Wegner DA, Hastings H III. Effect of proximal phalangeal fracture deformity on extensor tendon function. J Hand Surg [Am] 1998;23(4): 673–81.
[22] Schenck RR. The dynamic traction method. Combining movement and traction for intra-articular fractures of the phalanges. Hand Clin 1994;10(2): 187–98.
[23] Buchler U, Aiken MA. Arthrodesis of the proximal interphalangeal joint by solid bone grafting and plate fixation in extensive injuries to the dorsal aspect of the finger. J Hand Surg [Am] 1988;13(4): 589–94.
[24] Steel W. Articular fractures. In: Barton N, editor. Fractures of the hand and wrist. New York: Churchill Livingstone; 1988.
[25] Nagle DJ, af Ekenstam FW, Lister GD. Immediate silastic arthroplasty for non-salvageable intraarticular phalangeal fractures. Scand J Plast and Reconstr Surg 1989;23(1):47–50.
[26] Kim WK, Lim JH, Han SK. Fingertip replantations: clinical evaluation of 135 digits. Plast Reconstr Surg 1996;98(3):470–6.
[27] Bell Krotoski JA. Flexor tendon and peripheral nerve repair. Hand Surg 2002;7(1):83–109.
[28] Nicholson OR, Seddon HJ. Nerve repair in civil practice; results of treatment of median and ulnar nerve lesions. BMJ 1957;33(5053):1065–71.
[29] Best TJ, Mackinnon SE, Midha R, Hunter DA, Evans PJ. Revascularization of peripheral nerve autografts and allografts. Plast Reconstr Surg 1999;104(1):152–60.
[30] Kelleher MO, Al-Abri RK, Eleuterio ML, Myles LM, Lenihan DV, Glasby MA. The use of conventional and invaginated autologous vein grafts for nerve repair by means of entubulation. Br J Plast Surg 2001;54(1):53–7.
[31] Wang KK, Costas PD, Bryan DJ, Eby PL, Seckel BR. Inside-out vein graft repair compared with

nerve grafting for nerve regeneration in rats. Microsurgery 1995;16(2):65–70.
[32] Karacaoglu E, Yuksel F, Peker F, Guler MM. Nerve regeneration through an epineurial sheath: its functional aspect compared with nerve and vein grafts. Microsurgery 2001;21(5):196–201.
[33] Giardino R, Nicoli Aldini N, Perego G, et al. Biological and synthetic conduits in peripheral nerve repair: a comparative experimental study. Int J Artif Organs 1995;18(4):225–30.
[34] Risitano G, Cavallaro G, Merrino T, Coppolino S, Ruggeri F. Clinical results and thoughts on sensory nerve repair by autologous vein graft in emergency hand reconstruction. Chir Main 2002;21(3):194–7.
[35] Ogun TC, Ozdemir M, Senaran H, Ustun ME. End-to-side neurorrhaphy as a salvage procedure for irreparable nerve injuries. Technical note. J Neurosurg 2003;99(1):180–5.
[36] Buchler U. Traumatic soft-tissue defects of the extremities. Implications and treatment guidelines. Arch Orthop Trauma Surg 1990;109(6):321–9.
[37] Sundine M, Scheker LR. A comparison of immediate and staged reconstruction of the dorsum of the hand. J Hand Surg [Br] 1996;21(2):216–21.
[38] Lister G. Local flaps to the hand. Hand Clin 1985;1(4):621–40.
[39] Chang SM, Hou CL, Zhang F, Lineaweaver WC, Chen ZW, Gu YD. Distally based radial forearm flap with preservation of the radial artery: anatomic, experimental, and clinical studies. Microsurgery 2003;23(4):328–37.
[40] McGregor IA, Jackson IT. The groin flap. Br J Plast Surg 1972;25(1):3–16.
[41] Lister GD, McGregor IA, Jackson IT. The groin flap in hand injuries. Injury 1973;4(3):229–39.
[42] Manktelow RT, Zuker RM, McKee NH. Functioning free muscle transplantation. J Hand Surg [Am] 1984;9A(1):32–9.

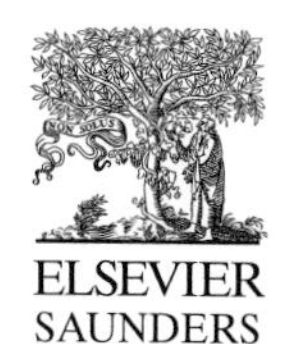

ELSEVIER
SAUNDERS

Hand Clin 21 (2005) 199–210

HAND
CLINICS

Clinical Outcomes Associated with Flexor Tendon Repair

Jin Bo Tang, MD*

Department of Hand Surgery, Hand Surgery Research Center, Affiliated Hospital of Nantong University, 20 West Temple Road, Nantong 226001, Jiangsu, China
Boston University School of Medicine, 715 Albany Street, Boston, MA 02118, USA
Surgical Research and Gene Therapy, Roger Williams Medical Center, 133 North Campus, 825 Chalkstone Avenue, Providence, RI 02908, USA

Flexor tendon injuries in the hand are a frequent clinical problem. Restoration of function after flexor tendon injuries has long been a challenge and a frustration to hand and orthopedic surgeons. In recent decades, laboratory and clinical investigations focused on flexor tendon biomechanics, refinement of repair methods, and optimization of rehabilitation regimens have remarkably improved functional outcomes [1–8]. Repair ruptures and adhesion formation are still unpredictable in some cases [8–15], however, and are believed to be attributed to inherent weakness in the healing capacity of tendons, particularly those in intrasynovial areas.

Worldwide, repair rupture occurs in 4%–10% of repaired fingers. Another 10% are estimated to develop restrictive adhesion requiring secondary tenolysis or a tendon graft. Stiffness of the interphalangeal joints occurs to some extent in more than half of patients. Repair rupture, adhesions, and joint stiffness after primary tendon surgery require secondary operations, and functional disability remains (which may persist even after secondary surgery), affecting patients' ability to work and their daily lives. Optimal treatment of tendon injuries and achieving a satisfactory outcome after surgery and postoperative care remain topics of debate and challenge to hand surgeons.

Outcomes of flexor tendon repair: an overview of experience over the past 15 years

The past 15 years have seen more than 20 major reports in English language journals on outcomes of primary flexor tendon repair from hand surgery centers worldwide [9–33].

A series of reports by Small et al [9], Cullen et al [10], and Savage and Risitano [11] were published 15 years ago, documenting clinical outcomes of controlled active finger flexion exercise after flexor tendon repairs. These promising preliminary reports summoned the expenditure in the years following to more aggressive exercise incorporating active finger flexion to the motion regimen. Small et al [9] presented 114 patients with 138 zone II flexor tendon injuries treated over a 3-year period. Early active mobilization of the fingers was commenced within 48 hours after surgery. Ninety-eight patients with injuries of 117 fingers were followed and graded using the total active range of motion (TAM) method. The active range of motion was graded excellent or good in 77% of the digits, fair in 14%, and poor in 9%. Repair rupture occurred in 11 digits (9.4%). The ruptures were re-repaired immediately and a similar early motion program was applied. Cullen et al [10] treated 34 adult patients with 70 zone II tendon lacerations in 38 fingers. Seventy-eight percent of fingers were rated excellent or good by Strickland criteria after a mean follow-up of 10 months. Two tendons ruptured during controlled active finger flexion exercise. Savage and Risitano [11] used a six-strand method of repairs to treat 36

* Correspondence. Department of Hand Surgery, Affiliated Hospital of Nantong University, 20 West Temple Road, Nantong 226001, Jiangsu, China.
E-mail address: jinbotang@yahoo.com.

doi:10.1016/j.hcl.2004.11.005

fingers with flexor tendon lacerations followed by protective active mobilization. Sixty-three percent of lacerations were zone II and 27% were zone I; 69% and 100%, respectively, achieved an excellent or good result using Buck-Gramcko's assessment method. Tang and Shi [14] reported the results of treatment of 72 flexor tendon injuries in zone II primarily or at the delayed primary stage. In 80.4% of the fingers, excellent or good results were achieved, as evaluated using Strickland and Glogovac criteria. Silfverskiöld and May [15] reported outcomes of use of cross-stitch epitendinous sutures combined with a modified Kessler core suture in treatment of flexor tendon injuries in zone II in 46 consecutive patients with 55 injured digits. For the first 4 weeks after operation, fingers were mobilized with a combination of active extension and passive and active flexion. Two tendons were reported as having ruptures. In the remaining fingers, the mean active distal interphalangeal (DIP) and proximal interphalangeal (PIP) range of motion was 63° and 94° 6 months after surgery, respectively. Elliot et al [19] reported a series of 233 patients with complete divisions of the flexor tendons in zones I and II. These included 203 patients with 317 divided tendons in 224 finger injuries and 20 patients with 30 complete divisions of the flexor pollicis longus (FPL) tendon of the thumb. The patients underwent a controlled active motion regimen postoperatively. Thirteen (5.8%) fingers and five (16.6%) thumbs suffered tendon rupture during the mobilization. Follow-up of the patients treated during the last year of the study showed that 10 of 16 (62.5%) fingers with zone I repairs, 50 of the 63 (79.4%) fingers with zone II repairs, on assessment by Strickland and Glogovac criteria.

Emphasis on the needs and application of four- or six-strand core repairs in clinical tendon repairs appeared first in Savage and Risitano's report [11] in the late 1980s, followed by the report of Tang et al [20] in 1994, and then a series of reports in *Atlas of Hand Clinics* by Taras [21], Sandow and McMahon [22], and Lim and Tsai [23] in 1996. Tang et al [20] reported using double- or multiple-looped sutures for primary tendon repairs with combined early active and passive mobilization for 3 weeks. In 51 fingers from 46 patients with zone II flexor tendon lacerations, doubled threads of the looped suture were placed to repair injured flexor digitorum profundus (FDP) or superficialis (FDS) tendons, or three threads of the looped suture to repair the FDP tendons. The results were good or excellent in 76.5% using White's criteria, with two repair ruptures (4%) during the postoperative motion program. Taras et al [21] applied double-grasping and cross-stitch peripheral sutures in 21 flexor tendon repairs of 14 digits. These included three FPL, four FDP zone I, and 14 FDS or FDP zone II repairs. The postoperative therapy regimen included active motion initiated on the first postoperative day, including place-hold exercise three times weekly under supervision. Between therapy sessions, a standard elastic-thread traction passive flexion and active extension program was maintained. Overall recovery of digital motion was graded as excellent in 12 and good in 2. The seven fingers with FDP and FDS repairs in zone II averaged 83% recovery of motion. Sandow and McMahon [22] reported 37 consecutive FDP tendons in zones I to V using a modified single-cross six-strand repair based on the original Savage method. Of 23 zone II tendon injuries in 18 patients, 78% were rated as good or excellent using Strickland and Glogovac criteria. There were no ruptures or secondary surgery in any patient in their series. Lim and Tsai [23] used six-strand tendon repairs with looped suture to repair the tendon injuries in zone II with good functional outcomes.

There were two reports on the outcomes of the largest series of flexor tendon injuries in this period, both of which came from England. Kitsis et al [25] treated 339 divided flexor tendons affecting 208 fingers. The tendons were repaired with a modified Kessler core and a Halsted peripheral stitch. Overall results by Strickland and Glogovac criteria were 92% excellent or good, 7% fair, and 1% poor. There were 43 complications in 31 patients, including five zone II ruptures (5.7%) and one rupture in zone V. Harris et al [27] reviewed results of 440 patients with 728 primary zone I and zone II flexor tendon repairs in 526 fingers. Overall, 23 patients ruptured 28 tendon repairs. A total of 129 fingers with zone I injuries had a rupture rate of 5% (6 fingers). A total of 397 fingers with zone II injuries had a rupture rate of 4% (17 fingers) (Table 1).

Sirotakova and Elliot [31] analyzed the results of primary repairs of the FPL tendon followed by early active motion with only the thumb splinted. The first 30 patients were repaired with a Kessler suture and simple epitendinous suture. The last 49 patients underwent repair with a Kessler suture and a reinforced epitendinous suture, but in a splint with the thumb position altered and the fingers also splinted. More recently, they reported 0% rupture rate in 48 patients with strengthened

Table 1
Summary of the reports of primary finger flexor tendon repairs in the past 15 years

Year	Authors	Number of digits	Zones	Excellent and good[a]	Rupture rate
1989	Small et al	117	II	77% (TAM)	9.4%
1989	Cullen et al	38	II	78%	6.4%
1989	Savage and Risitano	36	I,II,III,IV	81% (Buck-Gramcko)	2.8%
1989	Pribaz et al	43	II	70% (White)	7.0%
1992	Tang and Shi	54	II	80%	—
1994	O'Connell et al	95 (children)	I,II	69%[b]	0%
1994	Silfverskiold and May	55	II	90%[b]	3.7%
1994	Grobbelaar and Hudson	38 (children)	All zones	82% (Lister)	7.9%
1995	Berndtsson and Ejeskar	46 (children)	II	77%[b]	—
1994	Elliot et al	244	I,II	79%	5.8%
1994	Tang et al	51	II	77% (White)	4.0%
1996	Baktir et al	88	II	81%	4.5%
1996	Sandow and McMahon	23	II	78%	0%
1998	Kitsis et al	208	All zones	92%	2.9%
		(87	II	88%	5.7%)
1998	Yii et al	161	V	90% (TAM)	0%
1999	Harris et al	526	I,II	—	4.0%
		(129	I	—	5.0%)
		(397	II	—	4.0%)

[a] The criteria of evaluation was Strickland and Glogovac criteria unless otherwise specified.
[b] The percent return active motion range judged by the Strickland and Glogovac criteria.

core and peripheral sutures [7]. Other reports include those from Percival and Sykes [28], Noonan and Blair [29], Nunley et al [30], Fitoussi et al [32], and Kasashima et al [33]. Reported results of FPL repairs are detailed in Table 2.

Review of the outcomes of clinical flexor tendon repairs reported over the 15 years showed excellent or good functional return in more than three-fourths of primary tendon repairs followed by a variety of postoperative passive/active mobilization treatment. Repair ruptures nevertheless were documented in most of the reports and rupture rates ranged from 4%–10% in the finger flexors (see Table 1) and from 3%–17% in FPL of thumbs (Table 2). Most of these reports came from the finest hand surgery centers in the world and these teams were supervised by at least one expert hand surgeon with experience in treating flexor tendon injuries. One may reasonably assume that the outcomes in a general hospital setting might have actually reflected a lower level of success. In other words, flexor tendon repairs might have been unsatisfactory in a larger proportion of patients.

Factors affecting outcome of flexor tendon repair

Adhesion formation

Adhesion formation, like scar formation in cutaneous wounds, was believed to be inevitable after tendon surgery and postoperative

Table 2
Summary of the major reports of flexor pollicis longus tendon repairs

Year	Authors	Number of digits	Zones	Excellent and good	Rupture rate
1989	Percival and Sykes	51	I–III	53% (White)	8%
1991	Noonan and Blair	30	All zones	IP 71%, MP 82% normal	—
1992	Nunley et al	38	I,II	Average IP 35°	3%
1996	Thomazeau et al	20	All zones	85% (Tubiana)	5%
1999	Sirotakova and Elliot	30 (1st period)	I,II	70% (White) 73% (Buck-Gramcko)	17%
		39 (2nd period)	I,II	67% (White) 72% (Buck-Gramcko)	15%
		49 (3rd period)	I,II	76% (White) 80% (Buck-Gramcko)	8%
2002	Kasashima et al	29	I–III	63% (Japanese for surgery of the hand)	0%

immobilization [34,35]. The early motion regimen advocated in the past decades substantially decreased adhesions around repaired tendons and restored smoother gliding surface to the tendon. Tendon healing, though not ideally strong, satisfied the tendon motion program. In many instances, it is unrealistic to expect a tendon to heal without any adhesions, because some loose adhesions may develop after surgery even with exercise. Three distinct concepts are pertinent to healing and function, intrinsic healing, participation of extrinsic cells in healing, and formation of restrictive adhesions. Tendon healing exclusively through intrinsic cellular-activity occurs only in in vitro experimental situations. Clinically, it is not extrinsic interference (through cell seeding or formation of filmy adhesions) but the formation of restrictive adhesions that affects the outcomes of tendon repairs. The goals of a postoperative motion program are to disrupt or prevent adhesions that restrict tendon motion and to prevent joint stiffness, both vital to recovery of active range of finger motion.

Adhesions influence tendon movement depending on their density, which is determined by the tissues from which the adhesions arise. Adhesions are generally categorized as either loose or dense adhesion. As the preservation of the sheath becomes a consideration in tendon repairs, adhesions arising from the sheath structures are of a density between loose and dense. Three types of adhesions therefore can be seen in tenolysis: (1) loose adhesions arise from the subcutaneous tissue and are largely movable; repaired tendons glide fairly easily within such adhesions; (2) adhesions of moderate density arise from the synovial sheath or pulleys and are remarkably restrictive of tendon motion; and (3) dense adhesions arise from the bony floor or volar plates, and penetrate to the dorsal aspect of the tendons. Dense adhesions allow minimal tendon motion and severely jeopardize the healing of the tendon and the intratendinous structures. With an appropriate rehabilitation program, loose adhesions can be disrupted or modified so as to avoid reducing the amplitude of motion. Moderate or dense adhesions, however, should be prevented through careful surgical manipulation or postoperative treatments, because it is difficult to alter once they have developed.

Repair rupture

Among all the consequences of flexor tendon surgery, repair ruptures are of prime concern to hand surgeons, because they require secondary operations. If ruptures occur soon after primary repair, direct resuture of the ruptured tendons may be attempted; if ruptures occur at the late period, a secondary tendon graft is indicated [36]. Rupture of the primary repairs occurred in 4%–10% of the fingers in the reports referenced earlier. Limited healing ability and consequent weakness in the post-healing strength underlay the failure of achieving solid union of intrasynovial flexor tendons. The following factors may trigger the ruptures: (1) Overload of the repaired tendons: active flexion or extension of the fingers may subject the repaired tendons to a load exceeding the limit of the tensile resistance of the repairs. (2) Tendon edema or bulky tendons: edema of the tendons is inevitable after surgery, though severity varies among patients. Severely traumatized wounds, extensive soft tissue injuries, long duration of surgery, and poor surgical repair maneuvers all contribute to postsurgical edema. Edema makes the tendon bulky. In addition, excessive suture materials also contribute to bulkiness. A bulky tendon increases the pressure of the tendon on the surrounding tissues and its friction against the sheath or pulleys during tendon mobilization after surgery. A greater force must be applied to the finger to move the bulky tendons within the sheath, increasing the likelihood of ruptures. (3) Triggering in pulleys or edges of opened sheath: annular pulleys, particularly those of the distal and middle portions of the A2 and A4, are narrow and compress the tendon gliding beneath. Edematous or bulky tendons are easily entrapped by these pulleys. Incising the sheath leads to a certain measure of tendon bowstringing. At the edge of sheath openings, the tendons assume a greater degree of angulation during motion. Edematous and bulky tendons can be triggered at the edge of the sheath openings, halting the finger flexion or extension and causing patients to feel a sudden increase in resistance to finger motion. A forceful pull to overcome the resistance frequently leads to rupture of the repairs. (4) Unexpected finger motion: during the period of wearing protective splints or casts, patients may have some unexpected finger actions, such as falling down on outstretched hands and sudden gripping. These actions impose a sudden increase in the force transmitted through the repaired tendons and may subject tendons to a higher risk for ruptures. (5) Misuse of the fingers: analysis of the causes of ruptures in previous reports indicates that in approximately half of patients with ruptures, the rupture followed an ill-advised action [19,27]. Misuse of the repaired fingers, such as using the hand to lift a heavy object, may exceed the repair strength of the tendon and cause rupture. (6) Unprotected active motion: it is not an appropriate and accepted way of postoperative care after primary tendon repairs. Only some surgeons indicate the possibility of using this sort of exercise regimen. There are not sufficient data to justify the use of this type of regimen and its effect on strength of tendon healing. Active motion of the repaired fingers can cause ruptures if not properly applied or if used without protection. Surgical repairs and tendon healing are not sufficiently strong to accommodate unprotected active motion at present.

Joint stiffness

Stiffness of the DIP and PIP joints frequently is observed during the rehabilitation after primary flexor tendon repair. Stiffness of small joints after trauma to the joints is a troublesome disorder for hand surgeons. Clean-cut flexor tendon injuries themselves, however, usually do no trauma to finger joint structures. It is the postoperative protective finger position that causes joint contracture. It is obvious that modifications in the postoperative motion regimen, in particular the position of protective splints or casts and the maneuvers to move the joints, might lessen the chance of developing joint stiffness. Return of function to the tendons depends on sufficient gliding amplitude of the tendons and normal passive range of motion of the joints. To improve the outcome of tendon repair, greater emphasis should be placed on moving the joint. More specific physical therapeutic procedures to prevent or correct joint stiffness need to be incorporated in future motion protocols.

Original Kleinert traction frequently leads to loss of PIP joint extension. The fingers of patients were protected by rubber bands, and the PIP joint was flexed for long periods. With modified rubber band traction or with modification of dorsal splint with no protective palmar bars, larger degrees of PIP joint extension were achieved, but achieving full extension of the PIP joint and elimination of contracture of the volar plate remain an unsolved problem in rehabilitation after primary flexor tendon repairs in zone II. At present, eliminating joint stiffness is still an essential goal of physical therapy after removal of protective fixation 3–4 weeks after surgery.

Extent of injuries

The relative severity of injuries to peritendinous soft tissues affects the outcome of tendon repair. Extensive soft tissue destruction and epitendinous abrasion are associated with poorer functional outcome. A primary surgical repair is clearly indicated in clean-cut tendon injury. It is difficult to judge whether primary tendon repairs are justified for wounds that do not involve clean cuts, but in which direct approximation of the severed stumps is still possible. These wounds, which are typified by loss of soft tissues (sometimes with a short segment of flexor tendons and a portion of pulleys) over a limited area of the fingers or palm and defects of soft tissues, should be repaired with a local or distant flap, and have as borderline indication primary flexor tendon repairs. Are primary repairs of the tendons indicated in these wounds? Some surgeons (including this author) may prefer to repair the tendons followed by secondary tenolysis rather than wait for secondary free tendon grafts. In case reconstruction of multiple pulleys in these wounds is called for, however, primary tendon repairs are not justified. Digital nerve injuries are a frequent complication of tendon injuries in zone II. In the author's clinic, digital nerves are directly repaired when there are no defects or reconstructed with a vein conduit when there is a small (<3.0 cm) gap.

Surgical skills

Adequate surgical skills are a factor that cannot be overemphasized. The flexor tendon system is made of anatomic structures in an intricate biomechanic relationship. Simply reconnecting severed tendons is a simple procedure, but satisfactory repairs of the tendons and associated structures, particularly those in the intrasynovial regions, remain a challenge even to an experienced surgeon. In practice, these difficult injuries are treated not infrequently by residents or general orthopedic (or plastic) surgeons without sufficient expertise in flexor tendon surgery. With currently available knowledge and technical advances, favorable outcomes may be achieved by an experienced surgeon, but an individual who lacks expertise may effect repairs no better than those seen decades ago. Surgery based on poor mastery of anatomic knowledge and repair techniques can destroy the tissue structures and make delayed primary tendon repairs by an expert surgeon impossible. When no surgeons experienced in tendon surgery are available, patients should be

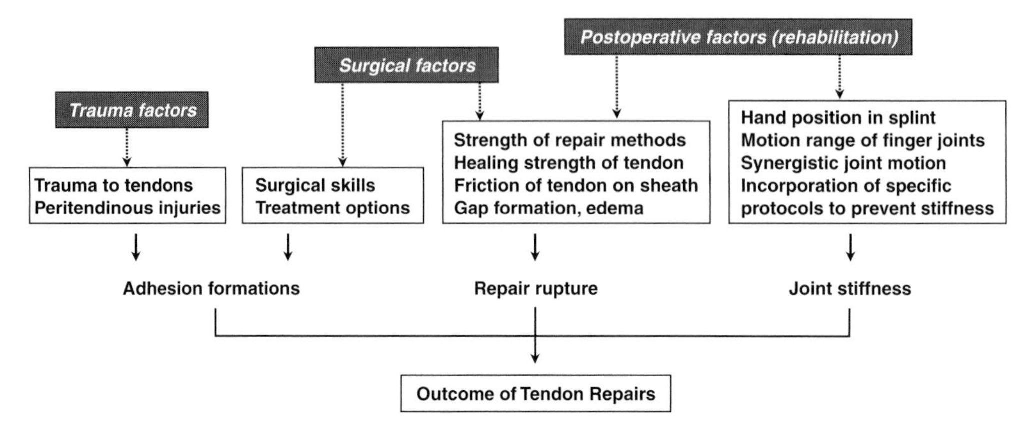

Fig. 1. Relation between factors affecting clinical outcome of flexor tendon repairs.

referred to hand centers with more experience in dealing with flexor tendon injuries. Alternatively, after primary closure of the skin wounds, tendon injuries may be repaired at a delayed primary stage by an experienced surgeon.

Adhesion formation, repair rupture, and joint stiffness ultimately determine the measure of outcome of the repair, whereas the latter two, extent of injuries and surgical skills, relate to the wound and surgical factors. Relation between these factors and outcomes is illustrated in Fig. 1.

Evaluation of outcome and possible modifications

Three methods of evaluating outcome after flexor tendon repair are used popularly: Strickland and Glogovac criteria [37] (Table 3), the TAM method, proposed by the American Society for Surgery of the Hand [38], and the Buck-Gramcko method [38], used largely by German-speaking hand societies. Most investigators have adopted the Strickland and Glogovac criteria in their documentation of outcome of flexor tendon repair in zones I and II. The author found these criteria (in fact, a modified TAM method) more practical than the TAM method. In the original TAM method, only the fingers whose total range of active motion is the same as that of the contralateral hand can be rated as excellent. The author has found that varying degrees of joint stiffness are invariably present after tendon repair and protective motion exercise; patients who entirely satisfy the criteria as excellent are extremely rare. The Strickland and Glogovac criteria give a more practical assessment of finger function than the original TAM method. Excellent functional status requires a sufficiently ample total range of active motion, but not necessarily a range of active motion equal to that of the contralateral side. TAM of the joints over 80% of the normal motion range usually gives excellent function to the fingers. Exclusion of the motion range of the metacarpophalangeal (MP) joint also gives more accuracy of documentation of motion ranges of the PIP and DIP joints in the Strickland and Glogovac criteria than the original TAM method. Among the less popular methods currently used are White's criteria, the Tubiana method, and tip-to-palm distance method. White's criteria and tip-to-palm distance were popular 15–20 years ago, and the Tubiana method is used mostly in France.

Table 3
Strickland and Glogovac criteria of evaluation

Grade	Total active range of motion[a] (degrees)	Functional return (%)
Excellent	>150	85–100
Good	125–149	70–84
Fair	90–124	50–60
Poor	<90	0–49

[a] Sum of the active range of motion of the DIP and PIP joints.

The length of follow-up affects the recorded outcome of the flexor tendon repair. Flexor tendon healing and collagen remodeling usually take longer than 2–3 months, and correction of interphalangeal joint contracture may require even longer. Outcome of flexor tendon repair should be determined appropriately not earlier than 3 months after surgery, when postoperative therapy is complete and before most patients would return to work.

Several questions remain in identifying an evaluation system that best reflects the performance of hands following repair of the flexor tendon or in developing a universally acceptable methodology for comparison of surgical repair results: (1) Which of the existing methods is the evaluation system best reflecting outcome of tendon repair? Currently, no specific studies on this point are seen in the literature. It thus would be meaningful to carry out studies to evaluate or compare assessment systems. (2) Would it be more informative to record the result of flexor tendon repair within the sheath area by subdivisions of the tendons in the fingers? Moiemen and Elliot [39] subdivided zone I into three subdivisions and recorded the results of the FDP tendon repair in these areas. Tang et al [40,41] subdivided zone II into four subdivisions and reported the results of repairs of the FDS and FDP tendons in these regions. Both systems use pulleys and FDS insertion as landmarks (Fig. 2). Recording results of the flexor tendon repair in subdivisions of the finger flexor tendons may facilitate more precise evaluation of the results and thereby provide valuable information about the outcome in specific regions and for specific components of the flexor tendon system. (3) Would it be more reasonable to evaluate separately the motion of all finger joints (TAM) and function of a single joint most pertinent to a tendon cut? Moiemen and Elliot [39] proposed evaluating the results of zone I tendon injuries with the original Strickland criteria and with a method to record only the range of motion of the DIP joint separately. They suggested the addition of an evaluation of function in the motion of the joint most relevant to the flexor tendon injury. (4) Are current evaluation items sufficient? The existing assessment systems include items regarding tip-to-palm distance and active range of joint motion, which relate to angulation of finger joints only. The function of the flexor tendon includes grip and pinch strength, however. Clinically, the repair of both of the FDS and FDP tendons in fingers would produce greater grip strength. In addition, digital flexor tendons contribute to deviation of the fingers. Existing criteria reflect none of the functions of the tendon except range of finger flexion-extension. A question therefore is whether these functions should be considered in evaluating repair results. (5) Should coordinated finger motion or wrist motion be considered? In flexor tendon injuries involving multiple fingers or multiple sites, injuries in zones III, IV, and V, or secondary tendon transfer, coordinated motion of multiple fingers or of fingers with the wrist often are disturbed. Coordination of the motion of multiple fingers and joints is important to the function of the entire hand; however, disturbance on this aspect is not reflected in the existing evaluation systems. For a more precise evaluation, such functional loss might be included as an integral part of the evaluation system in selected patient groups to reflect postoperative functional performance.

Approaches to improve outcome

Stronger surgical repairs

Pursuit of a stronger yet less strangulating tendon suture configuration has been a focus of

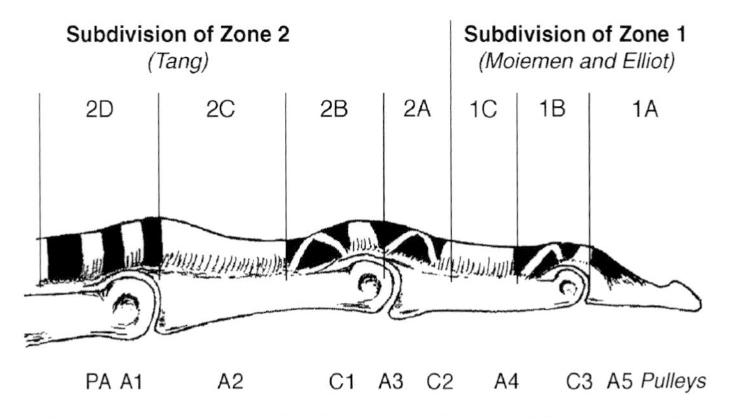

Fig. 2. Subdivisions of flexor tendon systems in digital sheath area by Tang, Moiemen, and Elliot using major pulleys and FDS insertion as landmarks. The area covered by the A2 pulley is zone IIC, the area of FDS insertion zone IIA, from the A4 pulley to the DIP joint zone IB.

biomechanic studies over the past decade [3–6, 42–48]. The conventional two-strand repair methods withstand a tension of 20–30 N, with the force to produce remarkable gaps (>2 mm) less than 20 N. It is true that most tendons repaired with the conventional two-strand repairs survived early postoperative exercise. Though the studies identified earlier seem to reflect a recent declining trend in rupture rates of repaired tendons after use of multiple strand repairs, however, there is no direct evidence of such a correlation, and no randomized prospective clinical trails have been performed on this particular issue. Early reports of active motion of the tendons repaired with conventional two-strand repair documented rupture rate of nearly 10% [9,10,12]. Such high rupture rates were not seen in more recent reports. The merits of multiple-strand tendon repair include increasing the safety margin to withstand the tension of postoperative motion exercise. This does not mean that most tendons repaired with two-strand techniques necessarily fail during motion or that multistrand repairs completely prevent repair ruptures. Rather, increasing repair strength through multistrand repairs decreases the likelihood of rupture in cases that may rupture when repaired conventionally with two-strand techniques. In addition, an increase in baseline surgical repair strength might allow one to apply a more aggressive exercise regimen and disrupt more adhesions, thus resulting in a better return of tendon motion and mobile joint range to the injured fingers.

In the author's experience, four-strand repairs seem to be the most appropriate choice for the tendon from zones I to IV. In addition, the author has performed six-strand repairs in zone II of the flexor tendon and in fact does not use conventional two-strand repair technique in zones I and II flexor tendon repair. Eight-strand repairs seem unnecessary, because four- or six-strand repairs already provide sufficiently high tensile strength to the tendon and eight-strand repairs are technically more difficult within the digital sheath area. The variety of multistrand repair techniques the author used over the past 15 years are illustrated in Fig. 3. In the last 2 years, a modified six-strand looped (M-Tang) method and a modified four-strand looped repair have become the methods of choice in the author's clinic. Over the past 2 years, we repaired FDP tendons in 36 fingers with zone II flexor tendon lacerations with the M-Tang method. We achieved 90% excellent or good recovery rate by Strickland and Glogovac criteria with combined protective active and passive motion for 3 weeks after surgery, with no repair rupture.

Sheath/pulley management

There is no longer controversy among hand surgeons regarding whether the synovial sheath should be closed after tendon repairs. Closure of the synovial sheath is not vitally required to tendon healing and gliding function [49–51]. Closure of the synovial sheath may be attempted in clean-cut injury without presence of sheath defects or abrasion. It is now agreed that the integrity of major pulleys is critical to tendon function, and avoiding compression of the edematous tendons by the sheath after surgery is important to tendon healing [51–53]. With major annular pulleys and a major part of the synovial sheath intact, opening a part of synovial sheath

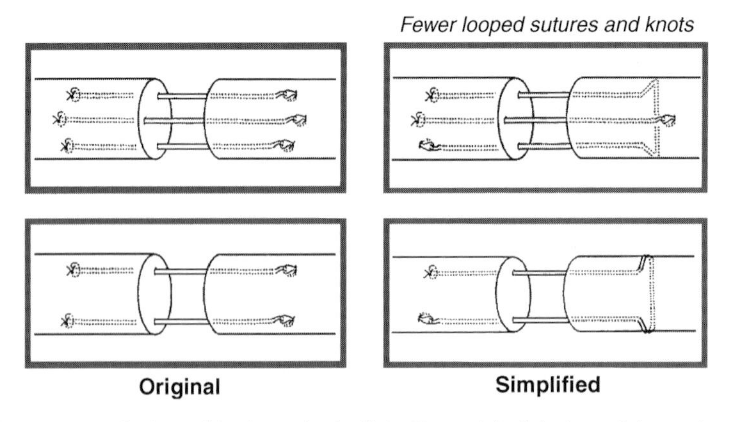

Fig. 3. Four tendon suture methods used in the author's clinic. Two original designs of 4-strand and 6-strand repairs using independent looped sutures (*left*) and two more recent modifications using fewer looped sutures and knots (*right*).

has no significant effects on tendon function and healing. On the other hand, when other pulleys or synovial sheaths are intact, incision of one single annular pulley or a critical part of the major annular pulley (A2 or A4 pulleys) does not significantly affect tendon gliding, but may release the compression of an edematous tendon by these constrictions, thus fostering the tendon healing process [53–58].

Clinically, the A4 or A2 pulley occasionally constitutes an obstacle for the repaired tendon to glide through, which is likely a cause of repair rupture during postoperative motion exercise. Releasing the A4 pulley entirely and releasing part of the A2 became accepted clinical practice in recent years. In the author's clinic, when the repaired FDP tendons are found tightly entrapped by the A4 pulley after testing during surgery, we completely release the A4 pulley (Fig. 4). Part of the A2 pulley, either proximal or distal (approximately one half to two thirds of the entire length of theA2 pulley), is cut when the FDS and FDP tendon are repaired in the area overlapping the A2 pulley.

Optimization of rehabilitation regimen

Optimization of the rehabilitation regimen has been a focus of clinical investigations. There seems to be a long way to go, however, before general agreement is reached. More likely, as understanding of the intricate relationship between tension on the flexor tendons during finger motion increases, the hand posture that affords the best postoperative protection with the least possible tension on the tendon will be identified, ultimately revolutionizing rehabilitation. Unprotected active motion of the fingers does not seem likely to be generally accepted in the near future, because even protected motion can cause certain repair ruptures. Science cannot yet bring about the healing necessary to support unprotected active motion. Protected combined active/passive motion is the option that most surgeons currently

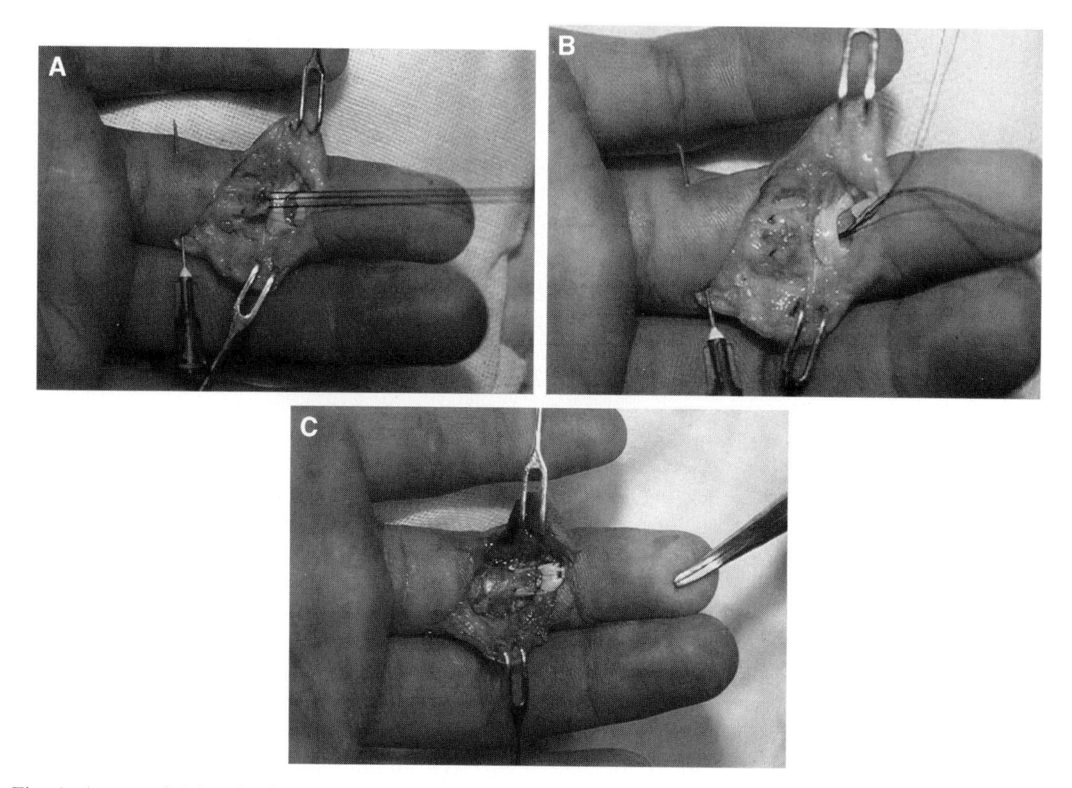

Fig. 4. A case of delayed primary repair of FDP tendon injury of the ring finger. (*A*) The FDP tendon stump was repaired with 3 groups (6-strand) of looped sutures. (*B*) The tendon was lead to pass beneath the narrow A4 pulley. (*C*) This pulley was vented and the repair was completed. Note the sheath proximal to the A4 pulley was maintained to avoid lengthy loss of sheath integrity.

adopt. The use of rubber bands is no longer a requirement and is known to cause contracture and extension lag of the joints. The trend is toward a rehabilitation regimen combining an ideal protective position of the hand, with intermittent active–passive finger flexion–extension, using no rubber bands.

Another area in which there is not yet agreement is the timing of rehabilitation and frequency of finger motion, either in a particular day or during each exercise episode. Theoretically, tendon adhesion develops starting from 2–3 weeks after surgery. Rehabilitation can begin anytime within 1 week following repair. Most studies report the initiation of rehabilitation as immediate or starting the first day after surgery. No studies have yet proven the need of starting the exercise on the first day after surgery. It seems equally reasonable to commence the exercise later, though within 1 week after surgery. Commencement of rehabilitation at the third or fourth day causes less pain and likely does not affect results compared with starting on the first day. We have not yet identified optimal frequency of motion in each exercise episode or whether more frequent exercise leads to better results. Similarly, we also do not know what sequences of active and passive motion are best for the tendons and whether the range of each motion cycle affects the outcome. Answering these questions is essential for optimization of rehabilitation programs for repaired tendons.

Biologic approaches

Flexor tendons, particularly those in the intrasynovial area, lack sufficient cellularity and generally have low growth factor levels. These are the basic reasons that adhesions or ruptures occur after surgery and that outcomes are less than perfect. Delivery of growth factors to proliferating tenocytes in vitro significantly enhanced their proliferation rate and collagen production [59–65]. Growth factors generally have a short biologic half-life, however, and continuous supplementation of exogenous growth factors to healing flexor tendons is not practical. Transfer of growth factor genes therefore would provide the tendons with continuous supplementation of the growth factors critical to the healing process. Delivery of growth factor genes through plasmid vectors has been shown to promote the expression of type I collagen gene in the tenocytes [66]. What systems are the safest and most efficient to deliver growth factor genes to healing tendons? How do we augment tenocytes' capacity to produce collagen to the healing process while limiting the occurrence of adhesions? Answering these questions is likely to be among the critical steps in future in vivo investigation. In addition, transplantation of stem cells to the healing tendons would provide sources of progenitor cells to promote the healing process of the tendon. Gene therapy and stem cell transplantation are two emerging fields of modern biology that offer new approaches to difficult problems in flexor tendon repairs. Future efforts to combine stem cell therapy and gene therapy would provide the tendons not only with a fresh source of progenitor cells (which may differentiate into tenocytes to aid in healing) but also with the growth factors required to promote the healing process.

Summary

Review of the outcomes of clinical flexor tendon repairs reported over the past 15 years showed advances in the outcomes with excellent or good functional return in more than three fourths of primary tendon repairs following a variety of postoperative passive/active mobilization treatments. Strickland and Glogovac criteria are the most commonly adopted methods to assess function. Repair ruptures (4%–10% for zone II finger flexors and 3%–17% for the FPL tendon), adhesion formations, and stiffness of finger joints remain frustrating problems in flexor tendon repairs and rehabilitation. Four approaches are suggested to improve outcomes of the repairs and to solve these difficult problems, which include stronger surgical repairs, appropriate pulleys or sheath management, optimization of rehabilitation regimens, and modern biologic approaches.

References

[1] Strickland JW. Flexor tendon injuries. Part I. Anatomy, physiology, biomechanics, healing, and adhesion formation around a repaired tendon. Orthop Rev 1986;15(10):632–42.

[2] Boyer MI, Strickland JW, Engles DR, Sachar K, Leversedge FJ. Flexor tendon repair and rehabilitation. J Bone Joint Surg [Am] 2002;84(9):1684–706.

[3] Angeles JG, Heminger H, Mass DP. Comparative biomechanical performance of 4-strand core suture repair for zone II flexor tendon repairs. J Hand Surg [Am] 2002;27(3):508–17.

[4] Xie RG, Zhang S, Tang JB, Chen F. Biomechanical studies of 3 different 6-strand flexor tendon repair techniques. J Hand Surg [Am] 2002;27(4):621–7.
[5] McLarney E, Hoffman H, Wolfe SW. Biomechanical analysis of the cruciate four-strand flexor tendon repair. J Hand Surg [Am] 1999;24(2):295–301.
[6] Tang JB, Wang B, Chen F, Pan CZ, Xie RG. Biomechanical evaluation of flexor tendon repair techniques. Clin Orthop 2001;386:252–9.
[7] Sirotakova M, Elliot D. Early active mobilization of primary repairs of the flexor pollicis longus tendon with two Kessler two-strand core sutures and a strengthened circumferential suture. J Hand Surg [Br] 2004;29(6):531.
[8] Elliot D. Primary flexor tendon repair—operative repair, pulley management and rehabilitation. J Hand Surg [Br] 2002;27(4):507–13.
[9] Small JO, Brennen MD, Colville J. Early active mobilization following flexor tendon repair in zone II. J Hand Surg [Br] 1989;14(4):383–91.
[10] Cullen KW, Tolhurst P, Lang D, Page RE. Flexor tendon repair in zone II followed by controlled active mobilization. J Hand Surg [Br] 1989;14(4): 392–5.
[11] Savage R, Risitano G. Flexor tendon repair using a "six strand" method of repair and early active mobilization. J Hand Surg [Br] 1989;14(4):396–9.
[12] Pribaz JJ, Morrison WA, Macleod AM. Primary repair of flexor tendons in no man's land using the Becker repair. J Hand Surg [Br] 1989;14(4):400–5.
[13] May EJ, Silfverskiöld KL, Sollerman CJ. The correlation between controlled range of motion with dynamic traction and results after flexor tendon repair in zone II. J Hand Surg [Am] 1992;17(6): 1133–9.
[14] Tang JB, Shi D. Subdivision of flexor tendon "no man's land" and different treatment methods in each sub-zone. A preliminary report. Chin Med J 1992;105(1):60–8.
[15] O'Connell SJ, Moore MM, Strickland JW, Frazier GT, Dell PC. Results of zone I and zone II flexor tendon repairs in children. J Hand Surg [Am] 1994; 19(1):48–52.
[16] Silfverskiöld KL, May EJ. Flexor tendon repair in zone II with a new suture technique and an early mobilization program combining passive and active flexion. J Hand Surg [Am] 1994;19(1):53–60.
[17] Grobbelaar AO, Hudson DA. Flexor tendon injuries in children. J Hand Surg [Br] 1994;19(6):696–8.
[18] Berndtsson L, Ejeskar A. Zone II flexor tendon repair in children. A retrospective long term study. Scand J Plast Reconstr Hand Surg 1995;29(1):59–64.
[19] Elliot D, Moiemen NS, Flemming AFS, Harris SB, Foster AJ. The rupture rate of acute flexor tendon repairs mobilized by the controlled active motion regimen. J Hand Surg [Br] 1994;19(5):607–12.
[20] Tang JB, Shi D, Gu YQ, Chen JC, Zhou B. Double and multiple looped suture tendon repair. J Hand Surg [Br] 1994;19(6):699–703.
[21] Taras JS, Skahen JR, Raphael JS, Marzyk S, Bauerle W. The double-grasping and cross-stitch for acute flexor tendon repair. Atlas Hand Clin 1996;1(1):13–28.
[22] Sandow MJ, McMahon MM. Single-cross grasp six-strand repair for acute flexor tendon tenorrhaphy. Atlas Hand Clin 1996;1(1):41–64.
[23] Lim BH, Tsai TM. The six-strand techniques for flexor tendon repair. Atlas Hand Clin 1996;1(1): 65–76.
[24] Baiktir A, Turk CY, Kabak S, Sahin V, Kardas Y. Flexor tendon repair in zone II followed by early active mobilization. J Hand Surg [Br] 1996;21(5): 624–8.
[25] Kitsis CK, Wade PJF, Krikler SJ, Parsons NK, Nicholls LK. Controlled active motion following primary flexor tendon repair: a prospective study over 9 years. J Hand Surg [Br] 1998;23(3):344–9.
[26] Yii NW, Urban M, Elliot D. A prospective study of flexor tendon repair in zone 5. J Hand Surg [Br] 1998;23(5):642–8.
[27] Harris SB, Harris D, Foster AJ, Elliot D. The aetiology of acute rupture of flexor tendon repairs in zones 1 and 2 of the fingers during early mobilization. J Hand Surg [Br] 1999;24(3):275–80.
[28] Percival NJ, Sykes PJ. Flexor pollicis longus tendon repair: a comparison between dynamic and static splintage. J Hand Surg [Br] 1989;14(3):412–5.
[29] Noonan KJ, Blair WF. Long-term follow-up of primary flexor pollicis longus tenorrhaphies. J Hand Surg [Am] 1991;16(4):651–62.
[30] Nunley JA, Levin LS, Devito D, Goldner RD, Urbaniak JR. Direct end-to-end repair of flexor pollicis longus tendon lacerations. J Hand Surg [Am] 1992;17(1):118–21.
[31] Sirotakova M, Elliot D. Early active mobilization of primary repairs of the flexor pollicis longus tendon. J Hand Surg [Br] 1999;24(6):647–53.
[32] Fitoussi F, Mazda K, Frajman JM, Jehanno P, Pennecot GF. Repair of the flexor pollicis longus tendon in children. J Bone Joint Surg [Br] 2000; 82(8):1177–80.
[33] Kasashima T, Kato H, Minami A. Factors influencing prognosis after direct repair of the flexor pollicis longus tendon: multivariate regression model analysis. Hand Surg 2002;7(2):171–6.
[34] Potenza AD. Tendon healing within the flexor digital sheath in the dog. J Bone Joint Surg [Am] 1962; 44(1):49–64.
[35] Potenza AD. Critical evaluation of flexor-tendon healing and adhesion formation within artificial digital sheaths. J Bone Joint Surg [Am] 1963;45(4): 1217–33.
[36] Liu TK, Yang RS. Flexor tendon graft for late management of isolated rupture of the profundus tendon. J Trauma 1997;43(1):103–6.
[37] Strickland JW, Glogovac SV. Digital function following flexor tendon repair in zone II: a comparison of immobilization and controlled passive

motion techniques. J Hand Surg [Am] 1980;5(6): 537–43.

[38] Kleinert HE, Verdan C. Report of the committee on tendon injuries. J Hand Surg [Am] 1983;8(Suppl): S794–8.

[39] Moiemen NS, Elliot D. Early active mobilization of primary flexor tendon repairs in zone 1. J Hand Surg [Br] 2000;25(1):78–84.

[40] Tang JB. Flexor tendon repairs in zone IIC. J Hand Surg [Br] 1994;19(1):72–5.

[41] Tang JB, Xu Y, Chen F. Impact of flexor digitorum superficialis on gliding function of the flexor digitorum profundus according to regions in zone II. J Hand Surg [Am] 2003;28(5):838–44.

[42] Barrie KA, Tomak SL, Cholewicki J, Merrell GA, Wolfe SW. Effect of suture locking and suture caliber on fatigue strength of flexor tendon repairs. J Hand Surg [Am] 2001;26(2):340–6.

[43] Grill RS, Lim BH, Shatford RA, Toth E, Voor MJ, Tsai TM. A comparative analysis of the six-strand double-loop flexor tendon repair and three other techniques: a human cadaveric study. J Hand Surg [Am] 1999;24(6):1315–22.

[44] Goldfarb CA, Harwood F, Silva MJ, Gelberman RH, Amiel D, Boyer MI. The effect of variations in applied rehabilitation force on collagen concentration and maturation at the intrasynovial tendon repair site. J Hand Surg [Am] 2001;26(5):841–6.

[45] Boyer MI, Gelberman RH, Burns ME, Dinopoulos H, Hofrm R, Silva MJ. Intrasynovial flexor tendon repair. An experimental study comparing low and high levels of *in vivo* force during rehabilitation in canines. J Bone Joint Surg Am 2001;83(6):891–9.

[46] Winters SC, Gelberman RH, Woo SL, Chan SS, Grewal R, Seiler JG. The effects of multiple-strand suture methods on the strength and excursion of repaired intrasynovial flexor tendons: A biomechanical study in dogs. J Hand Surg [Am] 1998;23(1): 97–104.

[47] Choueka J, Heminger H, Mass D. Cyclical testing of zone II flexor tendon repairs. J Hand Surg [Am] 2000;25(6):1127–34.

[48] Wang B, Xie RG, Tang JB. Biomechanical analysis of a modification of Tang method of tendon repair. J Hand Surg [Br] 2003;28(4):347–50.

[49] Gelberman RH, Woo SL, Amiel D, Horibe S, Lee D. Influences of flexor sheath continuity and early motion on tendon healing in dogs. J Hand Surg [Am] 1990;15(1):69–77.

[50] Tang JB, Ishii S, Usui M, Yamamura T. Flexor sheath closure during delayed primary tendon repair. J Hand Surg [Am] 1994;19(4):636–40.

[51] Tang JB, Shi D, Zhang QG. Biomechanical and histologic evaluation of tendon sheath management. J Hand Surg [Am] 1996;21(6):900–8.

[52] Manske PR, Lesker PA. Palmer aponeurosis pulley. J Hand Surg [Am] 1983;8(3):259–63.

[53] Lister G. Indications and techniques for repair of the flexor tendon sheath. Hand Clin 1985;1(1): 85–95.

[54] Tang JB. The double sheath system and tendon gliding in zone IIC. J Hand Surg [Br] 1995;20(3):281–5.

[55] Tomaino M, Mitsionis G, Bastidas J, Grewal R, Pfaeffle J. The effect of partial excision of the A2 and A4 pulleys on the biomechanics of finger flexion. J Hand Surg [Br] 1998;23(1):50–8.

[56] Kwai Ben I, Elliot D. Venting or partial release of the A2 and A4 pulleys after repair of zone II flexor tendon injuries. J Hand Surg [Br] 1998;23(4):649–54.

[57] Tang JB, Xie RG. Effect of A3 pulley and adjacent sheath integrity on tendon excursion and bowstringing. J Hand Surg [Am] 2001;26(4):855–61.

[58] Tang JB, Wang YH, Gu YT, Chen F. Effect of pulley integrity on excursions and work of flexion in healing flexor tendons. J Hand Surg [Am] 2001; 26(2):347–53.

[59] Khan U, Kakar S, Akali A, Bentley G, McGrouther DA. Modulation of the formation of adhesions during the healing of injured tendons. J Bone Joint Surg [Br] 2000;82(7):1054–8.

[60] Abrahamsson SO. Similar effects of recombinant human insulin-like growth factor I and II on cellular activities in flexor tendons of young rabbits: experimental studies in vitro. J Orthop Res 1997;15(2): 256–62.

[61] Chan BP, Chan KM, Maffulli N, Webb S, Lee KH. Effect of basic fibroblast growth factor. An in vitro study of tendon healing. Clin Orthop 1997;342: 239–47.

[62] Klein MB, Yalamanchi N, Pham H, Longaker MT, Chang J. Flexor tendon healing in vitro: effects of TGF-β on tendon cell collagen production. J Hand Surg [Am] 2002;27(3):615–20.

[63] Tang JB, Xu Y, Ding F, Wang XT. Tendon healing in vitro: promotion of collagen gene expression by bFGF with NF-κB gene activation. J Hand Surg [Am] 2003;28(2):215–20.

[64] Tang JB, Xu Y, Ding F, Wang XT. Expression of genes for collagen production and NF-κB gene activation of in vivo healing flexor tendons. J Hand Surg [Am] 2004;29(4):564–70.

[65] Tang JB, Xu Y, Wang XT. Tendon healing in vitro: activation of NIK, IKKα, IKKβ, and NF-κB genes in signal pathway and proliferation of tenocytes. Plast Reconstr Surg 2004;113(6):1703–11.

[66] Wang XT, Liu PY, Tang JB. Tendon healing in vitro: genetic modification of tenocytes with exogenous PDGF gene and promotion of collagen gene expression. J Hand Surg [Am] 2004;29(5): 884–90.

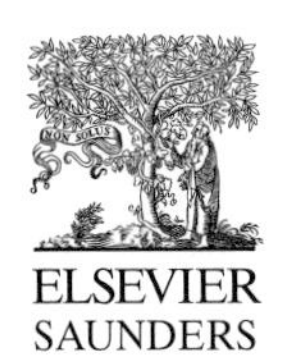
ELSEVIER
SAUNDERS

Hand Clin 21 (2005) 211–217

HAND
CLINICS

Flexor Tenolysis

Kodi K. Azari, MD[a,*], Roy A. Meals, MD[b]

[a]*Division of Plastic Surgery, 3550 Terrace Street, 6B Scaife Hall, University of Pittsburgh Medical Center, Pittsburgh, PA 15261, USA*

[b]*Orthopaedic Surgery, University of California–Los Angeles, 100 UCLA Med. Plaza, #305, Los Angeles, CA 90024-6970, USA*

To function properly, flexor tendons must glide through tight pulleys and move smoothly under the skin and over the bones and joints of the hand. Any damage to the bony [1] and soft tissue structures or to the tendon surface itself, be it laceration, crush, or infection, can result in tendon scarring with resultant adhesion formation [2]. When adhesions limit digital function and an ample course of hand therapy has reached maximal usefulness, surgical intervention should be considered. The concept of surgical tendon liberation from post-traumatic cicatrix has been in existence for more than 60 years [3]. Although the efficacy of tenolysis originally was questioned [4], it is now considered a procedure with valuable clinical usefulness in the restitution and enhancement of digital function [4–8].

This purpose of this article is to offer preoperative, operative, and postoperative considerations for flexor tenolysis with particular emphasis on the authors' personal preferences.

Preoperative consideration

Indication and timing

Tenolysis is indicated when the passive range of motion (ROM) is significantly greater than the active ROM at the same joint following fracture, flexor tendon repair, grafting, or tendon sheath infection [7]. Before embarking on conceivably the most challenging flexor tendon operation [4], however, several criteria must be strictly satisfied to provide the best prognosis [7,9]. These time-tested prerequisites include (1) well healed fractures that are in anatomic alignment, (2) coverage of all wounds with stable soft scar and supple skin, (3) intact tendon systems, (4) good muscle strength, (5) mobilization of joint contractures to near full passive ROM, and (6) a compliant, motivated patient who has access to an experienced hand therapist [7,8].

The exact timing of tenolysis has been historically open to controversy. From experiments in chicken tendons, Wray et al [10] attempted to define the optimal time for tenolysis by evaluating the blood supply, rupture rate, and the tensile strength of tenolysed and control tendons. They conclude that tenolysis at 12 weeks after tendon repair did not weaken the tendon and resulted in an increased blood supply. Other investigators have advocated waiting 3 months after primary flexor tendon operations and 6 months following flexor tendon grafting before tenolysis [9]. Contemporary wisdom holds that 3 months wait is adequate for embarking on the tenolysis pathway [6,7], however, provided that the previously mentioned preoperative tenolysis criteria are satisfied. The patient must have been active in a vigorous hand therapy regimen incorporating passive and active ROM exercises for approximately 3 months [6] and have reached a plateau in which there has been no quantifiable progress in the preceding 4–8 weeks [4,11]. This time frame in a therapy program allows for elongation of the tendon adhesions that have formed [10] and adequate time for wound healing and scar maturation. Proceeding with tenolysis earlier than 3 months is believed to jeopardize the nutritional supply and increase the rupture risk, whereas delay is believed to decrease this incidence [12].

* Corresponding author.
E-mail address: Kodiazari@yahoo.com (K.K. Azari).

0749-0712/05/$ - see front matter
doi:10.1016/j.hcl.2004.11.008

If the desired ROM is not achieved after 3 months of therapy, it is reasonable to consider tenolysis. In this consideration, the importance of patient selection and cooperation cannot be overemphasized. It is as much a key to success as is the operative procedure itself, because it is unlikely that tenolysis in an unmotivated or uncooperative patient will result in a successful outcome. There are no absolute indications for tenolysis and the advisability of surgery should consider subjectively the patient's age, occupation requirements, and global functionality. In the surgeon's considerations, a rational and pragmatic goal must be depicted for the patient. Each patient needs to be approached individually with unique requirements, limitations, and goals. For example, patients who are elderly or who have low functional demands may accept diminutive ROMs, whereas global functional improvement will not be attained in a cold and insensate replanted digit despite recovery of full ROM after tenolysis [6].

Flexor tenolysis is considered a technically difficult operation [12] and is considered by Strickland [7] as the most demanding of all flexor tendon procedures. Consequently the operation must be approached as a major surgical effort [7]. Preoperatively and as a matter of routine, the authors' patients are informed that intraoperative findings may be incompatible with proceeding with tenolysis efforts. For example, the authors may find a devascularized tendon or a ruptured pulley or flexor tendon. In this scenario, the authors proceed with the first step of staged tendon reconstruction and abort the tenolysis procedure.

Surgical technique

Anesthesia

Since the mid 1970s Hunter and Schneider [13] have popularized surgical lysis of tendon adhesions under local anesthesia with intravenous analgesic and sedative supplementation [14]. This anesthetic approach allows for active involvement of the patient at the conclusion of tenolysis to ensure that the tendon is adequately liberated from scar and that the motor unit powering the tendon is of sufficient strength to generate full digital flexion [4,6,7,12]. Local anesthetic (without epinephrine) is infiltrated in the local subcutaneous tissues or alternatively used as a regional block [13], such as a digital block or wrist block. During the operation, the anesthesia personnel titrate the analgesic medication as necessary for patient comfort, and at the conclusion, reduce it to a level that allows for awakening so that the patient can actively move the fingers. Performing this procedure (which may last more than an hour) under local anesthetic can have the liability of ischemic tourniquet discomfort and muscular paralysis [7]. To address these issues, circumferential subcutaneous infiltration of the local anesthetic can be administered about the distal forearm to anesthetize the superficial sensory nerves [12]. To reduce muscle paralysis and increase the time that the tourniquet is tolerated, Strickland [4,7] advocates the application of a sterile pediatric tourniquet to the mid-forearm, which can be inflated before the proximal arm tourniquet is released. This allows for preservation of a bloodless field and restoration of extrinsic flexor muscle activity within 5 minutes [4]. Feldscher and Schneider [6] perform the procedure under 1% or 2% lidocaine local anesthetic and intravenous sedation. When tourniquet paralysis ensues, the tourniquet is released, hemostasis is achieved with pressure and cautery, and the adequacy of their tenolysis is evaluated. The tourniquet then is reinflated and the remainder of the operation is performed until tenolysis is complete.

Alternatively, general anesthesia or axillary block should be used if the surgeon preoperatively expects an extensive operation (such as multiple digits) or a restless patient, to a degree that local anesthetic with intravenous sedation will not be tolerated [4]. Following tenolysis under these anesthetic modalities, a proximal wrist or palmar incision should be made, and, as described by Whitaker et al [15], the involved tendons passively pulled on. This "traction flexor check" maneuver allows for evaluation of the potential digital ROM and allows for further division of adhesions that were neglected [12]. One potential disadvantage of this technique is that the patient is unable to participate actively in the procedure; hence, the function of the tendon's motor unit cannot be ascertained. Another potential disadvantage of performing tenolysis under general anesthesia or axillary block is that the patient does not directly observe the improved digital ROM gained during the operation and therefore does not have the added inspiration necessary to preserve that gained ROM during the demanding postoperative therapy program [7].

Technique

The operation is begun by wide exposure of the entire length of the flexor tendon. The exposure options are either through zigzag incision [16] as advocated by Schneider [2,6,8] or midlateral incisions as championed by Strickland [4]. The Bruner zigzag incision has the advantage of providing the best surgical exposure of the flexor tendon anatomy and digital pulley system (Fig. 1). On the other hand, the midlateral incision approach leaves the neurovascular structures dorsal and is believed to diminish skin scarring directly over the flexor tendon [4].

Dissection proceeds from the unaffected area to the affected area [5] and the borders of the flexor tendons are defined [12]. Both flexors are raised en block [5], and in a precise and methodic fashion tendon adhesions are lysed. Next, when possible, the flexor digitorum profundus and flexor digitorum superficialis tendons should be separated from one another [4]. The tendon can be trimmed slightly and previous suture and foreign material debrided [5]. Because of severe adhesions and dense scar it may be necessary to sacrifice the flexor digitorum superficialis [8] to allow for unrestricted tendon gliding through pulley systems. Great diligence and care must be used to preserve as much of the tendon sheaths and pulley systems as possible. This can be accomplished by prudently creating transverse windows in the flexor retinaculum at multiple levels [4]. It is imperative to retain at a minimum the essential A-2 and A-4 pulleys. If necessary part or all of the A-3 pulley may be sacrificed to get the appropriate exposure [8].

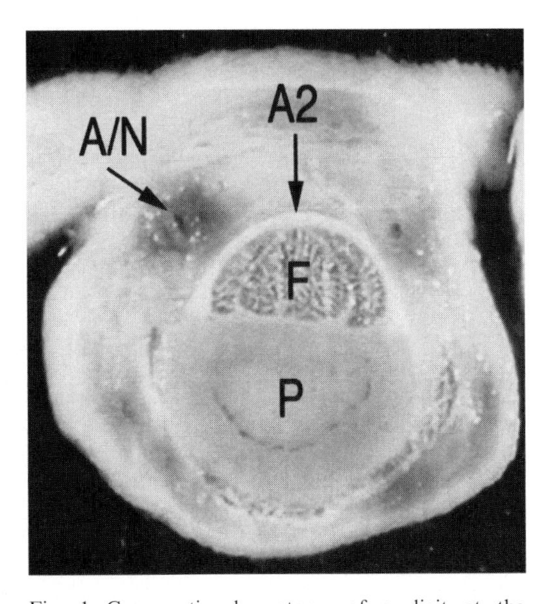

Fig. 1. Cross-sectional anatomy of a digit at the proximal phalanx. Notice the tight association between the flexor tendons (F), A2 pulley (A2), and phalanx (P). A/N, digital artery and nerve.

The dissection of scarred tendons from pulley systems can be a test of one's dexterity (Fig. 2). To aid in this potentially daunting task, hand surgeons have used a variety of instruments. McDonough and Stern [17] modified a 69 Beaver blade by applying a 45° angle to the flat surface. They report that this modification allows fewer incisions in the flexor sheath and comfortable angle for circumferential tendon dissection. Similarly, Schreiber [18] found that knee arthroscopic blades were small enough to fit within the confines of flexor sheaths and of adequate length to avoid incising the intervening sheaths. Following tenolysis, Strickland [4] slightly widens the annular pulleys with small pediatric urethral dilators to allow for smoother gliding of tendons. A simple method to separate the flexor digitorum profundus tendon from the volar surface of the proximal phalanx uses a strand of dental wire or a braided suture as a snare/saw (D.C. Ireland, MD, personal communication in American Society for Surgery of the Hand Correspondence Newsletter, 1988). The wire or braided suture is passed between the tendons and the bone. With steady traction and back and forth motion the dorsal surface of the tendon is liberated from adhesions. The same technique can be repeated to separate the flexor digitorum profundus and flexor digitorum superficialis tendons if intertendinous adhesions persist. A set of instruments specifically designed for tenolysis is available and many find it facilitates the procedure (Fig. 3). The necks of these

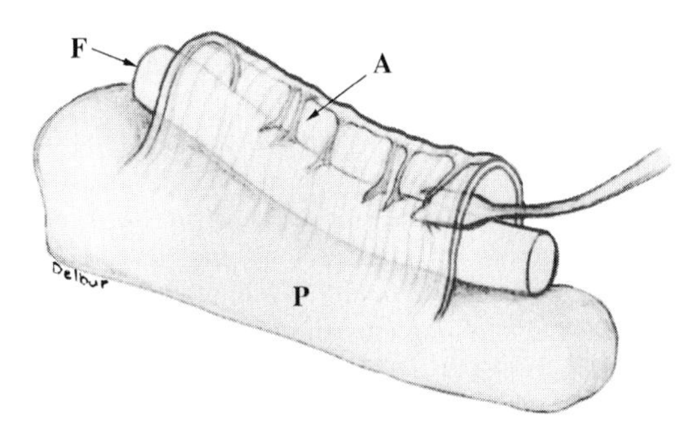

Fig. 2. Artist's rendition of tenolysis. Dense adhesions (A) formed between the flexor tendon (F), tendon sheath, and phalanx (P) are lysed with specifically designed tenolysis knives. The knife's concave leading edge captures and cuts, rather than slips off adhesions.

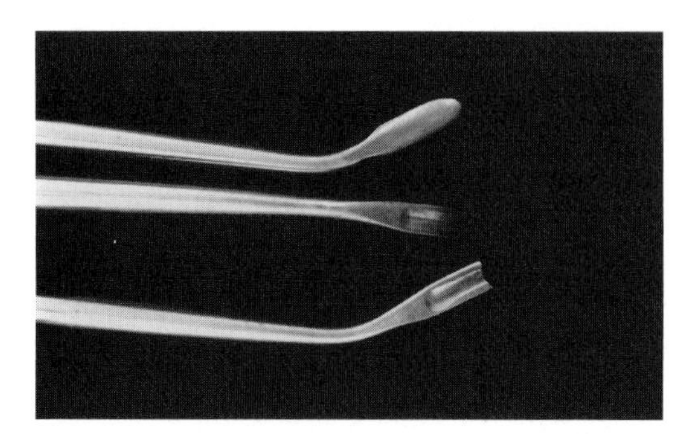

Fig. 3. Specifically designed tenolysis knives.

tenolysis knives follow the natural curvature of the finger. The knives have semisharp blades that conform on their cross-sections to the circumference of the tendon in all four quadrants within the sheath. The first knife has a convex leading edge to seek the original plane between the tendons and their surrounds. The other knives have a concave leading surface to capture and cut, rather than slip off, dense adhesions (see Fig. 2).

Although no clinical trials have been performed, Constantinescu et al [19] evaluated the efficacy of holmium:YAG laser to scalpel and CO_2 laser tenolysis in a rabbit model. Their study concluded that holmium:YAG laser tenolysis resulted in easier tendon gliding as compared with scalpel or CO_2 laser tenolysis at up to the 2-week time point and did not affect adversely intrinsic tendon strength.

Tenolysis is continued through the length of the digit and palm until the tendon is adequately freed of its restrictions. At this point, the adequacy of the procedure is assessed by pulling on the tendon through a separate proximal incision (traction flexor check) or by having the patient actively flex the digit. At this juncture, the quality and health of the tendon and the integrity of the essential pulley systems should be evaluated critically. If the tendon continuity is maintained only by a scar-filled gap [6] or if greater than 30% [4] of the tendon width is lost, tenolysis is unlikely to succeed. In this case, tenolysis should be aborted and staged tendon reconstruction with silicone rubber implant should be performed. Similarly, if the critical pulleys are attenuated or destroyed, tenolysis has a poor prognosis [8]. Here it is appropriate to proceed with immediate pulley reconstruction [4,5,20]. In the authors' experience this works best using a single strip of tendon wrapped around the phalanx and sutured securely to itself.

Adjunctive modalities

Steroids

In an effort to prevent the redevelopment of adhesions following tenolysis, many adjunctive measures have been used. Some investigators have advocated the use of steroid preparations [15, 21–24] at the conclusion of the operation to bathe the tendon bed. Although there is anecdotal evidence that steroid preparations may be useful in preventing recurrent adhesions [15], other investigators [9,25] doubt their efficacy in improving the final result. Because corticosteroids potentially carry inherent adverse wound healing and tendon healing liabilities, the authors do not use them in conjunction with tenolysis.

Interpositional devices

Interpositional materials have been used extensively to prevent recurrent adhesion formation. These materials have been used as mechanical barriers to separate the tendon from adjacent tissues. These barriers consist of biologic or artificial membranes, such as cellophane [26], polyethylene film, silicone sheeting, paratenon [27], amniotic membrane [28], and gelatin sponge [29], among many others. The use of these materials has been met with mixed results [4,30] and are believed by some investigators to function as foreign objects that hinder the revascularization process [30]. A potentially promising modality is the use of hyaluronic acid derivatives (Seprafilm Bioresorbable Membrane, Genzyme Corporation, Cambridge, Massachusetts), widely used to prevent adhesion formation in gastrointestinal surgery [31–33]. Karakurum et al [34] used Seprafilm Bioresorbable Membrane in a chicken flexor tendon model and demonstrated benefit in decreasing tendon adhesions after tenolysis. Clinical corroborating to this study is yet to be performed. The authors do not use interpositional substances.

Indwelling catheter

To minimize postoperative pain, several investigators [5,12,35] use transcutaneously placed local anesthetic catheters (polyethylene or silicone) in the area of tenolysis. For several days, patients can self-administer bupivacaine [4] on a periodic basis to relieve pain and allow active engagement in the postoperative therapy regimen. It should be emphasized that this adjunct should be reserved for the select patients who have low pain thresholds or extensive operations [4]. The authors have found that oral analgesics sufficiently alleviate pain in the postoperative period and that the risk for infectious wound complications does not warrant the use of this procedure.

Postoperative management

The postoperative hand therapy program is universally recognized as a crucial component of flexor tenolysis surgery to retain the ROM gained from operation. The timing of therapy initiation is, however, a source of contention. Some investigators advocate waiting for several days [5] or until the soft tissue inflammation and associated pain begin to subside. Others begin digital motion immediately in an effort to thwart the formation of new adhesions [4,6,7].

To a significant degree, postoperative treatment is dictated by intraoperative findings and these findings should be discussed directly with the therapist to tailor a closely supervised therapy program. Helpful referral information includes the procedures performed, tendon quality, digit vascularity, and intraoperative passive and active (if the patient was awake) ROM [6]. Furthermore, the surgeon's prognosis for motion may be of benefit to the therapist [6].

If the freed tendon is of poor quality with significant scarring and decreased caliber, the probability of rupture is considerable [6,7]. Protective splinting is required and a closely supervised therapy program should be designed to reduce the tensile loads of the tendon while maintaining the excursion achieved from surgery [7]. The "frayed tendon program" [4,7,11,36] is suggested in these instances and in other circumstances, such as postoperative synovitis [6] or palpable crepitus [6,7], in which the likelihood of rupture is increased. In this method, the tenolysed digit is manipulated passively into full flexion. Next, the patient is asked to hold the flexed position with their own muscle power and the manipulating digit is removed. This place and hold maneuver allows the tendon to pass through maximal excursion while minimizing tensile demands and decreasing the likelihood for rupture. In a closely supervised fashion, gentle active ROM exercises may be added gradually as the tendon heals with time.

If intraoperatively the tendon is deemed to be of good quality, then the patient may proceed immediately with more vigorous therapy. The treatment aims are to increase active and passive ROM, enhance muscle activity, and decrease edema and pain.

The active exercises should begin gently with the place and hold maneuvers [4,7,11,36] and advance to tendon gliding exercises [37,38] and blocking exercises [6]. Foucher et al [5] splint the hand and interphalangeal joints in flexion for the first 3 weeks with hourly removal to perform exercises. Passive ROM exercises are used if joint stiffness and inflexibility are present [6] and can be increased gradually [5] as required.

Postoperative edema is an expected consequence of tenolysis and measures must be taken to address it. Reduction of edema provides the patient with improved tendon excursion and ROM. The authors instruct the patient to maintain the hand elevated above the level of the heart until a time that he or she can comfortably leave it in a dependent position without pain. In addition, several times per hour the hand is raised overhead and 10 full fist pumps are performed. A particularly effective means of edema control is compression with the stipulation that there is satisfactory vascularity, intact sensation, and no wound compromise. For digits and the palm, elastic tape can be applied distally proceeding proximally without tension. For gentle compression of the hand, elasticized bandages or gloves may be used [11].

Continuous passive motion has been shown experimentally to increase the risk for tendon rupture, to increase the force required to flex the joints passively, and to result in less passive motion [39].

Results

Strickland [7] reports that in 64% of tenolysed digits there was a 50% improvement in active motion through the available passive arc at the proximal interphalangeal (PIP) and distal interphalangeal (DIP) joints. Fifteen percent of patients gained fair function; however, 20% did not benefit from the operation and 8% of fingers experienced tendon rupture.

Foucher et al [5] report the results of 78 tenolysed fingers with the introduction of two technical modifications. If required, robust pulley reconstruction with tendon graft was performed and the digit immobilized in a flexed position to maintain the tendon in a proximally migrated position. On postoperative day 2, the digits were extended passively to break adhesions. For 3 weeks thereafter, the digits were splinted continuously in some flexion with intermittent removal for extension exercises. Passive extension was gradually increased; however, no activity was allowed that required force for 5 weeks. The results of this study showed that active movement improved from 135° to 205° in 84% of the fingers. There was no improvement in four digits and nine digits were worse following tenolysis. There were two instances of tendon rupture.

Goloborod'Ko [40] studied 20 fingers that were followed 6 months to 1 year postoperatively. His protocol included tenolysis followed by immediate active flexion of the digit resulting in proximal excursion of the tendon. The digits were maintained in the flexed position until the first postoperative day when the digit was passively fully extended. The digits were again held in a flexed position and extended the following day for 5–6 days. The patients then began a regimen of tendon gliding exercises with flexion bandaging at night only for 10–12 days. He reports excellent results in 18 digits, fair in 1, and poor in 1 digit. Three patients sustained tendon ruptures.

Jupiter et al [41] reviewed their series of 37 replanted digits and four thumbs that had flexor tenolysis after replantation. The total active motion increased significantly from 72° to 130°. The results were rated as 13 excellent, 11 good, 6 fair, and 11 poor. The thumbs had two fair results and two poor results. They conclude that poor results were associated with crush or avulsion amputations, hands with more than two digits amputated, and those requiring PIP capsulotomy. There was no association with the number of arteries or tendons repaired and complications included tendon rupture and infection. They summarize that their study supports flexor tenolysis after replantation of fingers but not replanted thumbs.

Birnie et al [42] embarked on a study to determine if there is an age below which flexor tenolysis may not be beneficial and whether it is disadvantageous to wait for a more suitable age. In their study, patients in their first decade had minimal improvement in their active flexion after flexor tenolysis, whereas patients tenolysed more than 1 year after their original operation were not compromised by the prolonged interval between injury repair and tenolysis. They therefore conclude that after tenolysis, significant improvement in active flexion can be expected only in children older than the age of 11 years.

Complications

Similar to other reoperative procedures, complications are inherent to flexor tenolysis. Possibly the most frequent complication is the failure of the operation to improve ROM [8] and potentially to worsen it. Other complications include skin necrosis, dehiscence, and wound infection. Tendon rupture is an infrequent complication that carries potentially disastrous consequences [7]. If rupture occurs, the decision must be made as to whether to proceed with immediate repair or to allow time for wound healing with subsequent staged tendon grafting. Otherwise, consideration can be given to arthrodesis or amputation.

Summary

Flexor tenolysis is a challenging procedure with valuable clinical usefulness in the restitution and enhancement of digital function in the appropriate patient. In the absence of complications, improvement in digital flexion can be expected. The requisites for success are a skilled surgeon, a motivated and well informed patient, and a closely monitored hand therapy program.

Acknowledgments

The authors wish to thank Ms. Delbar Riahi for her illustration and photographs.

References

[1] Agee J. Treatment principles for proximal and middle phalangeal fractures. Orthop Clin N Am 1992; 23:35.

[2] Lindsay WK, Thomson HG. Digital flexor tendons: an experimental study. Part I. The significance of each component of the flexor mechanism in tendon healing. Br J Plast Surg 1960;12:289.

[3] Bunnell S. Surgery of the hand. Philadelphia: Lipincott; 1944.

[4] Strickland JW. Flexor tenolysis. Hand Clin 1985;1: 121.

[5] Foucher G, Lenoble E, Ben Youssef K, Sammut D. A postoperative regime after digital flexor tenolysis. A series of 72 patients. J Hand Surg [Br] 1993;18:35.

[6] Feldscher SB, Schneider LH. Flexor tenolysis. Hand Surg 2002;7:61.

[7] Strickland JW. Flexor tendon surgery. Part 2. Free tendon grafts and tenolysis. J Hand Surg [Br] 1989; 14:368.

[8] Schneider LH. Tenolysis and capsulectomy after hand fractures. Clin Orthop 1996;327:72–8.

[9] Fetrow KO. Tenolysis in the hand and wrist. A clinical evaluation of two hundred and twenty flexor and

extensor tenolyses. J Bone Joint Surg [Am] 1967;49: 667.
[10] Wray RC Jr, Moucharafieh B, Weeks PM. Experimental study of the optimal time for tenolysis. Plast Reconstr Surg 1978;61:184.
[11] Strickland JW. Flexor tendon injuries. Part 5. Flexor tenolysis, rehabilitation and results. Orthop Rev 1987;16:137.
[12] Schneider L. Flexor tendons—late reconstruction. In: Green D, Hotchkiss RN, Pederson WC, editors. Green's operative hand surgery. 4th edition. New York: Churchill Livingstone; 1999. p. 1898.
[13] Hunter JM, Schneider LH, Dumont J, Erickson JC III. A dynamic approach to problems of hand function using local anesthesia supplemented by intravenous fentanyl-droperidol. Clin Orthop 1974;104: 112–5.
[14] Hunter JM. Staged flexor tendon reconstruction. J Hand Surg [Am] 1983;8:789.
[15] Whitaker JH, Strickland JW, Ellis RK. The role of flexor tenolysis in the palm and digits. J Hand Surg [Am] 1977;2:462.
[16] Bruner JM. The zig-zag volar-digital incision for flexor-tendon surgery. Plast Reconstr Surg 1967; 40:571.
[17] McDonough JJ, Stern PJ. Modified 69 blade for tenolysis. J Hand Surg [Am] 1983;8:610.
[18] Schreiber DR. Arthroscopic blades in flexor tenolysis of the hand. J Hand Surg [Am] 1986;11:144.
[19] Constantinescu MA, Greenwald DP, Amarante MT, Nishioka NS, May JW Jr. Effects of laser versus scalpel tenolysis in the rabbit flexor tendon. Plast Reconstr Surg 1996;97:595.
[20] Schneider L, Hunter JM. Flexor tendons—late reconstruction. In: Green D, editor. Operative hand surgery. 3rd edition. New York: Churchill Livingstone; 1993. p. 1853.
[21] James J. The use of cortisone in tenolysis. J Bone Joint Surg [Br] 1959;41:209.
[22] James J. The value of tenolysis. Hand 1969;1:118.
[23] Ketchum LD, Martin NL, Kappel DA. Experimental evaluation of factors affecting the strength of tendon repairs. Plast Reconstr Surg 1977;59:708.
[24] Wrenn RN, Goldner JL, Markee JL. An experimental study of the effect of cortisone on the healing process and tensile strength of tendons. J Bone Joint Surg [Am] 1954;36:588.
[25] Brooks DM. Problems of restoration of tendon movements after repair and grafts. Proc R Soc Med 1970; 63:67.
[26] Wheeldon T. The use of cellophane as a permanent tendon sheath. J Bone Joint Surg [Am] 1939;21:393.
[27] Stark HH, Boyes JH, Johnson L, Ashworth CR. The use of paratenon, polyethylene film, or silastic sheeting to prevent restricting adhesions to tendons in the hand. J Bone Joint Surg [Am] 1977;59:908.
[28] Pinkerton M. Amnioplastin for adherent digital flexor tendons. Lancet 1942;1:70.
[29] Nichols H. Discussion of tendon repair with clinical and experimental data on the use of gelatin sponge. Ann Surg 1949;129:223.
[30] Bora FW Jr, Lane JM, Prockop DJ. Inhibitors of collagen biosynthesis as a means of controlling scar formation in tendon injury. J Bone Joint Surg [Am] 1972;54:1501.
[31] Altuntas I, Tarhan O, Delibas N. Seprafilm reduces adhesions to polypropylene mesh and increases peritoneal hydroxyproline. Am Surg 2002;68:759.
[32] Vrijland WW, Tseng LN, Eijkman HJ, et al. Fewer intraperitoneal adhesions with use of hyaluronic acid-carboxymethylcellulose membrane: a randomized clinical trial. Ann Surg 2002;235:193.
[33] Becker JM, Dayton MT, Fazio VW, et al. Prevention of postoperative abdominal adhesions by a sodium hyaluronate-based bioresorbable membrane: a prospective, randomized, double-blind multicenter study. J Am Coll Surg 1996;183:297.
[34] Karakurum G, Buyukbebeci O, Kalender M, Gulec A. Seprafilm interposition for preventing adhesion formation after tenolysis. An experimental study on the chicken flexor tendons. J Surg Res 2003; 113:195.
[35] Kirchhoff R, Jensen PB, Nielsen NS, Boeckstyns ME. Repeated digital nerve block for pain control after tenolysis. Scand J Plast Reconstr Surg Hand Surg 2000;34:257.
[36] Cannon NM, Strickland JW. Therapy following flexor tendon surgery. Hand Clin 1985;1:147.
[37] Wehbe MA, Hunter JM. Flexor tendon gliding in the hand. Part I. In vivo excursions. J Hand Surg [Am] 1985;10:570.
[38] Wehbe MA. Tendon gliding exercises. Am J Occup Ther 1987;41:164.
[39] McCarthy JA, Lesker PA, Peterson WW, Manske PR. Continuous passive motion as an adjunct therapy for tenolysis. J Hand Surg [Br] 1986;11:88.
[40] Goloborod'ko SA. Postoperative management of flexor tenolysis. J Hand Ther 1999;12:330.
[41] Jupiter JB, Pess GM, Bour CJ. Results of flexor tendon tenolysis after replantation in the hand. J Hand Surg [Am] 1989;14:35.
[42] Birnie RH, Idler RS. Flexor tenolysis in children. J Hand Surg [Am] 1995;20:254.

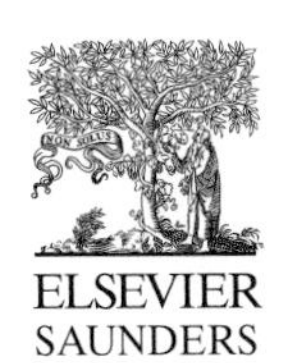
ELSEVIER
SAUNDERS

Hand Clin 21 (2005) 219–243

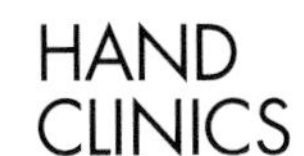
HAND
CLINICS

Delayed Treatment of Flexor Tendon Injuries Including Grafting

James W. Strickland, MD*

Department of Orthopaedic Surgery, Indiana University Medical Center, Indianapolis, IN, USA
Reconstructive Hand Surgeons of Indiana, 13421 Old Meridian Street, Suite 200, Carmel, IN 46032, USA

Tendon grafting to restore digital flexion is the treatment of choice in those cases in which the flexor tendons, divided in zone I or zone II, cannot be repaired directly or the interval following tendon division exceeds the time when delayed repair is possible. The indications and techniques for conventional free tendon grafting are described with consideration for the appropriate techniques to use in cases with interruption of the flexor digitorum profundus (FDP) and the flexor digitorum superficialis (FDS) and those with an intact FDS are described.

Tenolysis should always be considered as the potential final salvage procedure following tendon repair, conventional grafting, or staged reconstruction, for flexible fingers without active motion. The procedure must be approached as a major surgical effort with great consideration for patient selection, operative technique, and postoperative management. It is perhaps the most demanding of all flexor tendon operations with respect to attention to detail and patient–doctor cooperation. The surgical techniques for lysing adherent tendons are described with consideration for the important post-lysis rehabilitation program.

When digits are badly scarred as a result of injury or multiple failed efforts to restore continuity and excursion to badly damaged flexor tendons, staged reconstruction using the initial placement of a silicone implant in the tendon bed followed later by the replacement of that implant with a tendon graft can offer realistic salvage possibilities when few other options exist. An historical review of the development of staged methods of tendon reconstruction is discussed, together with the indications and surgical techniques for current methods for salvaging function in these difficult situations.

Free tendon grafts

In instances in which flexor tendons divided in zone I or zone II have not been or cannot be repaired directly, tendon grafting must be performed to restore digital flexion. Whether one selects conventional free tendon grafting or staged reconstruction depends on several factors unique to the involved digit, including the extent and magnitude of scar formation within the digital canal and the condition of the pulley system.

Division of the flexor digitorum profundus and superficialis

The first series in which free flexor tendon grafts were used in the hand was reported by Lexer in 1912 [1,2]. He used grafts to repair flexor tendons after rupture, old lacerations, infections, and "hopeless cases" of ischemic contracture [1]. In 1916, Leo Mayer published three articles that have served as the basis for the present day concepts of flexor tendon surgery [3–5]. He emphasized the need for exacting operative technique, with direct juncture of the tendon to bone, the use of an adequate muscle as a motor, and the necessity of peritenon around a flexor graft.

In January 1918, Sterling Bunnell published a classic article on tendon grafting in which he stressed atraumatic technique, a bloodless field,

* Corresponding author.
E-mail address: jim@docstrickland.com

doi:10.1016/j.hcl.2004.12.003

hand.theclinics.com

perfect asepsis, and the preservation of pulleys [6]. He preferred the palmaris longus tendon as the donor graft and described a modified cork borer that could be used as a tendon stripper [6]. Mason and Allen performed experiments in 1941 that indicated that tendon grafts should not be moved for 21–25 days [7]. In the first edition of his classic textbook on surgery of the hand in 1944, Bunnell [8] described the pullout wire suture technique, the success of which was confirmed by Moberg [9] in 1951.

The surgical methods and results of free flexor tendon grafting subsequently have been modified and reviewed by various leaders in the field of hand surgery, including Pulvertaft [10–12] in England; Graham [13], Littler [14], Boyes [15], Boyes and Stark [16], and White [17,18] in the United States; and Rank and Wakefield [19] in Australia. Important contributions also have been made by Verdan [20] in Switzerland and Tubiana [21] in France. Although few advances in tendon grafting have occurred in recent years, Boyes and Stark [16] and McClinton et al [22] have reported notable reviews of large clinical series and that good results have been obtained by grafting through an intact FDS for isolated profundus loss.

Indications

The indications for conventional free tendon grafting have been well established. Pulvertaft [12] stated that successful results from the standard grafting method are obtained only when certain rules are followed:

- The hand is in good overall condition. There is no extensive scarring. Passive movements are full or nearly full. The circulation is satisfactory. At least one digital nerve in the affected digit is intact.
- A precise and gentle surgical technique is used.
- The patient is cooperative. A child under three years of age is unlikely to assist in the after care and it is wise to postpone the operation until the child is older.

Schneider and Hunter [24] have emphasized that the surgeon must decide whether a conventional free tendon graft or a staged reconstruction is most appropriate in a particular situation. Some patients have experienced failed primary surgery or previous efforts at flexor tendon reconstruction, and the degree of scarring within the digit may preclude the realistic possibility of achieving a good result from free grafting. In these instances a staged reconstruction may be more appropriate. Tubiana [21] has detailed the principles for flexor tendon grafting, which include that only one graft should be placed in any one finger, that an intact superficialis tendon is never sacrificed, that the graft should be of small caliber, and that its ends should be fixed away from the tendon sheath. Tubiana also recommended the careful calculation of the tension of the graft and the sparing of at least one pulley to prevent bowstringing.

Although primary or delayed primary repair has now become the standard mode of treatment following acute severance of flexor tendons, free tendon grafting is applicable in those patients who for one reason or another have not had a timely repair. In such patients, severed tendon stumps are removed from the digital flexor sheath and replaced with a palm-to-distal phalanx graft. Almost all tendon surgeons agree that the procedure is applicable in patients older than 5 years of age following clean, sharp severance of the flexor tendons. The wounds should be well healed with a minimum of inflammatory reaction and the digits should be supple and free from swelling. A full range of passive motion should be achieved before the procedure and at least one and preferably both digital nerves should be functional. The patient should be well motivated and informed as to the rather rigorous postoperative therapy that is necessary.

Free tendon grafting usually is not appropriate for digits with fixed joint contractures or following severe phalangeal fractures. Crushing injuries or wounds with significant skin loss usually result in considerable scarring in or around the flexor tendon sheath, and a marked compromise of the performance of this technique can be expected. The procedure is contraindicated in insensate or poorly vascularized digits, in children younger than 3 years of age, and in elderly patients [25]. In some instances it is difficult for the surgeon to assess the amount of fibrosis within the digit or the condition of the pulley system before the actual operative procedure. Should the findings at surgery mitigate against free tendon grafting, the patient should be prepared for the possibility of staged flexor tendon reconstruction.

Although many surgeons including Bunnell [26,27] recommended excision of most of the flexor tendon sheath with retention of only small sections of the annular pulleys, it is now believed that one should strive to preserve as much of the sheath system as possible. Eiken [28] has even suggested transplanting synovial tissue from the toes or wrists as a sheath autograft to close open sections of the fibro-osseous canal. We have already seen that the wholesale ablation of sections of the flexor tendon sheath may have a detrimental effect on the efficiency of flexor tendons, and it is important to preserve most of the A_2 and A_4 annular pulleys. The reconstruction of pulleys at the time of free tendon grafting is rarely advisable, and in most instances the finding of a deficient pulley system should serve as an indication to proceed with staged reconstruction.

Donor tendons

Although there is some disagreement as to which donor tendons should be chosen for free flexor tendon grafting, the palmaris longus, when available, probably has the most advocates. The tendon is present in approximately 85% of all people [29], is of sufficient length and size, and is procured easily from the ipsilateral forearm by small incisions and gentle traction or the use of a tendon stripper. The plantaris tendon also may serve as a satisfactory tendon graft, particularly when the graft length is important. It is said to be present in approximately 93% of all individuals [30], although the author's personal experience indicates that its absence occurs somewhat more frequently. The plantaris tendon is usually 12–18 cm in length and may be garnered by an incision medial to the Achilles tendon and the use of a Brand tubular tendon stripper. Other tendons that may be used as grafts include the extensor digitorum longus tendons to the second, third, and fourth toes, the extensor indicis proprius, the extensor digiti quinti proprius, and the FDS tendon to the fifth finger [18]. The use of intrasynovial grafts has been advocated by Ark et al [31,32] and Noguchi et al, and the science behind their recommendations is compelling. Clinical evidence of the superiority of these grafts is awaited before they achieve common usage for these procedures.

Incisions for flexor tendon grafting may be the zigzag palmar incision advocated by Bruner [33] or the midaxial approach, which is favored by many surgeons [16,19,24,34–41]. The latter approach has the advantages of placing the scar away from the area of grafting and of providing a healthy bed of subcutaneous tissue over the sheath and graft. Continuous digital–palmar incisions as recommended by Tubiana [21] provide wide exposure of the flexor tendon system from the midpalm to the digital tip. Attempting to work through small incisions with limited exposure almost always necessitates blind dissection, which may endanger neurovascular structures and increase postoperative adhesion formation.

Surgical technique

Free tendon grafting is one of the most technically elegant of all hand surgery procedures (Fig. 1). Some surgeons prefer the use of a midaxial approach to the digit, using the method of Rank and Wakefield [19,40,41], in which the neurovascular bundle is left in its dorsal position and the flap is elevated across the flexor tendon sheath. This incision, however, cannot be used if a zigzag approach has been used previously. The neurovascular bundles must be carefully identified and protected, and dissection is carried from areas of normal anatomy toward the area of injury to provide the best identification of the tendon sheath with a minimum of additional injury. The annular portions of the sheath should be preserved carefully, but if they have collapsed, often they may be expanded by the use of pediatric urethral dilators (Fig. 2).

Small windows are fashioned in the cruciate–synovial areas of the sheath to identify the proximal and distal tendon stumps, and the distal stump of the profundus is mobilized. One centimeter of the profundus stump is preserved and reflected to its insertion in the distal phalanx. The profundus and superficialis stumps are withdrawn proximally if they still reside in the flexor sheath or if they are identified in the midpalm, where their ends will have enlarged. Distal traction then may be placed on the profundus tendon for several minutes to improve its excursion [42]. The bulbous profundus stump is trimmed back to good tendon and the lumbrical muscle is excised if it is scarred or adherent. The superficialis tendon is pulled forward and cut so that it retracts well away from the proximal graft juncture.

Whatever scarring exits at the site of the original injury then is excised meticulously, and if the scar proves to be excessive or if a great deal of the pulley system has been lost, it may be better to proceed with a staged reconstruction by implanting a silicone rod and reconstructing annular pulleys. It also is recommended that the distal portion of the superficial flexor be preserved to prevent recurvatum at the proximal interphalangeal joint, particularly when it has not been badly scarred by the initial injury.

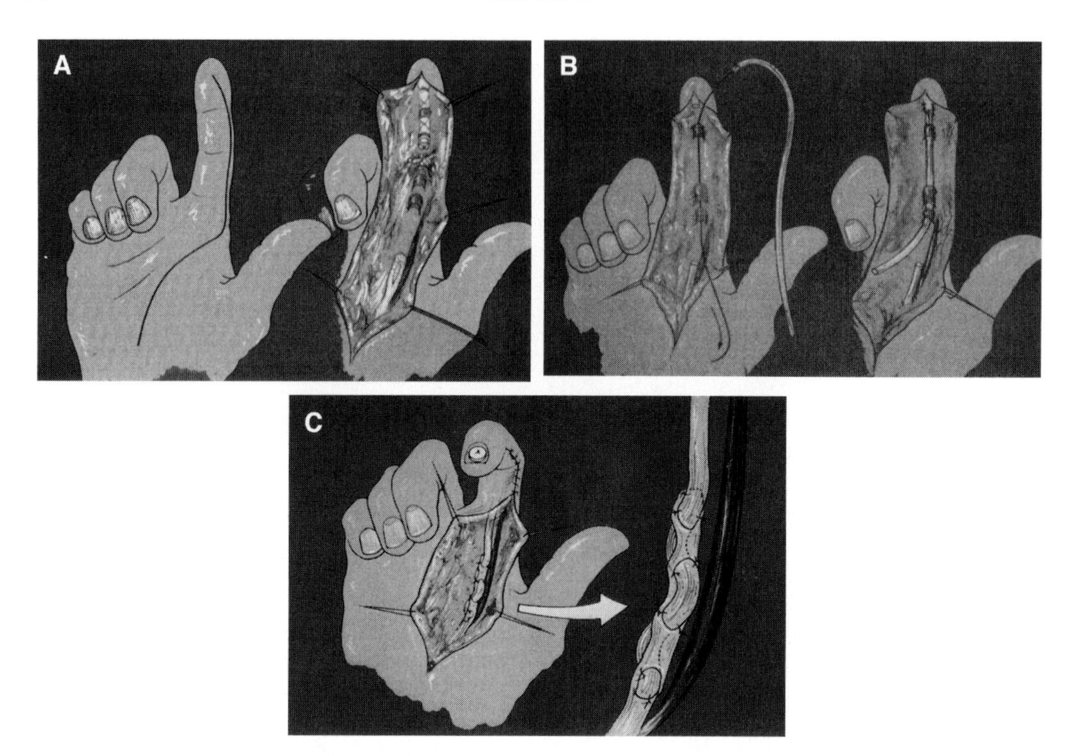

Fig. 1. Technique of free tendon grafting. (*A*) Surgical approach to the index finger using a radial midaxial incision turned across the distal palm to parallel the thenar crease. Following preparation of the digital canal by excision of scar tissue and careful retention of annular pulleys, a free tendon graft is attached to a suture and passed from the base of the distal phalanx into the palm. (*B*) The appearance of the tendon in the digital bed following completion of the distal tendon bone juncture. The profundus stump then is sutured to the graft to secure the juncture. (*C*) Following closure of the distal digital wound, a weave technique is used to join the proximal profundus stump to the graft. The juncture in the palm is under sufficient tension to place the index finger at slightly more than its normal resting posture.

Following preparation of the nail bed, a heavy suture is placed beneath the intact portions of the sheath by using a small blunt probe, and an oblique drill hole is fashioned in the base of the distal phalanx, directing the point of the drill from proximal–palmar to distal–dorsal. The surgeon should make an effort to minimize the dorsal cortical penetration by placing a finger over the proximal nail bed during the drilling process.

When the digital bed has been prepared, the donor tendon is procured. The palmaris longus, when present, is preferred. It is garnered by a transverse incision just proximal to the wrist, through which the distal tendon can be identified easily. A small hemostat is placed beneath the tendon to increase its tension and to allow the tendon to be palpated in the midforearm. A short transverse incision then is made directly over the tendon, and dissection is carried down to the proximal portion of the palmaris, which is withdrawn easily after it has been divided distally and freed of its attachments.

A 4-0 monofilament suture, armed at each end with straight needles, is twice passed through the distal end of the suspended graft, and an additional 4-0 suture is placed in the tendon before its release. The proximal graft suture is tied to the distal end of the suture in the digital bed and the tendon then can be drawn easily from distal to proximal beneath the intact portions of the tendon sheath. The straight needles then are passed through the distal phalangeal drill hole and usually exit over the proximal portion of the nail. The needles are taken through a gauze pad or a Kitner sponge and through the holes of a button. Distal traction on the suture pulls the tendon graft into the osseous defect in the distal phalanx and the suture may be tied over the button to anchor the graft. Additional sutures are used to secure the profundus stump to the graft and proximal

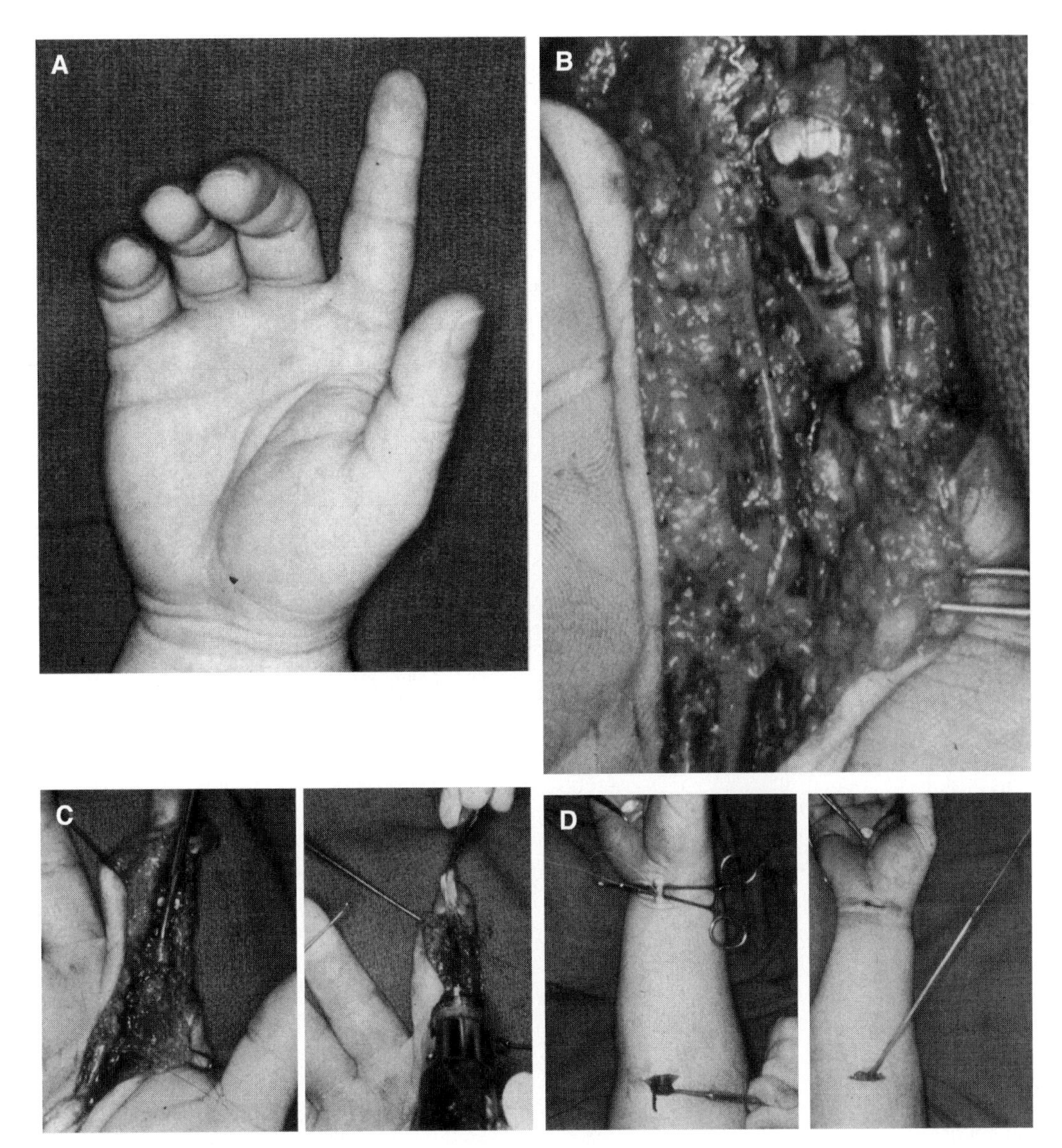

Fig. 2. Clinical photographs of free tendon grafting 3 months following interruption of the profundus and superficialis tendons in zone II of the right index finger. (*A*) Appearance of the hand with the loss of normal resting posture of the index digit resulting from interruption of both tendons. (*B*) The appearance of the flexor tendon bed following the resection of mid-digital scar with reflection of the proximal and distal profundus stumps. (*C*) The use of a urethral dilator to expand the A2 pulley, followed by passing a drill point just proximal to the insertion of the profundus tendon in the base of the distal phalanx. (*D*) The palmaris longus tendon has been withdrawn in the midforearm by the use of two transverse incisions. A double-armed suture on straight needles will be passed through the suspended distal tendon stump in preparation for the distal tendon bone juncture. (*E*) The tendon being drawn through the digital canal from distal to proximal using a suture previously placed beneath the pulleys. The double-armed straight needles are passed through the drill hole in the distal phalanx. (*F*) The appearance of the digital bed following completion of the distal tendon–bone insertion and suturing of the distal profundus stump to the graft. The weave juncture is completed in the palm following closure of the digital wound. (*G*) Appearance of the grafted index finger following completion of the proximal tendon weave and wound closure.

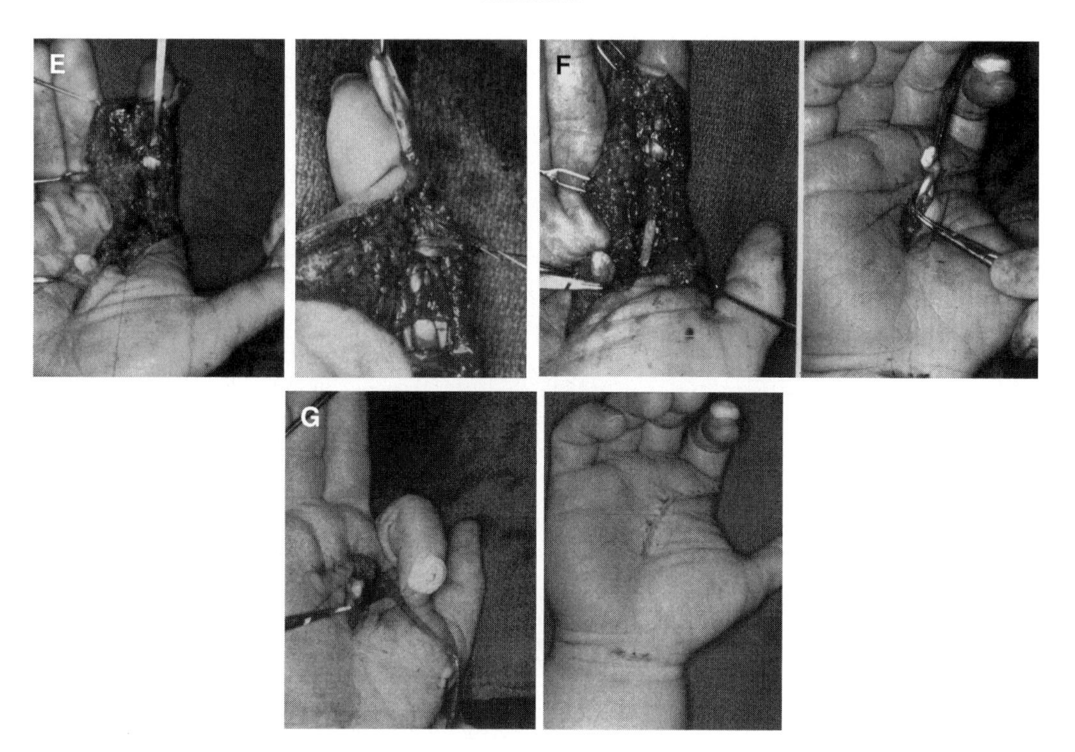

Fig. 2 (*continued*)

traction on the graft should demonstrate its excursion and produce full digital flexion.

In recent years, suture-anchors have been developed that can offer an excellent alternative method for strongly attaching a free tendon graft to the distal phalanx. There are several absorbable and nonabsorbable mini-anchors combined with varying suture sizes now available, and the use of one or even two anchors can produce a strong bone–tendon juncture with less damage to the distal phalangeal bone and fingernail bed than with the phalangeal drilling method. Again, a short flap of the remaining profundus insertion can be sutured over the graft to augment the juncture.

All wounds are closed and the proximal juncture of the graft to the profundus motor tendon is completed in the palm. A Pulvertaft [10–12] tendon weave is excellent for the proximal juncture and allows careful adjustment of the tension of the graft. In instances in which the caliber of the tendons is the same, one may prefer an end-to-end suture rather than the weave technique. Most surgeons agree that the tension placed on a tendon graft should result in a resting posture of the grafted digit that is slightly more flexed than it would be under normal circumstances. This is best achieved by placing the wrist in neutral and observing the posture of adjacent digits. In general, the posture of the grafted digit should be approximately the same as the adjacent ulnar digit, and in the fifth finger, a position of flexion somewhat greater than that of the fifth finger on the opposite hand would be appropriate. At the conclusion of the proximal tendon juncture, the digit is checked to be sure that it can be extended passively with the wrist in neutral.

Obviously certain variations in this technique may result from circumstances unique to the particular patient. The use of a drill hole at the base of the distal phalanx is not appropriate in children with open epiphyses; in such cases, direct tendon suture to the stump of the profundus is preferable. When a palmaris longus tendon is not present, one may select the plantaris, the superficialis tendon of the fifth finger, or one of the proprius tendons, with toe extensors reserved for those rare situations in which no other donors are available. In some instances, it is preferable to use the superficialis muscle as a motor for the tendon graft, particularly when it is less scarred than the profundus.

Postoperative care

Most surgeons are much more reluctant to use early motion programs following grafts than they are following flexor tendon repair. Although some surgeons are comfortable initiating a controlled early motion program after tendon grafting, most prefer to immobilize grafted digits for at least 3 weeks to avoid tension on the juncture sites and to allow for some graft revascularization [22]. Immobilization should be in a position midway between neutral and full wrist flexion with the metacarpophalangeal joints flexed to 60°–70° and the interphalangeal joints held in near full extension. This position relieves tension on the repair sites and provides the best safeguard against the development of interphalangeal joint flexion contractures. At 3–4 weeks, a gentle protective motion program that includes passive and active digital flexion and active extension is initiated. Full passive extension of the digit is not permitted for several additional weeks.

Intact flexor digitorum superficialis

The late treatment of FDP division or rupture with an intact superficialis tendon is controversial. If the patient has full, strong function of the superficialis, the functional impairment to the involved digit may not be great. Because a tendon graft brings with it the risk for compromising existing function, many surgeons have devised a conservative approach in this situation, with no treatment, tenodesis, or arthrodesis being preferred to free grafting [15,43–48]. Other surgeons have demonstrated satisfactory results with tendon grafts through an intact superficialis with varying indications in carefully selected patients [49–56]. The use of a tendon implant as a first stage, followed by grafting for isolated profundus loss, has been advocated by Versaci and Wilson [25,56,57]. Although generally in favor of free grafting for profundus division in selected cases, Pulvertaft expressed his concern when he stated that, "It should not be advised unless the patient is determined to seek perfection and the surgeon is confident of his ability to offer a reasonable expectation of success without the risk of doing harm" [53]. He further noted that the decision as to whether to carry out a graft in such circumstances depends on several factors, including the age of the patient, the condition of the finger and hand, and the occupation and wishes of the patient. At that time, he advised tendon grafting for the index and long fingers, but believed the procedure to be appropriate in the ring and little fingers only when the patient requires the action because of a special interest or occupation, as in the case of a musician or a skilled technician.

Pulvertaft [58] later changed his thinking and agreed that free tendon grafting is often appropriate in the small finger, particularly when the superficialis tendon is found to be weak, because in such patients the improvement of grip provided by the restoration of profundus function makes the procedure worthwhile. He favored the use of the plantaris tendon in such circumstances because it is "thin and thus the most rapidly revascularized and is of sufficient length to provide grafts for two digits." Stark and associates [55] believed that the prerequisites for grafting with an intact superficialis tendon include a superficialis tendon that is normal, full passive motion, minimal soft tissue scarring, and patient age of 10–21 years.

The procedure probably should be reserved for those few patients who have functional needs or a strong desire for the restoration of profundus function. Although a young age is not an absolute requirement, most of the author's patients have been younger than 25 years. Finally, the procedure should be performed only after a thorough and honest discussion with the patient about the details of the procedure and its possible complications.

Surgical technique

The technique for free flexor tendon grafting with an intact superficialis is similar to that used following the loss of both the profundus and the superficialis. Obviously one should take great care to avoid any damage to the normal superficialis or its decussation. The palmaris and plantaris tendons serve as the best donor tendons for this type of grafting because of their small size, although other small tendons, such as the extensor digitorum communis of the index finger, may prove effective for the small finger (Fig. 3). The graft should be gently passed through the decussation of the superficialis in an effort to restore its normal anatomic position. In such cases, when the chiasm has been closed and it is not possible to pass the graft between the superficialis slips, it may be passed around them. Distal and proximal graft junctures are the same as those already described for a combined tendon loss. Although some investigators have suggested that motion may be commenced earlier following grafting through an intact superficialis [59], the author's practice is to immobilize the involved hand for 3.5 weeks before permitting motion.

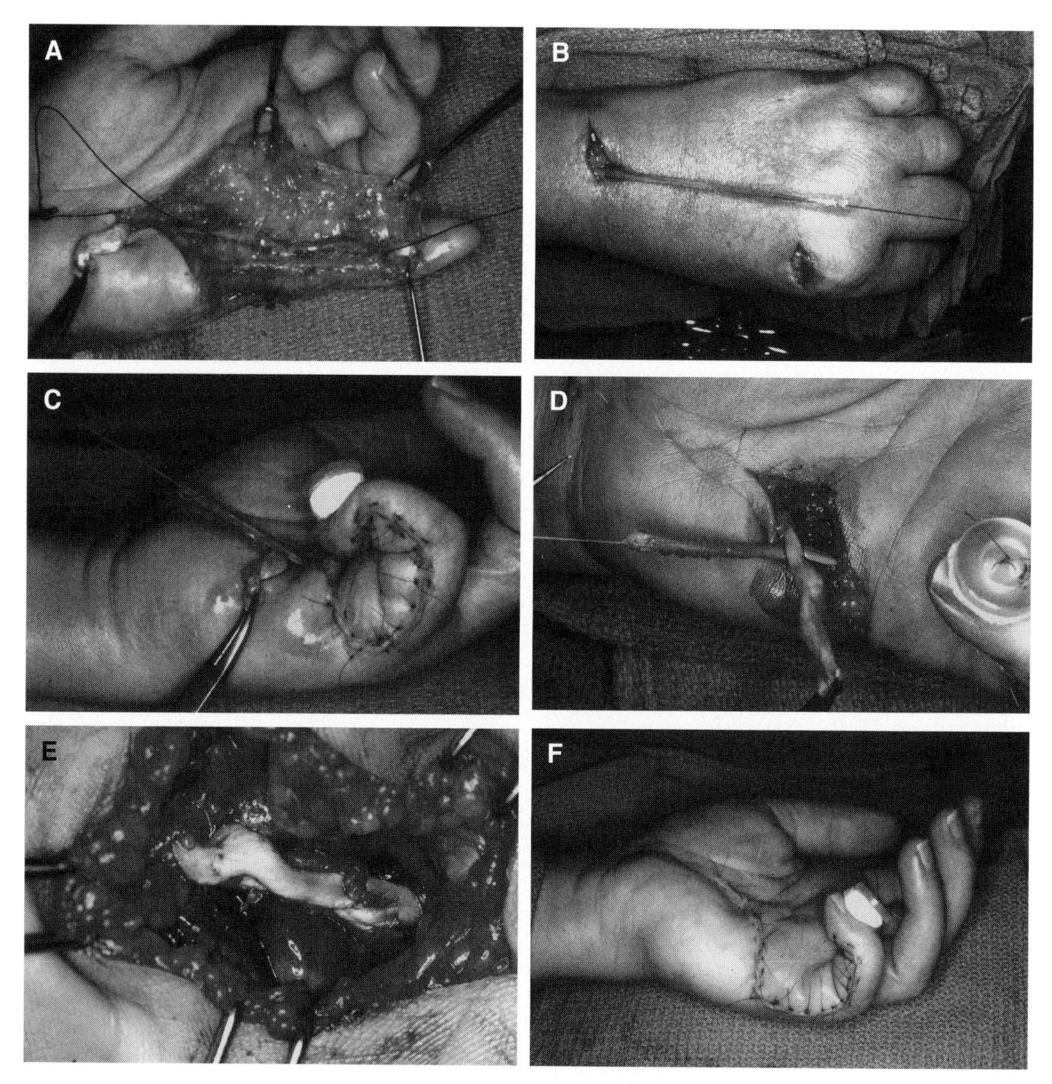

Fig. 3. (*A*) Appearance of a left small finger during a free tendon graft following severance and non-repair of flexor digitorum profundus tendon 6 months previously. A free tendon graft placed through an intact but weak flexor digitorum superficialis in an effort to improve grasp strength. The tendon bed has been prepared and a silk suture passed beneath the pulleys and through Camper's chiasma between the two superficialis slips to exit proximal to the A1 pulley. (*B*) In the absence of the palmaris longus, it was elected to use the extensor digitorum communis of the index finger as the donor graft for the small finger. (*C*) The graft has been withdrawn through the digit using the preplaced silk suture, attached distally through a distal phalangeal drill hole over a button over the digital nail. The digital wound has been closed, and the flexion of the digit produced by proximal traction on the graft is demonstrated. (*D*) The proximal weave of the tendon graft is initiated. (*E*) The appearance of the digit following wound closure is seen. Note the tension on the graft has been set so that the resting posture of the digit is slightly greater than normal. (*F*) The appearance of the digit following wound closure is shown.

Flexor tendon grafting summary

Free tendon grafting for flexor tendon severance that could not be repaired primarily is one of the most eloquent and technically demanding procedures in hand surgery. The techniques developed by the early masters of hand surgery remain largely unchanged today. When done with the correct indications and great attention to surgical detail and postoperative management, the procedure can yield surprisingly good results.

Flexor tenolysis

Despite the best efforts at flexor tendon repair, free tendon grafting, or staged reconstruction, adhesion formation with its obligatory restriction of tendon excursion occurs all too frequently. When satisfactory function cannot be restored, it may be necessary to proceed with tenolysis in an effort to surgically improve tendon movement. The biologic basis and clinical efficacy of this procedure has been questioned by some investigators [60–63], whereas others have indicated that, when performed properly, it is a worthwhile effort at restoring digital function [64–74]. Tenolysis must always be approached as a major surgical effort with careful patient selection and great attention to the details of the operative procedure and the postoperative mobilization program. Tenolysis is probably the most demanding of all flexor tendon procedures, and to be successful there must be close cooperation between the patient, the physician, and the therapist.

Indications

Tenolysis may be indicated following flexor tendon repair or grafting when the passive range of digital flexion significantly exceeds active flexion. The decision to carry out the procedure should be based on serial joint measurements that indicate there has been no appreciable improvement for several months despite a vigorous therapy program and the conscientious efforts of the patient. The prerequisites for tenolysis as set forth by Fetrow [64], Hunter et al [65], Schneider and Hunter [68], and Schneider and Mackin [69,70] should be adhered to closely. All fractures should be healed and wounds must have reached equilibrium with soft, pliable skin and subcutaneous tissues and minimal reaction around scars. Joint contractures must have been mobilized and a normal or near normal passive range of digital motion achieved. Satisfactory sensation and muscle strength should be regained and the patient must be informed carefully as to the objectives, surgical techniques, postoperative course, and pitfalls of the procedure. Many patients are content with less than normal active digital motion, whereas others who have returned a fairly good range may want near normal function, and in most circumstances should be offered the operation. When a patient elects to undergo tenolysis, he or she must understand that if the findings at surgery preclude the possibility of returning satisfactory function, it may be necessary to proceed with the implantation of a silicone rod as the first step of a staged flexor tendon reconstruction sequence.

Timing

The proper timing for tenolysis following tendon repair or graft is somewhat controversial. Wray et al [75] concluded from an experiment on chicken tendons that waiting 12 weeks seemed to be optimum, because it did not weaken the tendon and resulted in an increased blood supply. Fetrow [64] and Pulvertaft [76] have recommended waiting 3 months following a primary tendon repair and 6 months following a flexor tendon graft before performing tenolysis. Rank et al [63] advocated waiting 6–9 months following tendon grafting for those patients in whom serial examinations revealed no significant improvement. It is now generally accepted that one may consider tenolysis 3 months or more after repair or graft, providing the other criteria for the procedure have been satisfied and there has been no measurable improvement in active motion during the preceding 4–8 weeks.

Operative considerations

Lysing an adherent flexor tendon from a bed of scar tissue is perhaps the single most challenging in the spectrum of restorative procedures that follow injury to the complex interrelationship between the tendons and their enveloping sheath. It requires a thorough appreciation of the digitopalmar anatomy, extreme patience, and a willingness to persevere until it can be demonstrated that the tendon or tendons have been freed sufficiently to return flexion that is at least comparable to the presurgery passive range of motion.

Anesthesia and tourniquet

Schneider et al have popularized the use of local anesthetic supplemented by intravenous analgesia and tranquilizing drugs for tenolysis [65,67–70,77,78]. They contend that the method best allows the patient to demonstrate the completeness of the lysis by actively flexing the involved digit during surgery. They also believe it is important to allow the patient to observe the improved digital motion during surgery to provide motivation for the maintenance of that motion during the rigorous postoperative therapy program. Most surgeons now agree that the advantages of local anesthesia and active patient participation are enormous and recommend the use of this technique whenever possible [73]. Local-supplement anesthesias may not be appropriate for patients who are young, are uncooperative, have a low pain threshold, or in whom extensive surgery is anticipated. It then becomes the responsibility of the surgeon to demonstrate that a thorough release of all restraining adhesions has been achieved by the tenolysis procedure.

It must be remembered that although the use of local anesthesia does permit immediate evaluation of the effectiveness of tenolysis, tourniquet ischemia results in muscle paralysis in approximately 30 minutes, and although the active function returns after the tourniquet release, this delay is a surgical inconvenience [74]. In addition, the tourniquet may not be well tolerated after 20–40 minutes, depending on the effectiveness of supplementary analgesia. The use of a sterile pediatric tourniquet applied to the midforearm has proved to be an effective method of dealing with the problems of muscle paralysis and tourniquet pain. During the procedure it may be secondarily inflated, allowing for deflation of the upper arm tourniquet [73]. Hemostasis is preserved, tourniquet pain is minimized, and the function of the extrinsic forearm flexors usually can be restored following their revascularization. At the time of dressing application, the proximal tourniquet may be reinflated and the pediatric tourniquet removed.

The local anesthetic agent selected is at the discretion of the surgeon, and 1% or 2% lidocaine has been advocated by Hunter et al [65,67–70]. Bupivacaine (Marcaine) 0.5% is also a useful agent for tenolysis because of its longer duration (10–14 hours), which serves to minimize the immediate postoperative pain. Anesthesia administered by infiltration into the skin and subcutaneous tissues at the base of the finger usually is combined with a transmetacarpal digital block. The extent of the palmar dissection is anticipated at the time of injection, and when more than one finger is to undergo tenolysis or when extensive wrist-palm-digit exploration is likely, one may elect to use a wrist block. It should be remembered that this type of regional anesthetic results in paralysis of the intrinsic muscles and, to some extent, compromises the patient's ability to demonstrate normal digital kinetics following tenolysis [69,70]. Nonetheless, wrist block anesthesia permits full function of the extrinsic flexor system and is an excellent alternative to direct palmar injection in certain circumstances.

Although Schneider and Mackin [69,70] and Hunter et al [65] have stated a preference for the supplementary use of the agents Fentanyl-droperidol (Innovar) for tenolysis analgesia and sedation, other agents such as diazepam (Valium) may be substituted effectively when the anesthesiologist is unfamiliar with or reluctant to use this drug combination [65,73]. Whether the procedure is performed with the patient under local, regional, or general anesthesia, it is important that the condition and comfort level of the patient be monitored carefully by an anesthesiologist throughout the entire procedure.

Surgical technique

Flexor tenolysis requires wide surgical exposure. As with other digital procedures, the incision options are the midlateral or Bruner [79] zigzag exposures (Fig. 4). Schneider et al prefer the zigzag approach, believing that it provides the best exposure of the tendon anatomy and allows lysis of the adherent structures under direct visualization [65,67–70]. They also believe that this approach best preserves the vascular nutrition of the digits that have been injured or had previous surgical procedures. Other surgeons prefer a midlateral excision as described by Rank et al [63], in which the neurovascular bundles are left dorsalward [73]. The advantages of this approach are that it usually delivers a good bed of soft tissue back across the flexor tendons and sheath and that there is less wound tension produced by the early postoperative digital motion.

Despite the earlier recommendations by Verdan [80] that sheaths be widely excised at the time of tenolysis, most surgeons now prefer to preserve as much of the pulley system as possible [65,73]. If portions of the pulley system have been damaged by injury or previous surgery, the forces acting on the smaller remaining pulleys during active flexion are much greater, with an increase in the potential for pulley rupture [65]. It is therefore imperative to make every effort to maintain most of each of the annular pulleys.

Tenolysis is often a laborious procedure requiring the meticulous division of all limiting adhesions with great care taken to define the borders of the flexor tendons. When possible the profundus and superficialis tendons are separated to retain a two-tendon system (Fig. 5). In some instances, however, this cannot be done, and a single combined tendon is created and mobilized

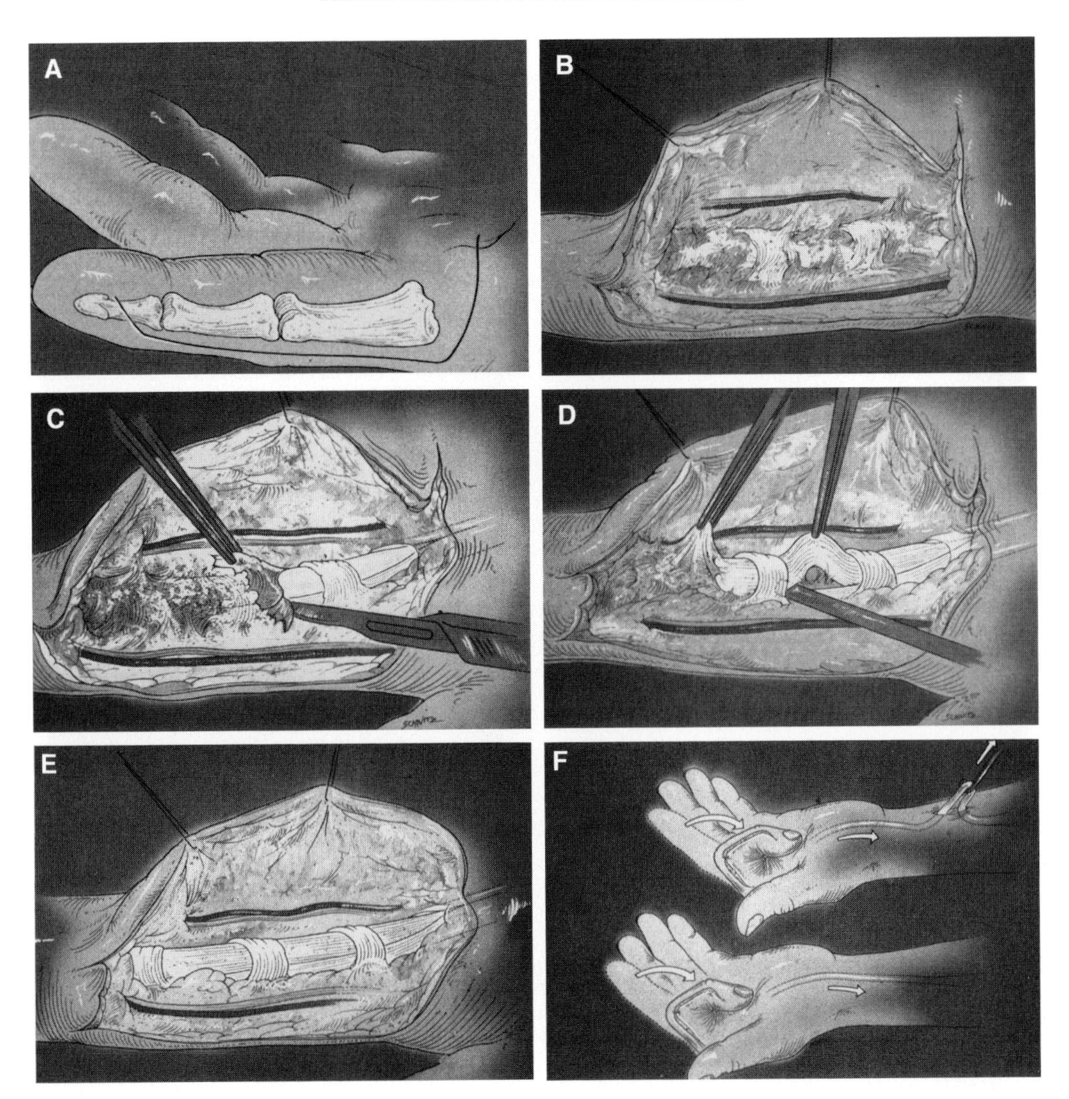

Fig. 4. Digital tenolysis of adherent flexor tendons is illustrated. (*A*) A long midlateral incision is depicted on the radial aspect of the index finger. The incision continues across the palm at the level of the distal palmar crease and can be turned proximally to gain the required palmar exposure of the flexor system. (*B*) The scarred digital sheath-flexor system at the time of surgery. Annular pulley remnants are visible and must be preserved. Meticulous surgical extrication of the flexor tendons is performed, preserving as much of the annular pulley restraints as possible. (*C*) Excision and release of peritendinous scar and separation of cross-adhesions between the profundus and the superficialis is shown. (*D*) Careful release of adhesions beneath the pulleys is facilitated by the use of small knife blades and elevators. (*E*) The appearance of the flexor tendons following tenolysis with the maintenance of three annular pulleys. (*F*) The procedure is concluded by demonstration that a complete release of all restraining adhesions has been achieved, either by a proximal traction check through a separate wrist incision (*top*), or preferably by the active participation of the patient under local anesthetic (*bottom*). (*From* Strickland JW. Flexor tenolysis. Hand Clin 1985;1:121–32 (GW Schnitz, artist); with permission.)

to its insertion. The judicious use of small knife blades, special tenolysis knives, and small elevators may help the surgeon to extricate the tendons from their scarred beds on the floor of the fibro-osseous canal and to divide connections to the annular pulleys. On occasion, small pediatric urethral dilators may be used to gently expand annular pulleys.

When the procedure is performed under local anesthesia, it should be possible to periodically ask the patient to actively flex the involved finger to determine the adequacy of the lysis.

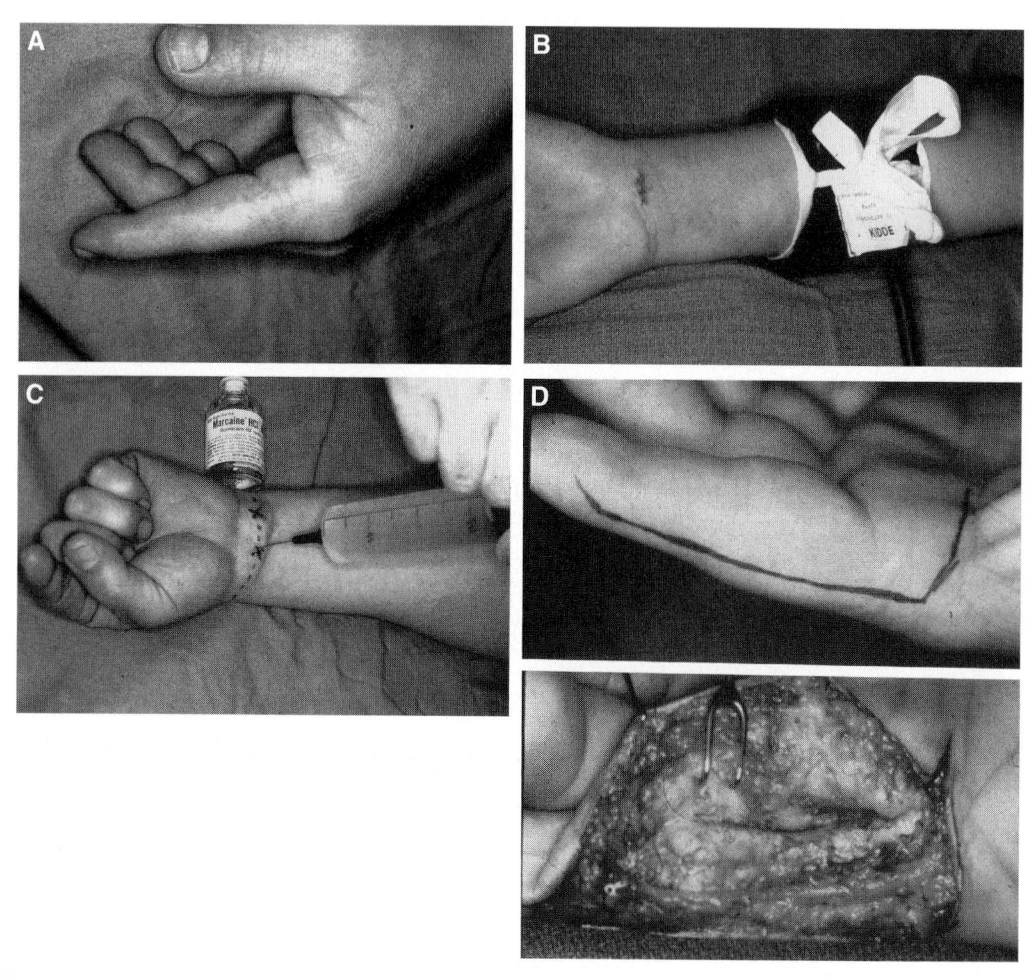

Fig. 5. The surgical technique of tenolysis is demonstrated clinically. (*A*) This patient lacked interdigital flexion of the index finger 5 months following division and repair of the profundus and superficialis tendons in zone II. (*B*) Use of sterile forearm tourniquet to relieve discomfort of upper arm tourniquet and return flexor muscle function during tenolysis under local anesthesia. This technique permits the patient to actively demonstrate the completeness of the lysis. (*C*) Wrist block anesthesia is administered to allow patient's active participation in digital flexion after the tendons have been extricated and are gliding well. (*D*) Midaxial approach to the badly scarred digital flexor bed. The appearance of the scarred flexor tendon bed with totally adherent flexor tendons at the time of tenolysis. (*E*) A small McIndoe elevator was used to release restraining adhesions with careful preservation of the annular pulleys. (*F*) A freer elevator is passed beneath the tendons and used to separate the tendons from the annular pulleys. (*G*) Appearance of the lysed profundus and superficialis tendons with preservation of the A1, proximal A2, and most of the A3, C2, and A4 pulley system. The pediatric urethral dilator shown can be used to gently dilate the annular pulleys if necessary. (*H*) Appearance of the digit following lysis and release of the tourniquet in preparation for active flexion by the patient. (*I*) If appropriate, the patient is allowed to observe the restoration of flexion that has been achieved by tenolysis. (*J*) The appearance of the digit following wound closure. The digit is held in flexion in the post-tenolysis dressing to facilitate the preservation of flexion during the early motion program that follows. (*K*) The continued satisfactory extension, and (*L*) flexion of finger is shown 3 months following tenolysis. (*From* Strickland JW. Flexor tenolysis. Hand Clin 1985;1:121–32 (G.W. Schnitz, artist); with permission.)

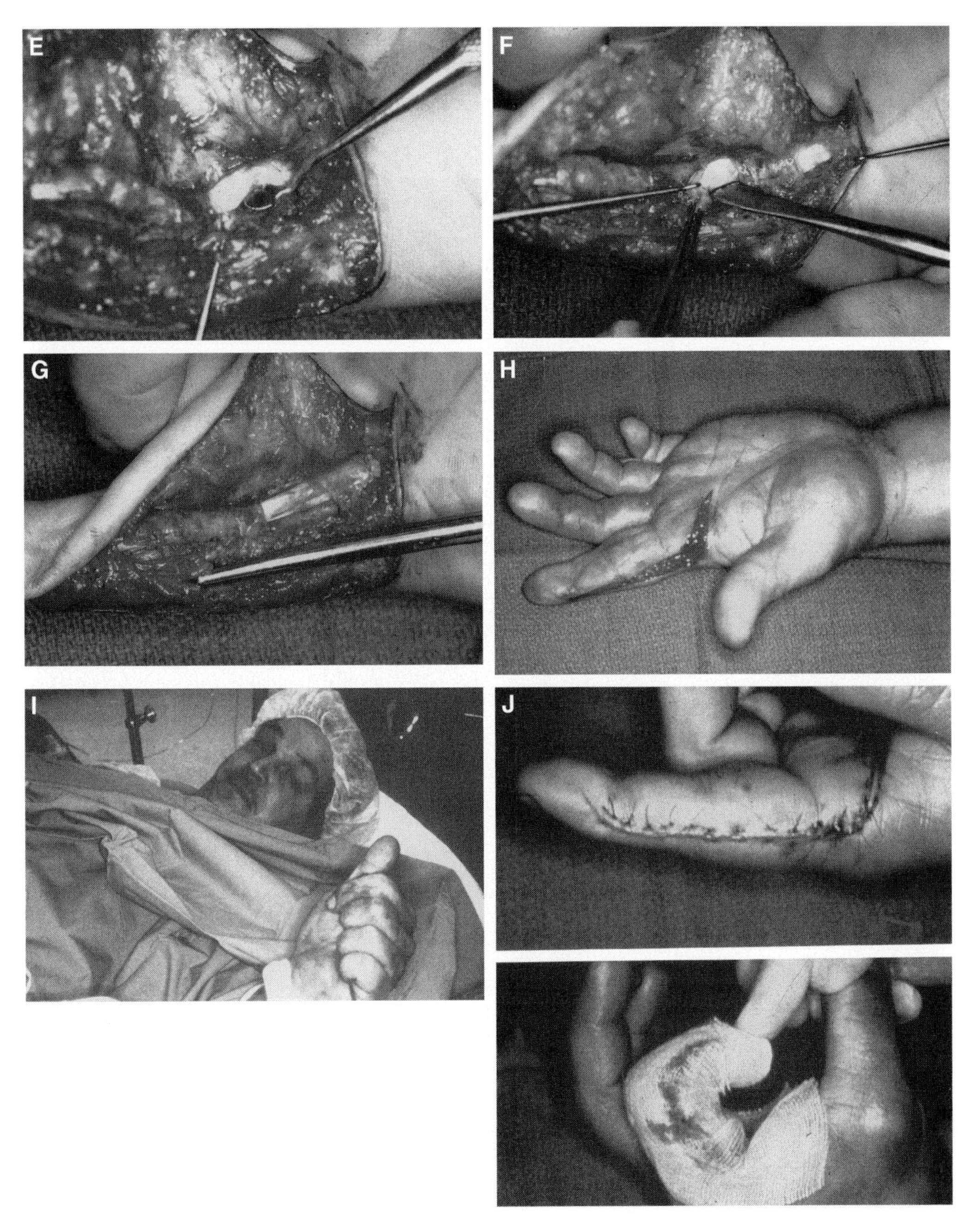

Fig. 5 (*continued*)

Occasionally this motion ruptures a few remaining adhesions and permits full excursion of the lysed tendon. At approximately 30 minutes, tourniquet paralysis precludes the ability of the patient to actively flex. At this point, the sterile pediatric tourniquet applied at midforearm may be inflated and the upper arm tourniquet released. Voluntary muscle function is restored and proximal tourniquet discomfort is relieved.

Dissection is continued until the adequacy of the release is demonstrated by active patient flexion or by a gentle proximal traction check in the palm. If the patient can fully flex the digit and if an adequate pulley system has been preserved,

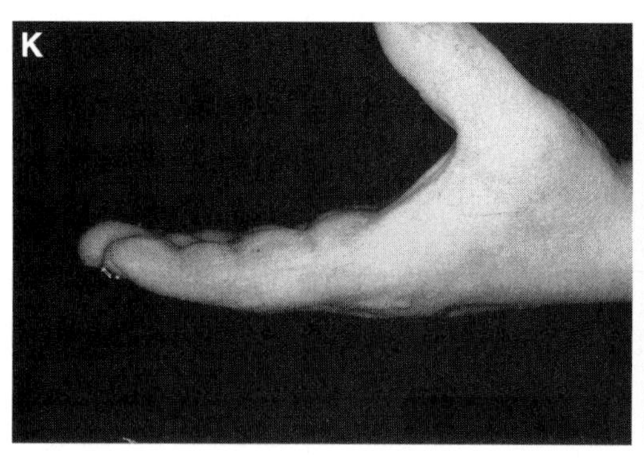

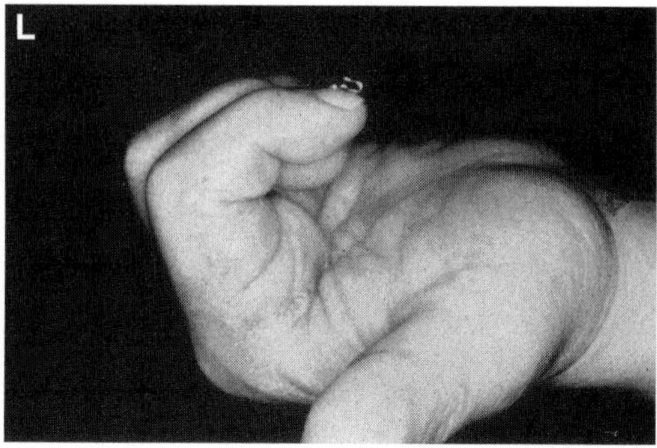

Fig. 5 (*continued*)

the wound is closed and the dressing applied. If annular pulleys are absent, attenuated, or inadequate, they must be rebuilt. The use of tendons passed circumferentially around the phalanges as described by Bunnell [61] is probably the most reliable method of pulley restoration during tenolysis. Pulleys may be protected by circumferential digital taping and their restoration should not alter substantially the postoperative tenolysis regimen [73]. Hunter et al [65] have emphasized the importance of assessing critically the quality of the flexor tendons at the time of surgery [78]. They state that if 30% of the tendon width has been lost or if the continuity of the tendon is through a small segment of scar tissue, it is questionable whether or not tenolysis should be performed. They suggest that when the quality of the tendon is seriously in doubt, it may be better to proceed with a staged reconstruction using an active or passive Hunter tendon implant. The final decision as to whether one should proceed with lysis when there is marginal tendon quality ultimately is left to the discretion of the individual surgeon. Fortunately there are methods of minimizing the tensile loading of the lysed tendons while preserving their excursion during the early postoperative therapy period, as described in the postoperative considerations section of this article. In certain circumstances, it may even be possible to combine the procedures by placing a Hunter tendon implant beneath the lysed tendon from the base of the distal phalanx to either the palm or distal forearm as suggested by Strickland [88]. The silicone rod then may serve as an underlay for the tendon and as a potential first stage reconstruction if tendon rupture should occur. When necessary, capsulectomy may be combined with flexor tenolysis and usually involves the resection of scar tissue or tightened check-rein extensions of the palmar plate at the level of the proximal interphalangeal joint. It should be emphasized, however, that every effort should be made to achieve full passive digital joint motion before surgery, because the concomitant lysis of tendons and joint release is prejudicial to the final result.

Various mechanical barriers have been used to limit the reformation of peritendinous adhesions following tenolysis. There is a conflicting opinion as to the usefulness of these materials. Boyes [81] advocated silicone inlays in certain instances, and Bunnell [61], Fetrow [64], and Verdan [80] have recommended peritenon and fascial inlays with satisfactory results reported. Bora et al [82] reviewed the results of fascia, vein, and cellophane around tenorrhaphy sites and stated that these materials failed to prevent the reformation of adhesions, and in fact acted as foreign bodies, promoting additional scarring and obstructing the revascularization process. The most common indications for silicone interposition at present are cases of repeat tenolysis in which the reformation of adhering scar tissue over a long distance would seem to be most inevitable [73]. The use of steroid preparations in an effort to modify the quality and quantity of tendon adhesions following tenolysis has provoked considerable debate. Wrenn et al [83], Rank et al [63], Carstam [84], James [85], and Whitaker et al [74] have indicated that locally instilled cortisone drugs may be of some value. Conversely, Fetrow [64], Brooks [60], and Verdan et al [80,86] believe that they do not improve the results of the tenolysis. The adhesion-limiting property of triamcinolone as demonstrated by Ketchum [87] makes this drug seem to be a logical adjunct to the preservation of tendon gliding. It is probably best to reserve the use of this medication for patients who have shown a propensity for the rapid and aggressive reformation of scar tissue or for those who are undergoing repeat lysis. In those instances, several milliliters of triamcinolone may be administered locally at the time of wound closure. One should be wary of the possibility of delayed wound healing or infection when using steroids in conjunction with this procedure.

Hunter et al [65] and Schneider and Mackin [69,70] have reported on the use of an indwelling polyethylene catheter to allow the administration of bupivacaine to the patient on a periodic basis in an effort to provide postoperative pain relief during the first few days of post-tenolysis therapy. Although this procedure is sometimes beneficial for patients with a low pain threshold or following extensive surgical procedures, it is rarely necessary for more routine procedures in which pain is not a major problem. Oral analgesics and the use of a transcutaneous nerve stimulator are usually effective in controlling discomfort and obviate the need for indwelling catheters with their attendant risks for inoculating the wound with infectious organisms.

At the conclusion of surgery a large compressive dressing is used, and one may elect to splint the digit in a position of flexion [73,88], because patients usually have much less difficulty bringing the finger from a flexed to an extended position. This motion also produces an obligatory gliding of the lysed tendon, which is more effective than that produced by passively flexing the digit.

Postoperative considerations

Although some investigators have advocated immediate motion following flexor tenolysis [62,63,65–70,73,74,86–89], others have recommended starting therapy in several days or "as soon as soft tissue healing permits" [62]. The rapid formation of new adhesions probably can be discouraged by methods that produce early tendon movement. Immediate motion compatible with wound healing is desirable. It is probably best to initiate digital motion within the first 12 hours following flexor tenolysis whenever possible [89]. Before initiating a postoperative therapy program, one must consider carefully many factors pertaining to the specific clinical situation presented by the patient. The surgeon and therapist should have direct communication regarding the patient's history, previous surgery, preoperative status, the condition of the tendon, and the status of the pulley system. An appreciation of the patient's motivation and tolerance for pain also add immeasurably. An effort also should be made to identify patients who have a tendency to develop excessive edema, those who have diminished vascularity resulting from previous injury or surgery, and those who have previously been infected. This information is useful in establishing realistic goals and in implementing an effective treatment program.

If the lysed tendon is of poor quality or if pulleys have been reconstructed, special postoperative methods are necessary in an effort to minimize the stress placed on the tendons, pulleys, or both. A strong, near normal-appearing tendon in a minimally scarred bed with an adequate pulley system is a candidate for an aggressive mobilization program. Some aspects of the therapy are dictated by the appearance of the involved digit and hand at the time of the removal of the surgical dressing. Excessive swelling, bleeding, infection, wound breakdown, or inordinate pain all may have a prejudicial effect on the initial efforts to regain motion. When possible, it is helpful if the surgeon is in attendance during the first therapy session to monitor carefully the initial attempts to mobilize the involved digit and to allay the apprehensions of the patient. An experienced therapist can, however, effectively commence the program if he or she is familiar with all aspects of the particular patient's injury and previous surgery and the findings at the time of tenolysis.

After the goals and methods of therapy have been discussed with the patient, the bulky compressive dressing is removed and a lighter dressing is applied that is compatible with the control of edema. When necessary, areas of pulley reconstruction are identified and protected by circumferential taping or the use of a thermoplastic ring [89]. This protection is continued for 10–12 weeks and should reduce the possibility of pulley rupture. Finger socks or Coban wraps may be applied to control digital edema. These small dressings are esthetically acceptable to the patient and tend to minimize the pain and bleeding that can sometimes hamper the early mobilization of the digit that has just undergone extensive surgery.

The initial exercise program consists of active and passive exercises designed to take the involved digit through the full range of motion that was passively present preoperatively. This session usually is not terminated until the patient can actively achieve the same flexion that was demonstrated at surgery. The patient is instructed to exercise with the wrist in various positions and to place equal emphasis on both extension and flexion. At the conclusion of the first effort at postoperative mobilization, the patient is instructed to continue the exercise program for 10–15 minutes each waking hour. The ability to carry out self-therapy is monitored carefully.

Postoperative splinting varies depending on the tendency toward joint stiffening in a given digit and the difficulty that the patient may have initiating motion from either a flexed or an extended position. Most post-tenolysis digits are managed by extension splinting between exercise sessions to place the digits at rest and diminish the tendency for proximal interphalangeal joint flexion contracture. When passive and active flexion are difficult to initiate and when full extension is achieved easily, it may be better to splint the digit in a flexed attitude.

If the tenolysed tendon has diminished caliber, is badly scarred, or has been judged to be of poor quality at the time of surgery, the risk for tendon rupture may be considerable. Impending rupture also may be suspected in some patients who develop palpable crepitation in the digit during the early mobilization program. In both instances, therapy should be designed to diminish the tensile strength demand on the involved tendon while preserving the excursion achieved at surgery. In those instances, a frayed tendon program has been suggested [73,89] and, it is hoped, will result in a reduced rate of rupture.

The frayed tendon program involves passively manipulating the digit into the fully flexed position and then asking the patient to actively maintain that flexion (Fig. 6). If the digit retains its flexed position following the removal of the manipulating finger, muscle contracture and tendon movement has been confirmed. In this manner, the tendon moves through its maximal excursion but with much less likelihood of rupture. In some instances, additional protection can be achieved by maintaining some element of wrist flexion or metacarpophalangeal joint flexion, although the full excursion of the tendon is not achieved in those positions. This program usually is continued for approximately 4–6 weeks following tenolysis.

Although the maintenance of the same active joint motion that was achieved at surgery often is compromised somewhat by the postoperative

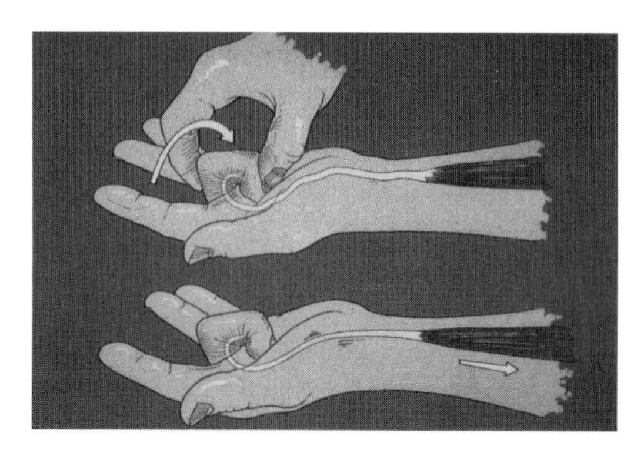

Fig. 6. Frayed tendon program: technique of postoperative movement of a digit following tenolysis. Full passive motion of all three digital joints is performed (*top*), followed by an active attempt by the patient to actively maintain that flexion with the wrist in extension (*bottom*). Tendon excursion is the same as that produced by composite active digital flexion with less tensile loading and less likelihood of tendon rupture. (*From* Strickland JW. Hand Clin 1985;1(1):121 (Gary Schnitz, artist); with permission.)

swelling of the involved digit, it is important that the therapeutic effort continue until the patient has achieved active motion that is equal to passive motion. Terminating the therapy session before that goal is accomplished can result in a gradual deterioration of active motion and a less than optimal final functional result. The use of a transcutaneous nerve stimulator (TENS) has been shown to be valuable in postoperative pain reduction, and the occasional use of an indwelling catheter for periodic instillation of a long-acting anesthetic also may be of benefit in the patient with a low pain threshold or a particularly complex situation [90]. Electrical stimulation may be beneficial when the flexor muscle of the tenolysed tendon is weakened and requires augmentation to produce full tendon excursion. For patients who protectively contract their antagonistic extensor muscle groups, the use of biofeedback may be of considerable value in overcoming this motion-defeating activity. Other adjunctive equipment, such as the use of continuous passive motion devices, is now proving to be helpful in maintaining joint motion and tendon motion, and their development and perfection may assist further in the sometimes difficult postoperative period.

Flexor tenolysis summary

The results of thorough tenolysis of the flexor tendons in the palm and digits in selected patients can be gratifying. Preoperative requirements include a well motivated patient with a supple digit and a wide discrepancy between active and passive ranges of digital motion. The surgical procedure consists of meticulous division of all restraining adhesions from one or both of the flexor tendons and a careful preservation or reconstruction of annular pulleys. One must demonstrate the adequacy of the lysis at the time of surgery by active flexion by the patient under local anesthesia or by a proximal flexor check in the patient under general anesthesia. Postoperatively every effort must be made to achieve active digital motion compatible with the passive motion as quickly as possible. The maintenance of the tendon excursion and joint motion achieved at surgery is difficult and challenging. A well designed treatment program usually can be implemented following careful consultation between surgeon and therapist, and special efforts may be necessary to modify pain, control edema, preserve passive motion, eliminate antagonistic muscle activity, protect pulleys, and, above all, maintain tendon excursion.

Flexor tendon reconstruction

Restoration of flexor tendon performance in badly scarred digits historically has been difficult. Several investigators have reported the use of single-stage tendon grafts in these situations [91,92] with only modest functional recovery. Tendon homografts and allografts have been used with varying degrees of clinical success [93–95], although a small number of composite sheath–tendon allografts were shown to provide a surprisingly good recovery [96,97]. Unfortunately, technical and logistic difficulties with the securing, preserving, and implanting of these grafts have been obstacles to their widespread use.

An ingenious staged flexor tendon repair was described by Paneva-Holevich [98]. In this technique, the severed flexor proximal ends of the profundus and superficialis tendons are sutured to each other in the palm. At the second stage, the flexor superficialis is divided at the musculotendinous junction, delivered distally through the flexor sheath, and sutured to the distal phalanx as a pedicle graft. Several surgeons have combined this technique with the use of a silicone prosthesis implanted in the digital sheath during the first stage to prepare a bed for the subsequent distal pedicle transfer [99,100]. The procedure apparently can provide satisfactory results in either acute or salvage conditions, although it has not been used widely in the United States.

In an effort to improve the biologic bed in which tendon grafts later may be placed, materials such as celloidin [101], glass [102], or metal [103] have been used, but these materials apparently led to joint stiffness because their rigidity did not allow for passive digital motion while a pseudosheath was being formed around the implant [104]. Bassett and Carroll [105] began using flexible silicone rubber rods to build pseudosheaths in badly scarred fingers in the 1950s and the method was later refined into a two-stage reconstruction of the digital flexor tendons by Hunter et al [106,107]. The implant and method that currently enjoys the most popularity has resulted largely from the work of Hunter et al [108,109], and LaSalle and Strickland [110] also have reported their results of the use of this method, and Wilson et al [57] have reported on the use of delayed two-stage reconstruction for isolated flexor profundus injuries. Hunter et al [111–113] also has pursued the development and clinical use of an active tendon implant, and in some instances the results of the use of these prostheses has been encouraging. Asencio et al [114] have demonstrated reasonable results from the use of human composite flexor tendon allografts for these difficult salvage situations.

Staged flexor tendon reconstruction with implantation of a silicone implant

Staged flexor tendon reconstruction involves the implantation of a silicone or silicone–Dacron-reinforced gliding implant into a scarred tendon bed, resulting in the formation of a mesothelium-lined pseudosheath around the implant. Following maturation of the pseudosheath, a tendon graft is inserted to replace the implant, with the hope that there is a minimum of adhesions formed around the graft. Schneider emphasizes that patients with severe neurovascular impairment are poor candidates for staged flexor tendon reconstruction. Some surgeons prefer to carry out staged tendon reconstruction by inserting the implant from the fingertip to the forearm, whereas others believe that when the palm has not been significantly involved in the original trauma or subsequent surgery, the procedure need only go from fingertip to the palm (Fig. 7).

Indications

Staged tendon reconstruction is a long process in which many factors must be carefully

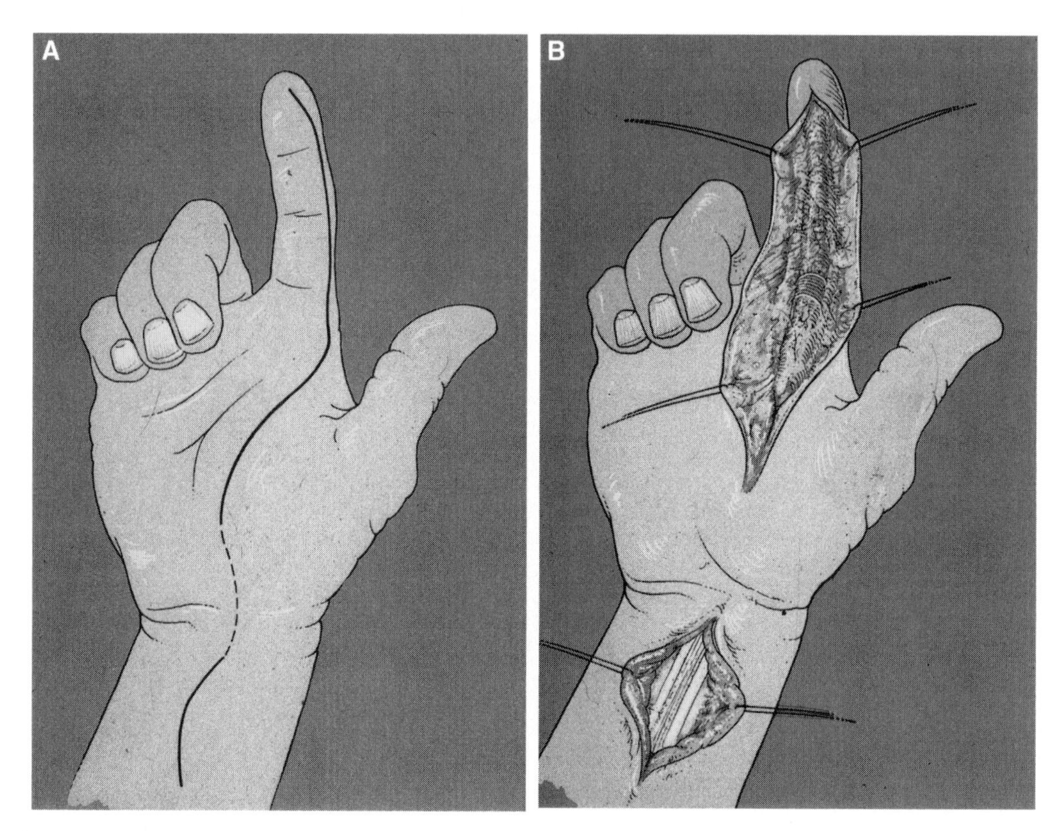

Fig. 7. The technique of staged flexor tendon grafting is illustrated. (*A*) Incisions used to expose scarred flexor tendon sheath and palm and prepare bed for passage of silicone rod from the fingertip to the distal forearm. (*B*) Appearance of the scarred flexor system. (*C*) The appearance of a silicone or silicone-Dacron implant placed in a scarred the digit, palm, and forearm. Preserved and reconstructed annular pulleys are shown over the implant. (*D*) Alternative method of distal insertion of the implant. (*E*) Emphasis on tendon gliding during interval between stages one and two. (*F*) At stage two, a tendon graft (usually plantaris) is attached to the distal end of the implant and pulled proximally with the implant through the digit, palm, and wrist into a distal forearm incision site. (*G*) After attaching the tendon graft to bone and tendon distally, the distal wound is closed and the proximal tendon weave is performed.

considered by physician and patient, and the status of the digital tissues including the skin, nerves, vessels, and joints weighs heavily in determining the appropriateness of proceeding with such a complex and multistaged restorative effort.

Surgery technique: stage one

The flexor system is exposed by palmar incisions that may be midaxial or zigzag, depending on the preference of the surgeon. Previous incisions must be recognized and respected to ensure satisfactory vascularity of the skin flaps. During dissection, care must be taken to preserve as much of the annular portions of the flexor sheath as possible. All tendon remnants are excised with a 1 cm stump of the flexor profundus carefully left attached to its insertion in the distal phalanx. When possible, long portions of the excised tendons should be preserved for use in pulley reconstruction. Joint flexion contractures are released by division of the check-rein extensions of the palmar plate and the accessory collateral ligaments. The profundus tendon then is transected in the midpalm, and through a curvilinear incision from the midforearm to the wrist, the superficialis tendon is withdrawn proximally and divided at its musculotendinous junction.

The selection of the appropriate size tendon implant is governed largely by the tightness of the digital pulleys and the expected size of the tendon graft to be used at stage two. A 4-mm implant is frequently satisfactory and it should be passed carefully through all remaining pulleys. It is

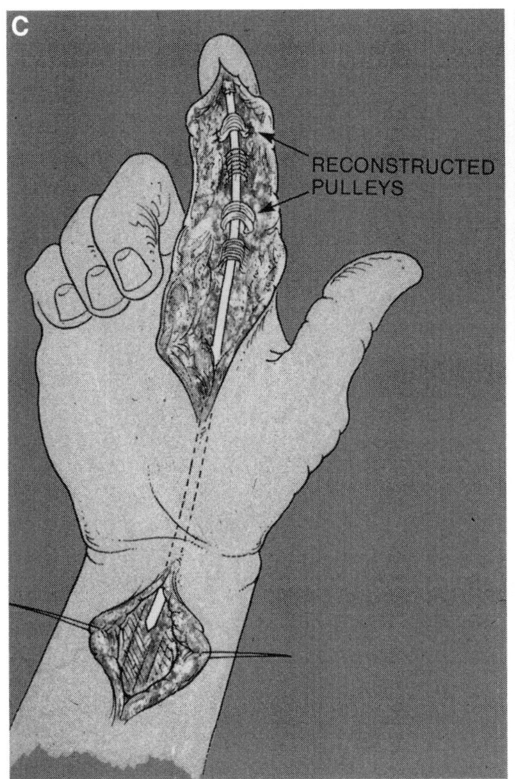

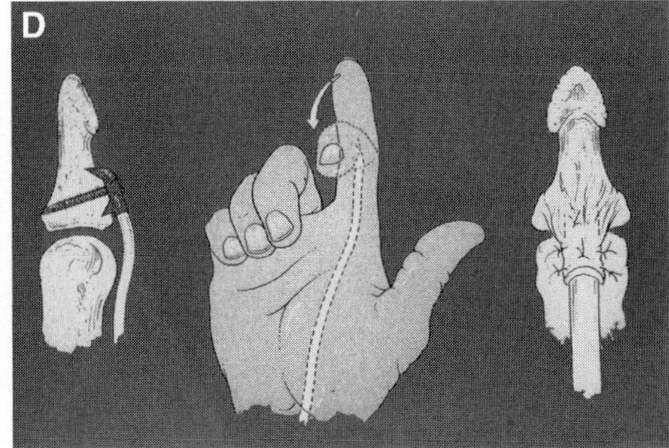

Fig. 7 (*continued*)

important to demonstrate that the implant glides freely in the tendon bed by pulling it back and forth and observing its movement. Distal insertion of the definitive implant then is performed, depending on the type of implant selected. One design (Holter-Houser) has a metal end piece that may be fixed to the distal phalangeal bone beneath the profundus stump with a small Woodruff self-tapping screw. The insertion preferred by most surgeons involves trimming the distal portion of the implant and suturing it strongly to the undersurface of the profundus stump with synthetic sutures. This implant–tendon juncture allows one to avoid the difficulties of passing the metal plate beneath the digital pulleys and the problems of accurate screw placement in the distal phalanx.

The implant then may be passed from the proximal palm to the distal forearm in the plane between the profundus and superficialis tendons by using a tendon passer (Fig. 8). Traction is placed on the proximal end of the implant to be sure that it glides smoothly beneath the preserved or reconstructed pulleys and to note the potential range of digital motion. The adequacy of the pulley system also may be observed at this time and additional pulleys should be reconstructed over the implant if necessary. The proximal end of the implant then is tunneled proximally to lie free over the profundus muscle in the midforearm, and it may be helpful to loosely tag the future profundus motor tendon to the implant. If the tendon to be used for graft attachment is independent and not held at length by its companion tendons (such as the common profundi to the middle, ring, and small fingers), it is probably a good idea to suture it down to the periosteum overlying the distal radius so that it does not undergo myostatic contracture during the interval between implant placement and free grafting. The wound is repaired and a compressive dressing applied, maintaining the wrist in slight flexion. Passive wrist and digital motion are commenced at 7–10 days, and small immobilization splints may be used to prevent digital joint stiffness.

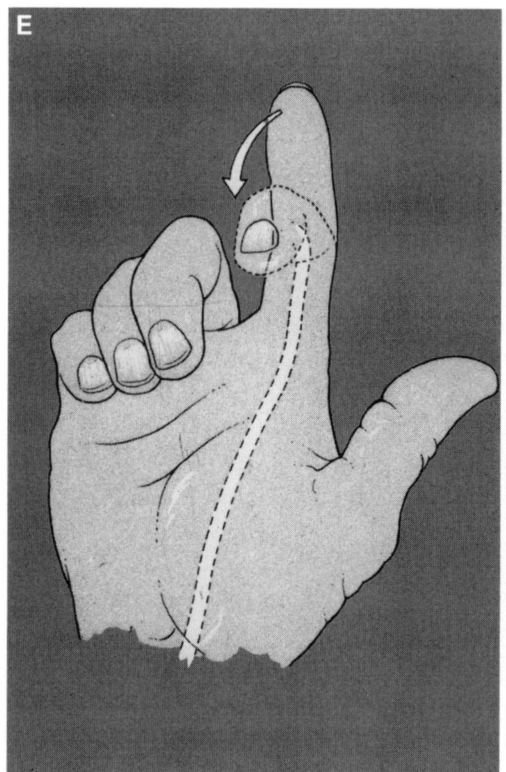

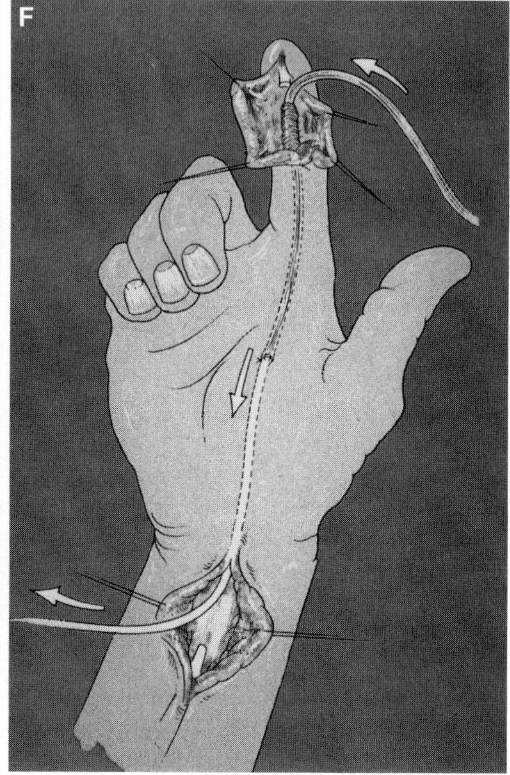

Fig. 7 (*continued*)

At approximately 3 months or after sufficient time for wound healing, scar maturation, and the formation of a pseudosheath around the implant, the second stage grafting procedure is considered. During the period between procedures, vigorous therapy programs are used in an effort to regain and maintain full passive digital motion.

Surgery technique: stage two

The replacement of the silicone implant by a free tendon graft may be performed by using the terminal portions of previous stage one digital and distal forearm incisions. Great care is taken not to open the pseudosheath proximal to the distal interphalangeal joint or to injure any of the middle phalangeal pulleys. The implant is identified and uncovered at its attachment to the stump of the flexor profundus tendon over the base of the distal phalanx and the connecting sutures are divided. The implant is tagged temporarily with a hemostat and the stump of the profundus is mobilized and retained at its insertion for suturing to the replacement free tendon graft. The proximal end of the implant is located through the forearm–wrist incision and any excess pseudosheath is resected to assure free gliding of the proximal graft juncture. The appropriate motor tendon is now selected, and most frequently the combined profundus mass is chosen for grafts to the middle, ring, and small fingers. The independent profundus to the index finger usually serves as the most appropriate motor for that digit. In certain circumstances, the superficialis muscle–tendons also can be used. Care is taken to mobilize fully the motor tendon unit, and the proximal end of the implant is tagged.

Unfortunately the palmaris longus usually is not of sufficient length to serve as a tendon graft for the forearm to digital tip technique of staged flexor tendon reconstruction. When present, the plantaris tendon makes a better graft for this procedure because of its small size and long length. An incision along the medial border of the Achilles tendon is used, and the graft is harvested from the posterior leg by the use of a long Brand stripper [23]. Other potential donor sources include the long toe extensors of the

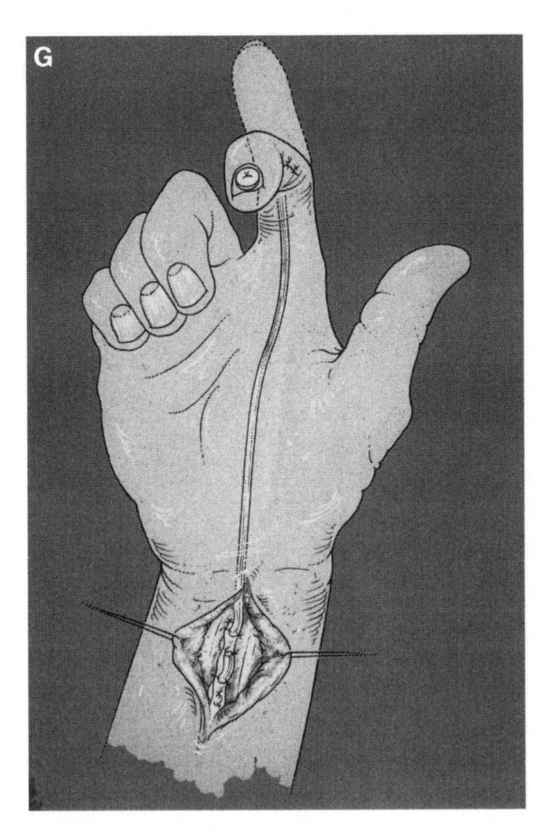

Fig. 7 (*continued*)

middle three toes, which are of sufficient length for use in this procedure but which are larger and more difficult to pass through the pseudosheath. The tendon graft is attached to the distal end of the implant and pulled proximally through the pseudosheath into the forearm incision. The implant then is removed and discarded, and the distal tendon juncture is secured in a manner identical to that described for free tendon grafting. The distal finger wound then is closed and the proximal motor tendon–graft juncture is performed in the forearm using a weave technique. Tension on the graft should be set so that the digit assumes a flexion posture slightly greater than its normal resting position with the wrist in neutral and all muscles relaxed. The proximal wound then is closed and the hand is immobilized in a bulky dressing with a posterior splint that maintains the wrist in mid-position between neutral and full flexion and maintains the metacarpophalangeal joints in 70° of flexion, with the fingers in near full extension.

Some surgeons believe the hand should be immobilized for 3–4 weeks given the salvage nature of the procedure, whereas others now favor an early protected motion program initiated at approximately 3 days following the second stage grafting procedure. In either event, therapy proceeds carefully through passive and light active motion stages until at least 6 weeks when the tensile strength of the tendon and its junctures are sufficiently strong to tolerate a more aggressive application of motion stress.

Complications of staged tendon reconstruction include synovitis around the implant, infection or wound breakdown, and disruption of the distal implant juncture after stage one. Stage two complications include rupture of the graft, a graft that is too loose or too tight, the development of an intrinsic plus phenomenon, and flexion deformities of the proximal or distal interphalangeal joints. Finally, adhesions of the graft may prevent a successful recovery of digital motion and may require tenolysis [110]. The complications of either stage of this complex reconstructive process may compromise severely the end result and must be dealt with promptly and appropriately.

Staged flexor tendon reconstruction: summary

When digits are badly scarred as a result of injury or multiple failed efforts to restore continuity and excursion to badly damaged flexor tendons, staged reconstruction using the initial placement of a silicone implant in the tendon bed followed later by the replacement of that implant with a tendon graft can offer realistic salvage possibilities when few other options exist. The procedure must be considered carefully by physician and patient, and the status of the digital tissues, including the skin, nerves, vessels, and joints, weighs heavily in determining the appropriateness of proceeding with such a complex and multistaged restorative effort. Nonetheless, this procedure has stood the test of time as a viable salvage option for the most difficult flexor tendon situations.

Summary

This article synthesizes an enormous amount of peer reviewed articles, book chapters, and anecdotal clinical information regarding the late management of flexor tendon injuries by free-tendon grafting, tenolysis, and staged reconstruction. Some of the most pertinent historical contributions to these subjects have been reviewed in concert with an update regarding the most widely used current clinical methods for

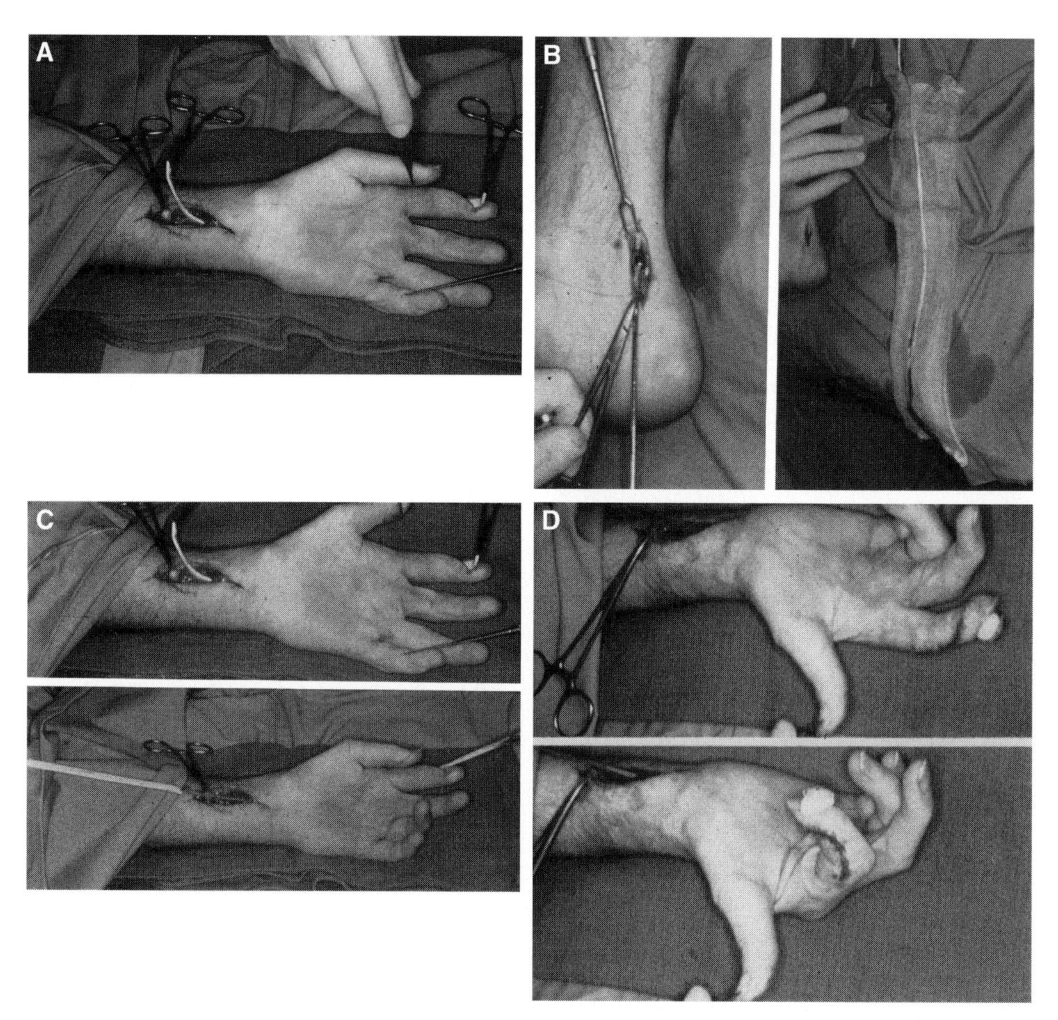

Fig. 8. (*A*) Appearance of a silicone tendon implant in a left index finger during stage two of flexor tendon reconstruction. Exposure of the silicone implant over the distal phalanx and in the distal forearm in preparation for graft passage. (*B*) Garnering of the plantaris tendon from the medial side of the Achilles tendon using a Brand tendon stripper. (*C*) Attachment of plantaris graft to the distal tip of the rod, followed by proximal traction on the implant to deliver it into the forearm. (*D*) Proximal traction of the graft after distal attachment through a drill hole in the distal phalanx and digital wound closure. The full composite flexion of the digit is demonstrated in preparation for the proximal weave into the selected motor tendon.

performing these procedures. This article points out areas of controversy and references the dissenting opinions from those presented here. The delayed treatment of flexor tendon injuries has advanced considerably in the last half century. Although much of the sage advice of the historic masters of flexor tendon surgery remains clinically applicable today, newer techniques and much improved therapy protocols have improved appreciably the results of the procedures described in this treatise. It is realistic and exciting to anticipate that the future will continue to improve the results of these methods through biologic manipulation of tendon healing and adhesion formation.

References

[1] Adamson JE, Wilson JN. The history of flexor tendon grafting. J Bone Joint Surg Am 1961;43A: 709–16.

[2] Lexer E. Did Verwehtung der freien Schnenstransplantation. Arch Klinic Chir 1912;98:818–25.

[3] Mayer L. The physiological method of tendon transplantation. I. Historical, anatomy, and physi-

ology of tendons. Surg Gynecol Obstet 1916;22:182–97.

[4] Mayer L. The physiological method of tendon transplantation. II. Operative technique. Surg Gynecol Obstet 1916;22:298–306.

[5] Mayer L. The physiological method of tendon transplantation. III. Experimental and clinical experiences. Surg Gynecol Obstet 1916;22:472–81.

[6] Bunnell S. Repair of tendons in the fingers and description of two new instruments. Surg Gynecol Obstet 1918;26:103–10.

[7] Mason ML, Allen HS. The rate of healing of tendons. Ann Surg 1941;133:424.

[8] Bunnell S. Surgery of the hand. Philadelphia: JB Lippincott Co.; 1944. p. 307.

[9] Moberg E. Experiences with Bunnell's pull-out wire sutures. Br J Plast Surg 1951;38:175.

[10] Pulvertaft RG. Repair of tendon injuries in the hand. Ann R Coll Surg Engl 1948;3:3–14.

[11] Pulvertaft RG. Tendon grafts for flexor tendon injuries in the fingers and thumb. A study of technique and results. J Bone Joint Surg Br 1954;38B:175.

[12] Pulvertaft RG. Indications for tendon grafting. AAOS Symposium on Tendon Surgery in the Hand. Philadelphia: CV Mosby Co; 1975. p. 123–31.

[13] Graham WC. Flexor tendon grafts to the finger and thumb. J Bone Joint Surg 1947;29:553–9.

[14] Littler JW. Free tendon grafts in secondary flexor tendon repair. Am J Surg 1947;74:315–21.

[15] Boyes JH. Why tendon repair? J Bone Joint Surg Am 1959;41A:577–9.

[16] Boyes JH, Stark HH. Flexor-tendon grafts in the fingers and thumb. A study of factors influencing results in 1000 cases. J Bone Joint Surg Am 1971;53A:1332–42.

[17] White WL. Secondary restoration of finger flexion by digital tendon grafts: an evaluation of seventy-six cases. Am J Surg 1956;91:662–8.

[18] White WL. Tendon grafts: a consideration of their source, procurement and suitability. Surg Clin N Am 1960;40:403–13.

[19] Rank BL, Wakefield AR. The repair of flexor tendons in the hand. Br J Plast Surg 1952;4:244–53.

[20] Verdan CE. Half a century of flexor-tendon surgery, current status and changing philosophies. J Bone Joint Surg Am 1972;54A:472–91.

[21] Tubiana R. Technique of flexor tendon grafts. Hand 1969;1:108–14.

[22] McClinton MA, Curtis RM, Wilgis EF. One hundred tendon grafts for isolated flexor digitorum profundus injuries. J Hand Surg Am 1982;7:224–9.

[23] Brand PW. Tendon grafting. J Bone Joint Surg Br 1961;43B:444.

[24] Schneider LH, Hunter JM. Flexor tendons, late reconstruction. In: Green DP, editor. Operative hand surgery, Vol. 2. New York: Churchill Livingstone; 1982. p. 1375–440.

[25] Wilson RL. Flexor tendon grafting. Flexor tendon surgery. Hand Clin 1985;1:97–107.

[26] Bunnell S. Repair of tendons in the fingers. Surg Gynecol Obstet 1922;35:88–97.

[27] Bunnell S. Surgery of the hand. 2nd edition. Philadelphia: JB Lippincott; 1948. p. 381–466.

[28] Eiken O, Holmberg J, Ederot L, et al. Restoration of the digital tendon sheath. Scan J Plast Reconstr Surg 1980;14:89–97.

[29] Reimann AF, Daseler E II, Anson BJ, Beaton LE. The palmaris longus muscle and tendon: a study of 1,600 extremities. Anat Rec 1944;89:495–505.

[30] Daseler MS, Anson BJ. The plantaris muscle. J Bone Joint Surg 1943;25:822–7.

[31] Ark JW, Gelberman RH, Abrahamsson SO, Seiler JG III, Amiel D. Survival and proliferation in autogenous flexor tendon grafts. J Hand Surg [Am] 1994;19(2):249–58.

[32] Noguchi M, Seiler JG III, Boardman ND III, Tramaglini DM, Gelberman RH, Woo SL. Tensile properties of canine intrasynovial and extrasynovial flexor tendon autografts. J Hand Surg [Am] 1997;22(3):457–63.

[33] Bruner JM. The zig-zag volar-digital incision for flexor tendon surgery. Plast Reconstr Surg 1967;40:571–4.

[34] Boyes JH, Stark HH. Flexor tendon grafts in the fingers and thumb: a study of factors influencing results in 1000 cases. J Bone Joint Surg [Am] 1971;53:1332–42.

[35] Littler JW. The digital extensor-flexor system. In: Converse JM, McCarthy JG, Littler JW, editors. Reconstructive plastic surgery: the hand and upper extremity, Vol. 6. 2nd edition. Philadelphia: WB Saunders; 1977. p. 3166–214.

[36] Peacock EE. Some technical aspects and results of flexor tendon repair. Surgery 1965;58:330–42.

[37] Pulvertaft RG. Suture materials and tendon junctures. Am J Surg 1965;109:346.

[38] Rank BK, Wakefield AR. Surgery of repair as applied to hand injuries. 2nd edition. Edinburgh: E & S Livingstone; 1960.

[39] Rank BK, Wakefield AR, Hueston JJ. Surgery of repair as applied to hand injuries. 4th edition. Baltimore: Williams & Wilkins; 1973.

[40] Tubiana R. Incisions and techniques in tendon grafting. Am J Surg 1965;109:339.

[41] Strickland JW. Flexor tendon injuries. Part III. Free tendon grafts. Orthop Rev 1987;16:56–64.

[42] Lister G. Pitfalls and complications of flexor surgery: flexor tendon surgery. Hand Clin 1985;2:133–46.

[43] Carroll RE, Match RM. Avulsion of the profundus tendon insertion. J Trauma 1970;10:1109.

[44] Leddy JP, Packer JW. Avulsion of the profundus insertion in athletes. J Hand Surg Am 1977;2:66.

[45] Littler JW. The physiology and dynamic function of the hand. Surg Clin N Am 1960;40:259.

[46] Nichols HM. The dilemma of the intact superficialis tendon. Hand 1975;7:85.
[47] Reid DAC. The isolated flexor digitorum profundus lesion. Hand 1969;1:115.
[48] Wakefield AR. The management of flexor tendon injuries. Surg Clin N Am 1960;40:267.
[49] Bora FW. Profundus tendon grafting with unimpaired sublimis function in children. Clin Orthop 1970;71:118.
[50] Chan W, Thoms OJ, White WL. Avulsion injury of the long flexor tendons. Plast Reconstr Surg 1972; 50:260.
[51] Goldner JL, Conrad RW. Tendon grafting of flexor profundus in the presence of a completely or partially intact flexor sublimis. J Bone Joint Surg Am 1969;51A:527.
[52] Jaffe S, Weckess E. Profundus tendon grafting with the sublimis intact. The end result of thirty patients. J Bone Joint Surg Am 1967;49A:1298.
[53] Pulvertaft RG. The treatment of profundus division by free tendon graft. J Bone Joint Surg Am 1960;42A:1363–80.
[54] Schneider LH. Treatment of isolated flexor digitorum profundus injuries by tendon grafting. In: Hunter JM, Schneider LH, Mackin EJ, editors. Tendon surgery in the hand. St. Louis: CV Mosby; 1987. p. 303–11.
[55] Stark HH, Zemel NP, Boyes JH, Ashworth CR. Flexor tendon graft through intact superficialis tendon. J Hand Surg Am 1977;2:456.
[56] Versaci AD. Secondary tendon grafting for isolated flexor digitorum profundus surgery. Plast Reconstr Surg 1970;45:57.
[57] Wilson RL, Carter MS, Holeman VA, et al. Flexor profundus injuries treated with delayed two-staged tendon grafting. J Hand Surg Am 1980;5:74–8.
[58] Pulvertaft RG. Tendon grafting for the isolated injury of the flexor digitorum profundus. Bull Hosp J Dis Orthop Inst Fall 1984;44(2):424–34.
[59] Honner R. Treatment of isolated flexor digitorum profundus injuries. In: Hunter JM, Schneider LH, Mackin EJ, editors. Tendon surgery in the hand. St. Louis: CV Mosby; 1987. p. 303–7.
[60] Brooks DM. Problems of restoration of tendon movements after repair and grafts. Proc R Soc Med 1970;63:67–8.
[61] Bunnell S. Surgery of the hand. 2nd edition. Philadelphia: JB Lippincott Co.; 1967.
[62] Peacock EE, Van Winckle W. Surgery and biology of wound repair. Philadelphia: WB Saunders Co.; 1970.
[63] Strickland JW. Flexor tenolysis: a personal experience. In: Hunter JM, Schneider LH, Mackin EJ, editors. Tendon surgery in the hand. St. Louis: CV Mosby; 1987. p. 216–33.
[64] Fetrow KW. Tenolysis in the hand and wrist. J Bone Joint Surg Am 1967;49A:667.
[65] Hunter JW, Seinsheimer F, Mackin EJ. Tenolysis: pain control and rehabilitation. In: Strickland JW, Steichen JB, editors. Difficult problems in hand surgery. St. Louis: CV Mosby Co.; 1982.
[66] James JIP. The value of tenolysis. Hand 1969;1:118.
[67] Schneider LH, Hunter JM. Flexor tenolysis. In: American Academy of Orthopaedic Surgeons: Symposium on Tendon Surgery in the Hand. St. Louis: CV Mosby Co.; 1975.
[68] Schneider LH, Hunter JM. Flexor tendon, late reconstruction. In: Green DP, editor. Operative hand surgery. New York: Churchill Livingstone; 1982.
[69] Schneider LH, Mackin EJ. Tenolysis. In: Hunter JM, Schneider LH, Mackin EJ, Bell JA, editors. Rehabilitation of the hand. St. Louis: CV Mosby Co.; 1978.
[70] Schneider LH, Mackin EJ. Tenolysis: dynamic approach to surgery and therapy. In: Hunter JM, Schneider LH, Mackin EJ, Callahan AD, editors. Rehabilitation of the hand. 2nd edition. St. Louis: CV Mosby Co.; 1984.
[71] Strickland JW. Functional recovery after flexor tendon severance in the finger: the state of the art. In: Strickland JW, Steichen JB, editors. Difficult problems in hand surgery. St. Louis: CV Mosby Co.; 1982.
[72] Strickland JW. Management of acute flexor tendon injuries. Orthop Clin N Am 1983;14:827.
[73] Strickland JW. Flexor tenolysis. Hand Clin 1985;1: 121–32.
[74] Whitaker JH, Strickland JW, Ellis RG. The role of tenolysis in the palm and digit. J Hand Surg Am 1977;2:462.
[75] Wray RC, Moucharafieh B, Weeks PM. Experimental study of the optimal time for tenolysis. Plast Reconstr Surg 1978;61:184.
[76] Pulvertaft RG. Experience in flexor tendon grafting in the hand. J Bone Joint Surg Br 1959;41B:629.
[77] Hunter JM, Schneider LH, Dumont J, Erickson JC. The dynamic approach to problems of hand function utilizing local anesthesia supplemented by intravenous fentanyl-droperidol. Clin Orthop 1974;104:112.
[78] Strickland JW. Results of flexor tendon surgery in zone II. Hand Clin 1985;1:167–80.
[79] Bruner JM. The zig-zag volar digital incision for flexor-tendon surgery. Plast Reconstr Surg 1967; 40:571.
[80] Verdan CE. Tendon surgery of the hand. Edinburgh: Churchill Livingstone; 1979.
[81] Boyes JH. The great flexor tendon controversy. In: Cramer LM, Chase RA, editors. Symposium on the hand, Vol. 3. St. Louis: CV Mosby Co.; 1971.
[82] Bora F, Lane JM, Prockop DJ. Inhibitors of collagen biosynthesis as a means of controlling scar formation in tendon injury. J Bone Joint Surg Am 1972;54A:1501.
[83] Wrenn RL, Goldner JL, Markee JL. An experimental study of the effect of cortisone on the heal-

ing process and tensile strength of tendons. J Bone Joint Surg Am 1954;36A:588.
[84] Carstam N. The effects of cortisone on the formation of tendon adhesions and on tendon healing: an experimental investigation in the rabbit. Acta Chir Scand 1953;182:1.
[85] James JIP. The use of cortisone in tenolysis. J Bone Joint Surg Br 1959;41B:209.
[86] Verdan CE, Crawford GP, Martini-Benkeddache Y. The valuable role of tenolysis in the digits. In: Cramer LM, Chase RA, editors. Symposium on the hand, Vol. 3. St. Louis: CV Mosby Co.; 1971.
[87] Ketchum LD. The effects of triamcinolone on tendon healing and function. Plast Reconstr Surg 1971;47:471.
[88] Strickland JW. Flexor tenolysis: a personal experience. In: Hunter JM, Schneider LH, Mackin EJ, editors. Tendon and nerve surgery in the hand. St. Louis: CV Mosby Co.; 1997. p. 443.
[89] Cannon NM, Strickland JW. Therapy following flexor tendon surgery. Hand Clin 1985;1(1):147.
[90] Cannon N, Foltz RW, Koepfer JM, et al. Control of immediate postoperative pain following tenolysis and capsulectomies of the hand with transcutaneous electrical nerve stimulation. J Hand Surg Am 1983;8:626.
[91] Butler B, Burkhalter WE, Cranston JP. Flexor-tendon grafts in the severely scarred digit. J Bone Joint Surg Am 1968;50A:452.
[92] McCormick RM, Demuth RJ, Kindling PH. Flexor tendon grafts in the less-than-optimal situation. J Bone Joint Surg Am 1962;44A:1360.
[93] Cameron RR, Sell K, Latham WD. The experimental transplantation of freeze-dried composite flexor tendon allografts. J Bone Joint Surg Am 1970;52A:1065.
[94] Potenza AD, Melone CW. Functional evaluation of freeze-dried flexor tendon grafts in the dog. J Hand Surg Am 1977;2:233.
[95] Potenza AD, Melone CW. Evaluation of freeze-dried tendon grafts in the dog. J Hand Surg Am 1978;3:157.
[96] Peacock EE. Restoration of finger flexion with homologous composite tissue tendon grafts. Am J Surg 1969;26:564.
[97] Peacock EE, Madden JW. Human composite flexor tendon allografts. Ann Surg 1967;166:624.
[98] Paneva-Holevich E. Two-stage tenoplasty in injury of the flexor tendons of the hand. J Bone Joint Surg Am 1969;51A:21.
[99] Chuinard RG, Dabezies EJ, Matthews RE. Two stage superficialis reconstruction in severely damaged fingers. J Hand Surg Am 1980;5:135.
[100] Kesler FB. Use of a pedicled tendon transfer with a silicone rod in complicated secondary flexor tendon repairs. Plast Reconstr Surg 1972;49:439.
[101] Mayer L. Celloidin tube reconstruction of extensor communis sheath. Bull Hosp Joint Dis Orthop Inst 1940;1:39.
[102] Milgram JE. Transplantation of tendons through preformed gliding channels. Bull Hosp Joint Dis Orthop Inst 1960;21:250.
[103] Thatcher HW. The use of stainless steel rods to canalize flexor tendon sheaths. South Med J 1939;32:13.
[104] Chang W, Thoms OJ, White WL. Avulsion injury of long flexor tendons. Plast Reconstr Surg 1972;50:260.
[105] Bassett CAL, Carroll RE. Formation of tendon sheaths by silicone rod implants. Proceedings of American Society for Surgery of the Hand. J Bone Joint Surg Am 1963;45A:884.
[106] Hunter JM. Artificial tendons. Early development and application. Am J Surg 1965;109:325.
[107] Hunter JM, Salisbury RE. Flexor-tendon reconstruction in severely damaged hands. A two-stage procedure using a silicone Dacron reinforced gliding prosthesis prior to tendon grafting. J Bone Joint Surg Am 1971;53A:829.
[108] Schneider LH. Staged flexor tendon reconstruction using the method of Hunter. Clin Orthop 1978;171:164–71.
[109] Schneider LH. Staged tendon reconstruction. Hand Clin 1985;1:109–20.
[110] LaSalle WB, Strickland JW. An evaluation of the two-stage tendon reconstruction technique. J Hand Surg Am 1983;8:263–7.
[111] Hunter JM, Jaeger SH. Flexor tendon reconstruction and rehabilitation using active tendon implants. In: Green DJP, editor. Operative hand surgery. 3rd edition. New York: Churchill Livingstone; 1993. p. 1900–14.
[112] Hunter JM, Singer DI, Jaeger SH, Mackin EJ. Active tendon implants in flexor tendon reconstruction. J Hand Surg Am 1988;13A:849–59.
[113] Hunter JM, Singer DI, Mackin EJ. Staged flexor tendon reconstruction using passive and active tendon implants. In: Hunter JM, Schneider LH, Mackin EJ, Callahan AD, editors. Rehabilitation of the hand: surgery and therapy. 3rd edition. St. Louis: CV Mosby; 1990. p. 427–57.
[114] Asencio G, Abihaidar G, Leonardi C. Human composite flexor tendon grafts. J Hand Surg Br 1996;21B:84–8.

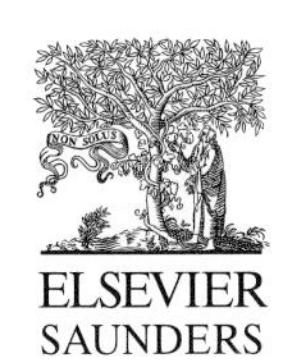

ELSEVIER
SAUNDERS

Hand Clin 21 (2005) 245–251

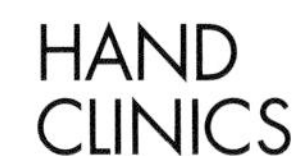

Flexor Tendon Pulley Reconstruction

Vishal Mehta, MD[a,*], Craig S. Phillips, MD[b]

[a]*Department of Surgery, Section of Orthopaedic Surgery, University of Chicago Hospital, 5841 S. Maryland Avenue, MC 3079, Chicago, IL 60637, USA*

[b]*Reconstructive Hand and Upper-Extremity Surgery, Microvascular Surgery, The Illinois Bone and Joint Surgery, 2401 Ravine Way, Glenview, IL 60025, USA*

Few parts of the human anatomy are more elegant than the flexor tendon pulley system. As striking as the elegance of this system is the efficiency by which it is able to convert tendon excursion into angular motion at the metacarpophalangeal (MCP) and interphalangeal joints. When severely injured, the pulley system often requires reconstruction to avoid ensuing disability. Reconstructing such an intricate system rarely yields results equivalent to the untouched, intact pulley system. Nevertheless, the results are better than performing no reconstruction at all. Many techniques have been developed and modified to reconstruct the pulley system, though the optimal technique remains controversial. This article provides a review of the anatomy and function of the pulley system and a discussion of several contemporary reconstructive options.

Anatomy of the pulley system

In 1975, Doyle and Blythe first described the anatomy of the flexor tendon pulley system as consisting of four annular and three cruciate pulleys [1]. A fifth annular pulley later was identified and today five annular and three cruciate pulleys are recognized (Fig. 1) [2]. Manske and Lesker proposed the existence of the palmar aponeurosis pulley proximal to the metacarpophalangeal joint, which was described further by the more recent work of Phillips and Mass [3,4]. The A1, A3, and A5 pulleys are located over the MCP, proximal interphalangeal (PIP), and distal interphalangeal (DIP) joints, respectively. Because of their location at the joint they take origin from the volar plate and from the bone itself. The A2 and A4 pulleys are located over the proximal and middle phalanges, respectively. These two pulleys take their origin exclusively from bone. Located between the second and fifth annular pulleys are three cruciate pulleys. As their names imply, the pulleys differ in shape, with the annular pulleys being ring shaped and the cruciate pulleys having a cross-like configuration. The C1 pulley overlies the distal portion of the proximal phalanx between the A2 and A3 pulleys. The C2 pulley is located at the base of the middle phalanx between A3 and A4, and the C3 pulley is located at the distal part of the middle phalanx just beyond the A4 pulley [5–8]. The annular pulleys are much more robust structures than the cruciate pulleys with the A1 and A4 pulleys being the strongest and the A2 pulley the weakest [9]. The average lengths of the A1, A2, A3, and A4 pulleys are 11 mm, 17 mm, 5 mm, and 8 mm, respectively. The location, strength, and lengths of the pulleys contribute directly to their function and are important considerations in pulley reconstruction, as is discussed later in this article [10].

Function of the pulleys

The primary function of the pulley system is to convert the available excursion of the flexor tendons into angular motion across the interphalangeal joints, thereby allowing flexion of the PIP and DIP joints. Additionally, the pulley system functions to transform the finite tendon excursion into power grip at the fingertips. The pulley system performs this function in an efficient manner, making prudent use of the power of the

* Corresponding author.
E-mail address: vishal@mehtas.com (V. Mehta).

0749-0712/05/$ - see front matter
doi:10.1016/j.hcl.2004.12.002

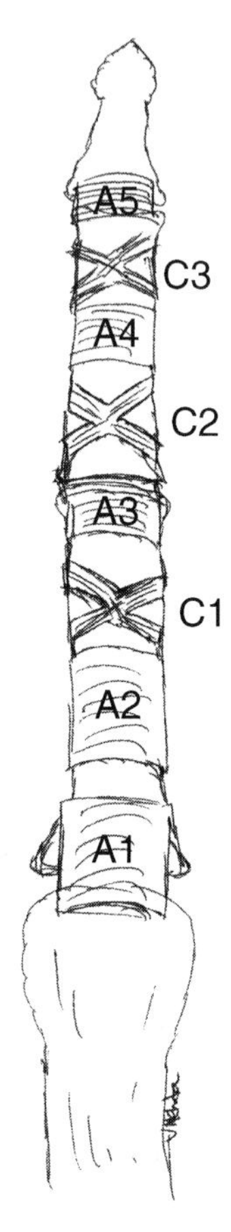

Fig. 1. An illustration of the volar aspect of the pulley system. Note the location of the pulleys and the differing shape of the annular and cruciate pulleys.

forearm musculature. The pulleys achieve these objectives by ensuring the flexor tendons remain close to the axis of rotation at the digital joints throughout the arc of motion, thus minimizing the amount of tendon excursion required to make a fist. The tendon is held in a position close to the bone, where it must pull out of plane with the desired direction of movement; as the joint angle increases, the force imparted by the flexor tendons becomes volarly directed, resisted exclusively by the pulley system, thereby allowing for improved flexion of the joint. In this manner, the pulley system decreases the amount of required tendon excursion, but does so at the expense of force generated at the fingertip and increases the friction required [11–13].

The function of the individual pulleys has been studied extensively. It is generally accepted that the A2 and A4 pulleys are the most important [5,6,11,14]. Peterson et al studied the effects of pulley loss on work of the flexor tendon system in cadavers. They found the A2 and A4 pulleys to be the most important and noted that these two pulleys had to be intact for near normal function to occur [12]. Doyle et al confirmed the importance of these two pulleys [5,6]. Other investigators also have confirmed the importance of the A2 and A4 pulleys but found the three-pulley system of A2, A3, and A4 to be more efficient [15,16]. Rispler et al reported that an intact three-pulley system of A2, A3, and A4 provided near normal efficiency and was statistically better than an intact two-pulley system of A2 and A4 [15]. Many investigators have reported the A2 pulley to be the single most important pulley. Even this is controversial, however, as others have demonstrated more detrimental effects from loss of the A4 pulley than loss of the A2 pulley. In fact, in a cadaver model, loss of the A2 pulley resulted only in decreased efficiency of excursion with no effect on work, whereas loss of the A4 pulley resulted in decreased efficiency of excursion and increased work [15]. Isolated loss of the A1 or A5 pulley results in no change in work or excursion efficiency [11,15]. Although areas of controversy exist, it is generally accepted that the A2 and A4 pulleys are the most important members of the pulley system and must be preserved or reconstructed when associated with extensive pulley loss. The A3 pulley is likely of some lesser importance, whereas A1 and A5 cause no detrimental effects to the system when removed in isolation. The cruciate pulleys have not been well studied and generally are not considered to be critical members of the pulley system. The cruciate pulleys assume a more important role with increased flexion of the digits. At high flexion angles the annular pulleys "concertina," assuming a triangular configuration, whereas the cruciate pulleys tend to unravel, allowing the crossed fibers to become parallel and taught. The reason for this phenomenon is as yet unknown but believed to play an important role in resisting tendon bowstringing while allowing smooth gliding during digital flexion. The concepts of pulley reconstruction flow directly from these observations. Most investigators recognize the importance of the A2 and A4 pulleys and attempt to reconstruct at least these two pulleys.

Reconstructive options

When reconstructing the annular pulley system, the literature is replete regarding the number

[1], size [17], height [9], strength [18,19], material [20–23], location [9,14,24], and technique options [9,17–28]. There is, however, a paucity of information regarding the pressure at which the reconstructed pulley should be tensioned [26–28].

Basic principles

Although many different philosophies and techniques exist regarding the reconstruction of the pulley system, certain basic principles should be followed. One should retain as much of the uninjured pulley system and sheath as possible. Attempts to repair damaged pulleys should be made and constricted pulleys should be dilated to accept the flexor tendon or implant. The sheath itself also should be preserved, because flexor tendons have been shown to have improved intrinsic healing if the tendon sheath is left intact [29–33]. When exposure of the flexor tendons is required, entering the sheaths through the cruciate pulleys is prudent as their role in digital mechanics seems to be less important. During reconstruction of the annular pulleys, every attempt should be made to replicate the intact pulley with special reference to length and location of the reconstructed pulley. Pulleys should be reconstructed with synovial-lined grafts whenever possible. This is preferable to the use of extrasynovial grafts, because an intrasynovial-lined graft decreases the amount of resistance and work in the tendon/pulley system and heals faster with less scar [20,21,34]. When completely deficient, the A2 and A4 pulleys should be reconstructed at the very minimum with consideration given to reconstructing a third pulley as dictated by the clinical situation. When the flexor tendon is severely injured in combination with a deficient pulley, reconstruction should be performed over a synthetic rod to allow for pulley healing and the formation of a pseudosynovial sheath before flexor tendon grafting. Unique to pulley reconstruction, the surgeon must decide as to what pressure the reconstructed pulley should be tensioned. Ideally the pulley should be tight enough to prevent any tendon bowstringing and loose enough to allow unimpeded tendon gliding. Some investigators have performed this procedure under sensory digital anesthesia to allow the patients to actively flex the digits to accurately assess the pulley function [26]. Others have proposed placing a Kirschner wire alongside the flexor tendon during pulley reconstruction to ensure adequate space available for tendon gliding. Lister proposed placing hemostats on all four corners of the reconstructed pulley to maintain sufficient tension to prevent bowstringing yet also permit free tendon gliding. Brand and Crannor advocated a simple method of assessing the efficiency of the newly constructed pulley by ensuring the tendon excursion from full extension to 30° flexion was the same as that from 60°–90° of flexion [27]. The best available technique of pulley reconstruction would reproduce the anatomic length and location of the pulley and also allow the surgeon to sequentially tension multiple loops or strands of the reconstructed pulley. It is for this reason that the authors tend to use either the three-loop technique described by Okutsu or the so called "shoelace interweave" described by Weilby and modified by Kleinert. When a loop technique is used to reconstruct the A2 or A3 pulleys, the loops must be passed volar to the extensor mechanism (between the extensor tendon/lateral bands and the proximal phalanx), whereas when used to reconstruct the more distal A4 pulley, the loop must be passed dorsal to the extensor mechanism (conjoint lateral bands, oblique retinacular bands and triangular ligament). Although every case of pulley reconstruction is unique, adherence to these principles improves outcomes and provides some basic guidelines for the treating surgeon.

Techniques

Kleinert/Weilby technique

Kleinert and Weilby advocated a technique involving weaving a tendon through the "always-present fibrous rim" of the pulley being reconstructed (Fig. 2A) [35]. Variations of this technique have been reported with minor modification and with the use of different tendon grafts. Usually the tail of the superficialis tendon is used, but if not available, a tendon graft may be used instead. As mentioned previously, one of the advantages of this technique is that it affords the surgeon good control over setting tension in the reconstructed pulley. A disadvantage is that it lacks immediate strength compared with the other reconstructive techniques [18]. Its effects on resistance and efficiency of the tendon system are unclear, as different studies have shown both increased and unchanged resistance and average and good efficiency of excursion [21,25].

Triple loop technique

Okutsu described this modification of the original Bunnell technique in which three tendon

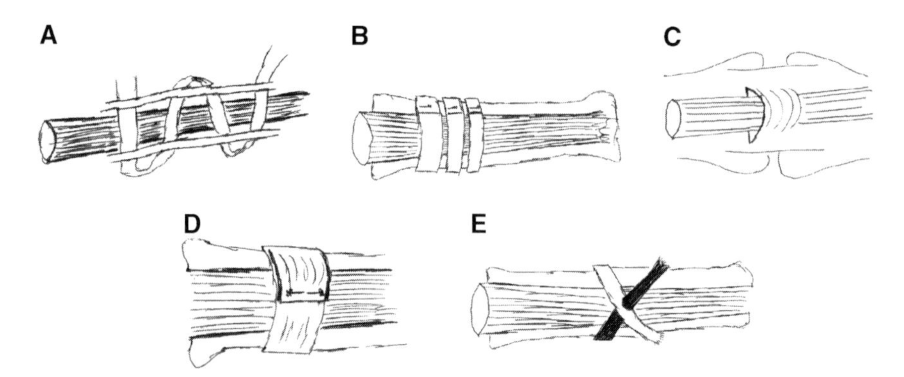

Fig. 2. (*A*) The Kleinert/Weilby technique weaves a tendon through the "always-present fibrous rim" of the pulley being constructed. (*B*) The triple loop forms a wide pulley reconstruction by individually passing three tendon grafts around the phalanx. (*C*) The Karev technique involves making two transverse incisions in the volar plate and sliding the tendon through the so called "belt-loop" that is formed. (*D*) Lister's technique wraps a segment of extensor retinaculum around the phalanx. (*E*) The loop and a half technique passes a tendon graft around the phalanx and then through the substance of one limb of the tendon graft.

grafts are individually passed around the phalanx, tensioned, and sutured to themselves (Fig. 2B) [26]. Okutsu believed the single loop technique described by Bunnell to be too narrow. He theorized that the narrow reconstruction would allow perpendicular movement that would lead to a reduction in postoperative function. The modified, wider reconstruction would eliminate this fault and provide increased strength for early postoperative motion. Indeed, this technique has been shown to be the strongest of the pulley reconstruction techniques and can stand as much load to failure as a normal pulley [19]. Nishida et al demonstrated the excursion resistance of this technique to be superior to that of the Kleinert/Weilby technique but inferior to Lister's or Karev's technique [21].

In a cadaver study, the authors compared the Lister, Karev, Kleinert/Weilby, loop, and a half and the triple loop technique to determine which had the best efficiency of digital flexion as determined by effects on excursion, load, and work. The authors found the triple loop and Kleinert/Weilby techniques to be superior to the other techniques (presented at the American Society for Surgery of the Hand, 54th Annual Meeting, Boston, Massachusetts).

Karev—belt-loop technique

The Karev technique involves making two transverse incisions in the volar plate and sliding the flexor tendon through the so called "belt loop" formed between the two incisions (Fig. 2C) [36]. Because the tendon must be passed through the belt loop, this technique can be used only in the presence of an adjunctive flexor tendon repair or tendon graft/implant and not for simple pulley reconstruction around an intact tendon. This technique has been shown to require the least amount of tendon excursion because of its advantageous position at the joint and significant tension exerted on the underlying flexor tendon [25]. It has average strength and is stronger than the Kleinert/Weilby and Lister techniques but weaker than the loop and a half and triple loop techniques [18]. The major disadvantage is that the stiffness of the volar plate causes an increase in total friction and work as the increased tension on the flexor tendon inhibits gliding. Additionally, the long-term effects of this technique on the metacarpophalangeal joint remain unknown.

Lister's technique

Lister's technique involves harvesting a segment of the extensor retinaculum, which is reversed and then passed around the phalanx (Fig. 2D) [37]. The major disadvantage of this technique is that a normal portion of the extremity must be violated to harvest the retinaculum. The main advantage is that the retinaculum provides a smooth gliding surface producing the lowest amount of resistance among the reconstructive techniques [21]. This technique also has been shown, however, to have the lowest mechanical efficiency because of difficulties associated with obtaining and maintaining tension on the pulley [25]. This technique also has been shown to have a low load to failure [18].

Loop and a half technique

This technique is performed by passing a tendon graft around the phalanx and then through the substance of one limb of the tendon graft (Fig. 2E). The two free ends then are sutured to their respective sides of the loop and then rotated away from the flexor tendon. The loop and a half technique was described initially by Widstrom in his article comparing the "mechanical effectiveness" of six different pulley reconstruction techniques [25]. He found it to have equivalent "mechanical effectiveness" to most of the other techniques but to be inferior to Karev's technique. In a follow-up article he compared the strengths of these six techniques and found the loop and a half to be the strongest [18]. The triple loop technique was not included in either of these studies, however. In a cadaver study, the authors found the loop and a half technique to be ineffective at preventing bowstringing because of the limited length of this technique. This bowstringing subsequently led to an increase in excursion required for digital flexion.

Synthetic materials

Numerous attempts have been made to use synthetic materials to reconstruct the flexor tendon pulley system. Dacron, silicone, nylon, and polytetrafluoroethylene (PTFE) have all been studied as potential pulley grafts [17,22,23,38–41]. The most promising of these materials is PTFE for several reasons. PTFE has been shown not to interfere with the normal tendon healing process in an in vivo chicken model [22]. The breaking strength of PTFE also has been studied and is strong enough to allow immediate mobilization of the digits without fear of pulley rupture [38]. Furthermore, PTFE is incorporated by host tissues, elicits no foreign body reaction, and causes no adhesions [39]. Fortunately the need for synthetic material during pulley reconstruction is a rare event. When the need does arise, it seems that PTFE is the most promising synthetic material available for use as a pulley graft.

Attempts have been made to reconstruct pulleys using free vascularized pulley grafts. Although this is an innovative and promising approach to the complex problem of pulley reconstruction, its place in clinical practice is yet to be established. At the current time, results remain anecdotal, with few surgeons experienced in this technique. Considering the amount of resources and time required and the paucity of data, most surgeons are best served by relying on the established methods of pulley reconstruction as outlined previously.

Clinical studies

Clinical outcome data on pulley reconstruction techniques are extremely limited. In fact, a review of the literature reveals only a single study [26]. This study reports the outcome of six pulley reconstructions using the triple loop technique at an average follow-up of 21 months. Total active motion was improved by an average of 30° and all patients achieved satisfactory grip function. This study is limited by its retrospective design, small size, and early follow-up period. The paucity of clinical studies is a testament to the difficulties in studying such a diverse and rare clinical problem. Unfortunately this forces the clinician to rely on cadaver studies and anecdotal accounts when attempting to determine the best reconstructive procedure. A cadaver hand is by no means an accurate representation of the intricate anatomy of the living, functioning human hand. Large prospective randomized clinical studies with long follow-up periods are needed to help determine the optimal pulley reconstructive technique and the clinical outcome that can be expected.

Complications

Reconstruction of the flexor tendon and its pulley system is fraught with potential complications. The most common complications after two-stage tendon reconstruction are flexion contracture (41%), synovitis (8%), and infection (4%) [42]. Synovitis following two-stage tendon reconstruction using a silicone prosthesis may or may not be a result of pulley reconstruction. The cause of synovitis is not clear, though excessively tight pulleys are believed to play a role. During pulley reconstruction, passive range of motion should be checked intraoperatively to ensure adequate gliding of the tendon through the reconstructed pulleys. Infection is of constant concern but can be minimized with careful attention to sterile technique and meticulous soft tissue management. Once infection has set in, any implant must be removed and the infection eradicated with antibiotics and debridement. Failure of the pulley itself may occur, although compliance and oversight by a hand therapist minimizes this complication. Use of a strong pulley reconstruction, such as the triple loop, helps decrease the incidence of this complication. Bone resorption with subsequent fracture also has been reported secondary to pulley reconstruction [43]. Although the complication rate is high, reconstruction of the pulley system almost always improves function and as a general rule is worth the risk for the aforementioned complications.

Summary

Pulley reconstruction remains a challenging intellectual and technical exercise. When performed correctly, however, it can be a gratifying procedure that provides much improved function of the digit. As described in this article, there are many different techniques by which the pulley can be reconstructed. Each of these techniques has distinct advantages and disadvantages. The hand surgeon should be familiar with each of these techniques and the general principles of pulley reconstruction as laid out in this article. With this knowledge base, the treating surgeon is able to tailor the procedure performed to the exact anatomy and clinical situation of each patient. Although great strides have been made over the past half century, more clinical research is needed to determine the best technique, not just in the cadaver model, but also in the complex model of the living human hand.

References

[1] Doyle JR, Blythe W. The finger flexor tendon sheath and pulleys: anatomy and reconstruction. AAOS Symposium on Tendon Surgery in the Hand. St. Louis: CV Mosby; 1975. p. 81–7.

[2] Hunter JM, Cook JF, Ochiai N, Konikoff JJ, Merklin RJ, Mackin GA. The pulley system. Orthop Trans 1980;4:4.

[3] Manske PR, Lesker PA. Palmar aponeurosis pulley. J Hand Surg [Am] 1983;8(3):259–63.

[4] Phillips C, Mass D. Mechanical analysis of the palmar aponeurosis pulley in human cadavers. J Hand Surg [Am] 1996;21(2):240–4.

[5] Doyle JR. Anatomy of the finger flexor tendon sheath and pulley system. J Hand Surg [Am] 1988; 13(4):473–84.

[6] Doyle JR. Anatomy of the flexor tendon sheath and pulley system: a current review. J Hand Surg [Am] 1989;14(2 Pt 2):349–51.

[7] Katzman BM, Klein DM, Garven TC, Caligiuri DA, Kung J, Collins ED. Anatomy and histology of the A5 pulley. J Hand Surg [Am] 1998;23(4):653–7.

[8] Strauch B, de Moura W. Digital flexor tendon sheath: an anatomic study. J Hand Surg [Am] 1985;10(6 Pt 1):785–9.

[9] Manske PR, Lesker PA. Strength of human pulleys. Hand 1977;9(2):147–52.

[10] Hume EL, Hutchinson DT, Jaeger SA, Hunter JM. Biomechanics of pulley reconstruction. J Hand Surg [Am] 1991;16(4):722–30.

[11] Lin GT, Amadio PC, An KN, Cooney WP. Functional anatomy of the human digital flexor pulley system. J Hand Surg [Am] 1989;14(6):949–56.

[12] Peterson WW, Manske PR, Bollinger BA, Lesker PA, McCarthy JA. Effect of pulley excision on flexor tendon biomechanics. J Orthop Res 1986;4(1): 96–101.

[13] Strickland JW. Flexor tendon injuries. Part 4. Staged flexor tendon reconstruction and restoration of the flexor pulley. Orthop Rev 1987;16(2):78–90.

[14] Barton NJ. Experimental study of optimal location of flexor tendon pulleys. Plast Reconstr Surg 1969; 43:125–9.

[15] Rispler D, Greenwald D, Shumway S, Allan C, Mass D. Efficiency of the flexor tendon pulley system in human cadaver hands. J Hand Surg [Am] 1996; 21(3):444–50.

[16] Goldstein SA, Greene TL, Ward WS, Matthews LS. A biomechanical evaluation of the function of the digital pulleys. Orthop Trans 1985;8:342.

[17] Wray RC Jr, Weeks PM. Reconstruction of digital pulleys. Plast Reconstr Surg 1974;53(5):534–6.

[18] Widstrom CJ, Doyle JR, Johnson G, Manske PR, McGee R. A mechanical study of six digital pulley reconstruction techniques: Part II. Strength of individual reconstructions. J Hand Surg [Am] 1989; 14(5):826–9.

[19] Lin GT, Amadio PC, An KN, Cooney WP, Chao EY. Biomechanical analysis of finger flexor pulley reconstruction. J Hand Surg [Br] 1989;14(3): 278–82.

[20] Nishida J, Seiler JG, Amadio PC, An KN. Flexor tendon-pulley interaction after annular pulley reconstruction: a biomechanical study in a dog model in vivo. J Hand Surg [Am] 1998;23(2):279–84.

[21] Nishida J, Amadio PC, Bettinger PC, An KN. Flexor tendon-pulley interaction after pulley reconstruction: a biomechanical study in a human model in vitro. J Hand Surg [Am] 1998;23(4):665–72.

[22] Semer NB, Bartle BK, Telepun GM, Goldberg NH. Digital pulley reconstruction with expanded polytetrafluoroethylene (PTFE) membrane at the time of tenorrhaphy in an experimental animal model. J Hand Surg [Am] 1992;17(3):547–50.

[23] Bader KF, Sethi G, Curtin JW. Silicone pulleys and underlays in tendon surgery. Plast Reconstr Surg 1968;41:157–64.

[24] Solonen KA, Hoyer P. Positioning of the pulley mechanism when reconstructing deep flexor tendons of the fingers. Acta Orthop Scand 1967;38:321–8.

[25] Widstrom CJ, Johnson G, Doyle JR, Manske PR, Inhofe P. A mechanical study of six digital pulley reconstruction techniques. Part I. Mechanical effectiveness. J Hand Surg [Am] 1989;14(5):821–5.

[26] Okutsu I, Ninomiya S, Hiraki S, Inanami H, Kuroshima N. Three-loop technique for A2 pulley reconstruction. J Hand Surg [Am] 1987;12(5 Pt 1):790–4.
[27] Brand PW, Cranor KC, Ellis JC. Tendon and pulleys at the metacarpophalangeal joint of a finger. J Bone Joint Surg 1975;57(6):779–84.
[28] Hunter JM, Cook JF Jr. The pulley system: rationale for reconstruction. In: Strickland JW, Steichen JB, editors. Difficult problems in hand surgery. St. Louis: CV Mosby; 1982. p. 94–102.
[29] Eiken O, Lundborg G, Rank F. The role of the digital synovial sheath in tendon grafting. An experimental and clinical study on autologous tendon grafting in the digit. Scand J Plast Reconstr Surg 1975;9(3):182–9.
[30] Lundborg G, Eiken O, Rank F. Synovium as a nutritional medium in tendon grafting. Handchirurgie 1977;9(3):107–11.
[31] Lundborg G, Myrhage R, Rydevik B. The vascularization of human flexor tendons within the digital synovial sheath region—structural and functional aspects. J Hand Surg [Am] 1977;2(6):417–27.
[32] Manske PR, Lesker PA, Bridwell K. Experimental studies in chickens on the initial nutrition of tendon grafts. J Hand Surg [Am] 1979;4(6):565–75.
[33] McDowell CL, Snyder DM. Tendon healing: an experimental model in the dog. J Hand Surg [Am] 1977;2(2):122–6.
[34] Gelberman RH, Mankse PR. Factors influencing flexor tendon adhesions. Hand Clin 1985;1(1):35–42.
[35] Kleinert HE, Bennett JB. Digital pulley reconstruction employing the always present rim of the previous pulley. J Hand Surg 1978;3:297–8.
[36] Karev A, Stahl S, Taran A. The mechanical efficiency of the pulley system in normal digits compared with a reconstructed system using the "belt loop" technique. J Hand Surg [Am] 1987;12(4):596–601.
[37] Lister GD. Reconstruction of pulleys employing extensor retinaculum. J Hand Surg [Am] 1979;4(5):461–4.
[38] Bartle BK, Telepun GM, Goldberg NH. Development of a synthetic replacement for flexor tendon pulleys using expanded polytetrafluoroethylene membrane. Ann Plast Surg 1992;28(3):266–70.
[39] Dunlap J, McCarthy JA, Manske PR. Flexor tendon pulley reconstructions—a histological and ultrastructural study in non-human primates. J Hand Surg [Br] 1989;14(3):273–7.
[40] Hanff G, Dahlin LB, Lundborg G. Reconstruction of flexor tendon pulley with expanded polytetrafluoroethylene (E-PTFE). An experimental study in rabbits. Scand J Plast Reconstr Surg Hand Surg 1991;25(1):25–30.
[41] Schneider LH. Staged flexor tendon reconstruction using the method of Hunter. Orthop Trans 1978;2:1.
[42] Wehbe MA, Hunter JM, Schneider LH, Goodwyn BL. Two-stage flexor-tendon reconstruction. Ten-year experience. J Bone Joint Surg 1985;68(5):752–63.
[43] Lin GT. Bone resorption of the proximal phalanx after tendon pulley reconstruction. J Hand Surg [Am] 1999;24(6):1323–6.

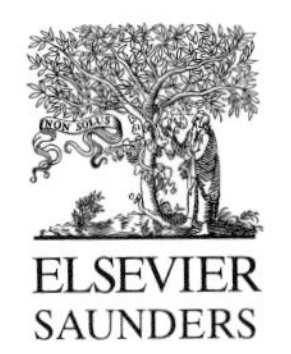

ELSEVIER
SAUNDERS

Hand Clin 21 (2005) 253–256

HAND
CLINICS

Pediatric Flexor Tendon Injuries

Timothy G. Havenhill, MD[a],
Roderick Birnie, MD, MB BCh, MMed[b,*]

[a]*Hand and Upper Extremity, Surgery Department of Orthopedic Surgery, Washington University School of Medicine, Suite 1130, 1 Barnes Hospital Plaza, St. Louis, MO 63110, USA*

[b]*Section of Orthopedic Surgery and Rehabilitation Medicine, The University of Chicago Hospitals, 5841 South Maryland Avenue, MC 3079, Chicago, IL 60637, USA*

In the pediatric hand, flexor tendon injuries are transected most commonly by glass or knives [1–3]. A physician may not recognize or appreciate the severity of the injury, and therefore a high index of suspicion should be maintained. In young children, parents and physicians may miss the tendon injury because of trapping with flexion, in which the child flexes the injured finger with the neighboring finger.

Pediatric flexor tendon injuries heal rapidly and contractures are rare, as long as the joint has not been injured. Flexor tendons in children are smaller and more delicate than those in adults, but there are no anatomic differences between them. The surgical approach and techniques of repair are the same as in the adult, but for obvious reasons the diagnosis and rehabilitation pose unique challenges. Unlike children, adults are able to recognize the injury, comply with the examination, and participate in a rehabilitation protocol. These differences also affect the identification of complications and their management. Although no specific age delineates when an injured patient can be treated as an adult, a general guideline of 10 years of age has been recommended [4]. Still, the decision should be made on a case-by-case basis.

Diagnosis

The examination begins with observation of the resting posture of the hand. A digit in extension and not resting in the usual cascade likely has a flexor tendon injury (Fig. 1). If the child permits, gentle wrist flexion and extension uses the tenodesis effect to generate flexor excursion. Alternatively, compression of forearm structures generates passive flexor excursion (Fig. 2). Compression over the flexor carpi radialis (FCR) tendon generates thumb flexion (Fig. 3), and compression ulnar to the FCR generates flexion of the other digits.

Radiographs of the extremity may be useful to show a retained foreign body or an associated fracture. Ultrasound has limited diagnostic accuracy, and MRI is expensive and requires a general anesthetic for young children. Both are unlikely to aid in the diagnosis, because they require a cooperative patient.

The possibility of an associated injury to the neurovascular structures should always be suspected. Arterial bleeding from a volar laceration of a digit presupposes a digital nerve injury because of the anatomic relationship of the nerve being more volar than the artery. Covering the hand and asking which finger is being touched is always equivocal in a young child. Loss of resistance to glide using a plastic pen can help in diagnosing loss of sweating in a nerve injury. The immersion test is useful for the very young child but may not be a practical option [5]. (The injured hand is immersed in room temperature water until skin wrinkling occurs. Because only innervated skin wrinkles, an area of unwrinkled skin indicates a likely nerve injury.)

The diagnosis of a tendon (or nerve) injury in a young frightened child is always difficult and the

* Corresponding author.
E-mail address: rbirnie@surgery.bsd.uchicago.edu (R. Birnie).

0749-0712/05/$ - see front matter
doi:10.1016/j.hcl.2004.11.004

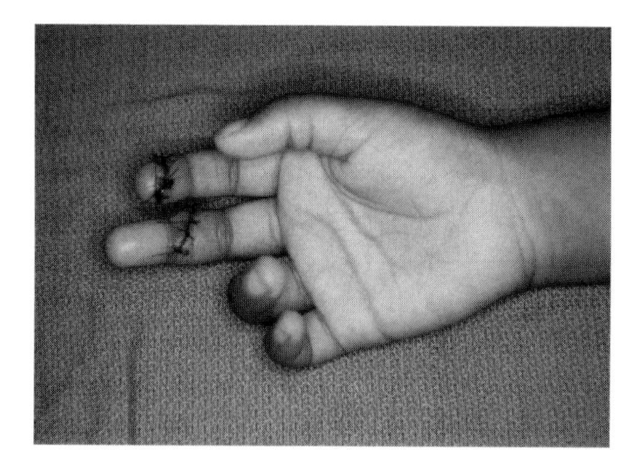

Fig. 1. Loss of normal finger cascade.

recommendation is a surgical exploration under general anesthesia and a bloodless field at the slightest suspicion.

Technique

The technique of suture repair in children is the same as in adults, with several exceptions. A zone I rupture with a distal profundus stump may be sutured using a tendon-to-tendon technique. If no stump exists, the profundus tendon may be sutured directly to bone using a nonabsorbable suture or over a button [5]. Small-core suture sizes are needed in small fingers, even as small as a 6-0 in a 2-year-old child. Additionally, absorbable sutures are recommended for wound closure to avoid another anesthetic exposure for suture removal.

Rehabilitation

In adults, protected early motion is the principle of flexor tendon rehabilitation. Such a protocol requires a child who can comprehend and comply

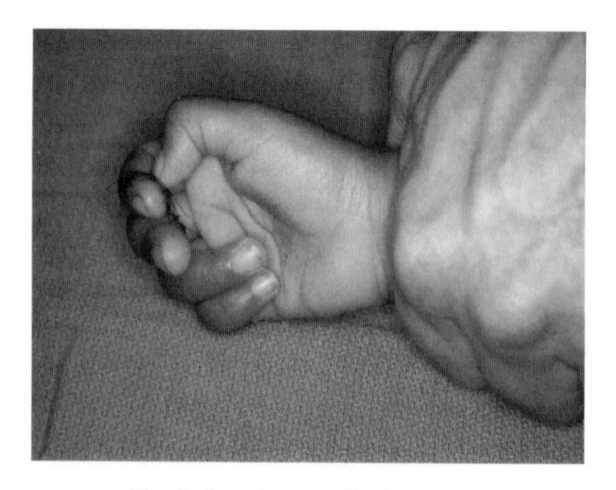

Fig. 2. Long finger FDP laceration.

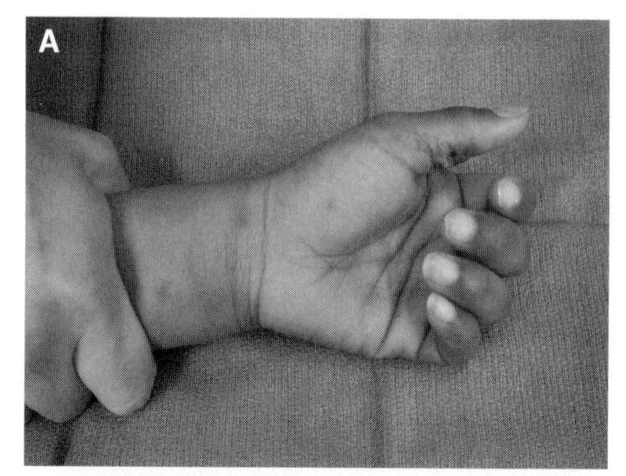

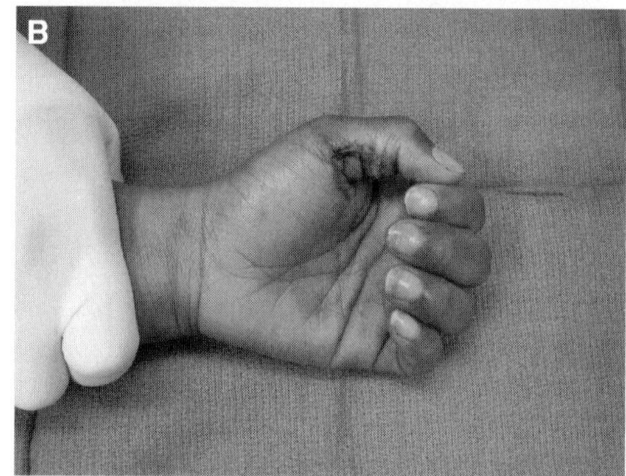

Fig. 3. (*A*) Before FPL repair. (*B*) After FPL repair.

with treatment [6–9]. Protected immobilization therefore is recommended for the pediatric patient unable to participate in an early motion protocol. Cast immobilization of repairs at all levels for 3–4 weeks [5] allows for immediate unsupervised use of the extremity without concern for tendon rupture. The use of removable day or night splints is unpredictable. Constant immobilization prevents use of the hand and protects the repair against spontaneous or voluntary muscle contractions.

In a cooperative older child, immobilization may consist of a short-arm cast or posterior splint. An uncooperative child necessitates a long-arm cast with the elbow at 90°, the wrist in 30–40° of flexion, and the metacarpophalangeal joints flexed 60–70° (Fig. 4). The interphalangeal joints are left in a resting position. The exception to this rule is the zone IV repair with release of the transverse carpal ligament. The wrist is kept in neutral with more digital flexion to protect the repair and to prevent bowstringing of the tendons in the carpal tunnel.

The extremity is immobilized for 3–4 weeks post-repair. In a child younger than 3 years of age,

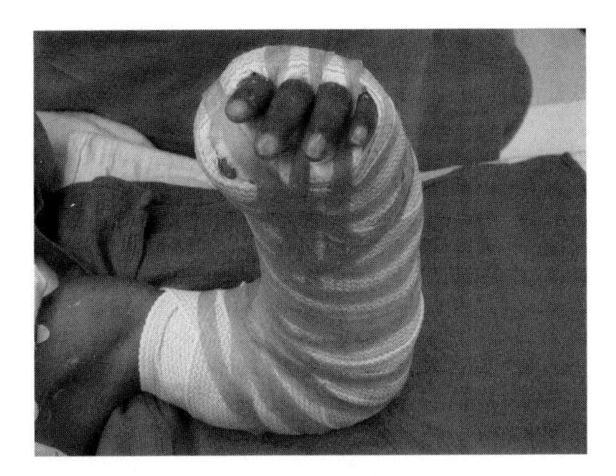

Fig. 4. Immobilization after FPL repair.

no further immobilization is necessary unless a concomitant neurovascular injury exists. For this, a dorsal blocking splint is used for 2 additional weeks. In a child older than 3 years of age, a daytime dorsal blocking splint is used for 2–3 weeks to prevent accidental forced passive finger extension. After immobilization, play therapy is used to encourage flexion and extension. Passive extension and resistive flexion exercises (putty) may begin 5–6 weeks post-repair. If the digit is unable to achieve full extension by 6 weeks, a nighttime extension resting splint is recommended.

Complications

Delayed diagnosis

One quarter of all pediatric flexor tendon injuries may be unrecognized on the initial evaluation [10–11]. The consequences of this include irreversible myostatic contracture of the musculoskeletal unit, loss of flexor sheath patency, and impairment of digital growth [12]. It has been recommended that all flexor tendon injuries, regardless of age, be surgically explored [13]. Delayed primary repairs up to 76 days postinjury have been reported [14]. Good results with primary repair have been seen in children up to 2 months postinjury [15]. Primary repair has been shown to be superior to free tendon grafting and staged reconstruction in children [1,13,16–18].

Free tendon grafting requires (1) a remaining, suitable flexor tendon sheath, (2) intact A2 and A4 pulleys, and (3) a proximal musculoskeletal unit with at least 3 cm of excursion. Potential donors include the superficialis tendon of the involved digit, palmaris longus, plantaris, and the toe extensor tendons. Tension is typically set the same as in adults. The extremity is immobilized for 4 weeks, the same as for a primary repair. The postoperative rehabilitation is the same as for a primary repair.

Postoperative tendon rupture

A postoperative tendon rupture is difficult to appreciate because of limited digital motion from the postoperative immobilization. If the rupture is recognized early and the digit has retained passive motion, then the site is re-explored and a primary repair is performed. If the age of the rupture is unclear, the tissues are inflamed, or the child or family are uncooperative with the postoperative management, planning a reconstruction at a later age may be prudent. In this situation, regaining and maintaining supple passive motion to prevent contracture is critical.

Tendon adhesions

In patients with nonfunctional active motion and passive motion restricted because of flexor adhesions and not joint contractures, tenolysis is recommended. Again, management requires a mature patient able to follow a postoperative rehabilitation protocol. Results of tenolysis are unpredictable [1,16]; however, when done in a manner identical to an adult—under a local anesthetic with early aggressive therapy—the results are far superior to a tenolysis performed with the child requiring a general anesthetic who is unable to participate in an immediate therapy program [4].

Repair results

Although the assessment of outcomes of flexor tendon repair optimally is done by objective means, the same obstacles to diagnosing the injury exist with attempting to measure the results of surgery. The simplest method is the technique of Boyes using the distance between the pulp of the distal phalanx and the distal palmar crease [19]. This still requires a cooperative patient, however, who can sustain maximal flexion. Additionally, transposing adult values on the pediatric hand is difficult. Furthermore, the results may change over time with growth.

Another system that has been applied to children is total active motion (TAM). Again, this system requires a cooperative patient able to maintain maximal digital flexion for measurement of angles at each joint. A study by O'Connell et al [14] evaluated zone I and II repairs in children using

TAM. Zone I repairs were shown to have better motion than zone II repairs, but within zones no significant differences were noted between early motion and 3–4 weeks of immobilization.

Summary

Flexor tendon injuries in children differ from adults in their diagnosis and postoperative rehabilitation principles. The child may be uncooperative, so indirect methods of tendon integrity must be used for diagnosis. Radiographs may be useful for associated fracture or retained foreign bodies. A high index of suspicion necessitates surgical exploration. Although surgical approach and repair techniques are identical to those in adults, postoperative immobilization for 3–4 weeks is used instead of an early motion protocol. Delayed diagnosis is more common in the pediatric population, and recognition and management of postoperative complications can be difficult, because the child may be unable to cooperate or comply with the treatment.

References

[1] Vahvanen V, Gripenberg L, Nuutinen P, et al. Flexor tendon injury of the hand in children. Scand J Reconstr Surg 1981;15:43.
[2] Bell JL, Mason ML, Koch SL, et al. Injuries to flexor tendons of the hands in children. J Bone Joint Surg 1958;40A:1220.
[3] Joseph KN, Kalus AM, Sutherland AB, et al. Glass injuries of the hand in children. Hand 1981;13:113.
[4] Birnie RH, Idler RS. Flexor tenolysis in children. J Hand Surg 1995;20A:254.
[5] Idler RS. Pediatric tendon injuries. In: Peimer CA, editor. Surgery of the hand and upper extremity. New York: McGraw-Hill; 1996. p. 2165–77.
[6] Chow JA, Thomes LJ, Dovelle S, et al. A combined regimen of controlled motion following flexor tendon repair in "no man's land." Plast Reconstr Surg 1987;79:447.
[7] Chow JA, Thomes LJ, Dovelle S, et al. Controlled motion rehabilitation after flexor tendon repair and grafting: a multi-center study. J Bone Joint Surg 1988;70B:591.
[8] Duran RJ, Houser RG, Coleman CR, et al. A preliminary report in the use of controlled passive motion following flexor tendon repair in zones II and III. J Hand Surg 1976;1:79.
[9] Strickland JW, Glogovac SV. Digital function following flexor tendon repair in zone II: a comparison of immobilization and controlled passive motion techniques. J Hand Surg 1980;5:537.
[10] Osterman AL, Bozentka DJ. Flexor tendon injuries in children. Oper Tech Orthop 1993;3:283.
[11] Gilbert A, Masquelet A. Primary repair of flexor tendons in children. In: Tubiana R, editor. The hand. Vol. III. Philadelphia: Saunders; 1998. p. 354–8.
[12] Hage J, Dupuis CC. The intriguing fate of tendon grafts in small children's hands and their results. Br J Plast Surg 1965;18:341.
[13] Glicenstein J, LeClerq C. Late treatment of injuries of the flexor tendons in children. In: Tubiana R, editor. The hand. Vol. III. Philadelphia: Saunders; 1988. p. 359–63.
[14] O'Connell SJ, Moore MM, Strickland JW, et al. Results of zone I and zone II flexor tendon repairs in children. J Hand Surg 1994;19A:48.
[15] Leddy JP. Primary and delayed primary repair of flexor tendon lacerations in zone II in children. J Hand Surg 1982;7:410.
[16] Amadio PC, Wood MB, Cooney WP, et al. Staged flexor tendon reconstruction in the fingers and hand. J Hand Surg 1988;13A:559.
[17] Boyes JH, Stark HH. Flexor tendon grafts in the fingers and thumb. J Bone Joint Surg 1971;53A:1332.
[18] Ejeskar A. Flexor tendon repair in no man's land. Scand J Plast Reconstr Surg 1980;14:279.
[19] McClinton MA, Curtis RM, Wilgis EFS. One hundred tendon grafts for isolated flexor digitorum profundus injuries. J Hand Surg 1982;7:224.

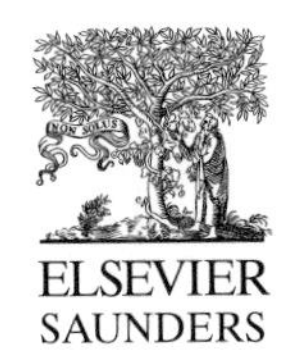

ELSEVIER
SAUNDERS

Hand Clin 21 (2005) 257–265

HAND
CLINICS

Rehabilitation after Flexor Tendon Repair, Reconstruction, and Tenolysis

Kathy Vucekovich, OTR/L, CHT*, Gloria Gallardo, OTR/L, Kerry Fiala, OTR/L

Hand Therapy Clinic, Occupational Therapy Department, DCAM4-A, The University of Chicago Hospitals, 5758 South Maryland, MC 9039, Chicago, IL 60637, USA

"A man's best friends are his ten fingers" [1]. Complete function and expressive use of one's "best friends" requires an intact flexor tendon system. Much attention and study therefore has been placed over the past several decades in reparation and rehabilitation after a flexor tendon injury. As flexor tendon surgery has advanced through scientific research and clinical investigation, rehabilitation of flexor tendon injuries has progressed right alongside. Immobilization protocols first advocated by Dr. Bunnell [2] evolved into early passive motion protocols, which have evolved most recently into early active motion protocols. The latter, however, has not replaced the former. All three programs still hold their place in hand rehabilitation clinics today. Critical clinical decision-making skills based on knowledge of tendon anatomy, evidenced-based healing concepts, and good communication with the surgeon are required for the hand therapist to guide the person with a repaired flexor tendon system to maximum hand and finger function. The following article reviews the advancement of rehabilitation of flexor tendon repair, reconstruction, and tenolysis.

Flexor tendon primary repair rehabilitation

Immobilization program

Using complete immobilization postoperatively is the most conservative approach to rehabilitation after a flexor tendon repair, and this method still holds a place in hand rehabilitation. "No matter how sophisticated our therapeutic and surgical care becomes, there probably will always be a need for immobilization of flexor tendon repairs in some circumstances" [3]. An immobilization program may be indicated after a flexor tendon repair for the following reasons: children and adults who are unable to comprehend and follow through with a complex mobilization protocol, associated injuries to the adjacent structures, such as fracture, and disorders and health conditions that affect tissue healing, such as rheumatoid arthritis. Collins and Schwarze developed an early progressive resistance program for the immobilized repaired tendon [4]. The immobilization cast or dorsal blocking splint positions the wrist and metacarpophalangeal (MCP) joints in flexion and the interphalangeal (IP) joints in full extension. In general, the cast is removed after 3–4 weeks and is replaced by a dorsal blocking splint. The patient begins passive flexion with the wrist held in 10° of extension and gentle differential tendon gliding exercises (Fig. 1).

During this phase, the difference between the digital total active motion and total passive motion is evaluated. A 50° difference indicates dense adhesion formation, which would lead the therapist to initiate early progressive resistance beginning with blocking exercises (Fig. 2).

If at 4.5 weeks extensive adhesions remain, light putty squeezing and putty extension looping is commenced. At 4–6 weeks the dorsal protective splint is discontinued during the day, but the

* Corresponding author.

E-mail address: kathrynjune@rcn.com (K. Vucekovich).

doi:10.1016/j.hcl.2004.11.006

hand.theclinics.com

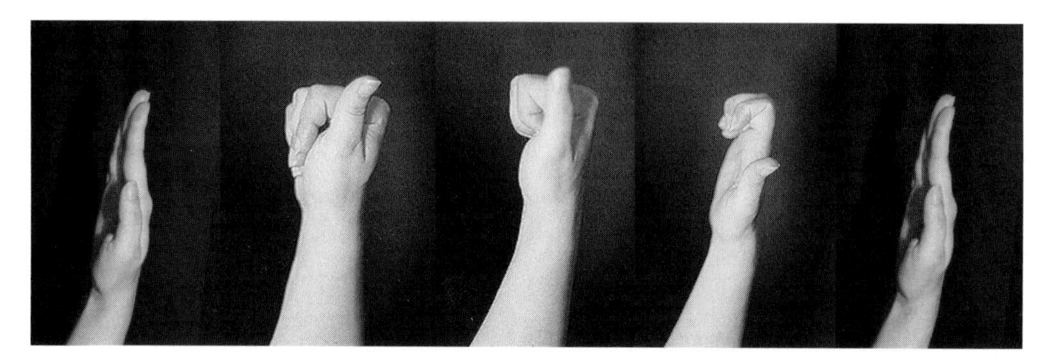

Fig. 1. Differential gliding exercises.

patient is advised to wear the splint when outdoors and during sleep for protection. Gentle active wrist and digital extension begins, together with blocking and fisting exercises. At this phase, if extrinsic flexor tightness is noted, a forearm-based splint holding the wrist and digits in comfortable maximum extension is worn at night. Typically, significant resistive exercise begins at 6–8 weeks. Timing and load intensity of the resistive exercise depends on the severity of adhesion formation (Table 1).

Controlled motion programs

Because of improvements in strong, gap-resistant suture techniques [5], a trend has developed in tendon rehabilitation from immobilization to early controlled motion protocols. Studies have shown that early controlled forces applied to the healing tissues improve recovery of tensile strength [6], decrease adhesions [7], improve tendon excursion [8], and promote intrinsic healing [9]. Controlled motion rehabilitation protocols were developed mainly for zone II flexor tendon repairs but also are used with adaptation for zones I, III, IV, and V. Zone II is the area from the metacarpal head to mid-middle phalanx. The flexor digitorum profundus (FDP) and flexor digitorum superficialis (FDS) are housed in zone II within a flexor tendon sheath. Repairs in this zone have the highest probability of adhesion development because of its unique anatomy, including Camper's chiasm, vincular anatomy, and the presence of the A2 and A4 pulleys. For the hand therapist, edema, scar formation, and patient compliance also contribute to the challenge of rehabilitation after a zone II flexor tendon repair.

There are two basic passive motion programs that stand as the basis for other passive motion protocols: the Kleinert method and the Duran method. Both approaches have been adapted, built on, and even combined by hand specialists, including the Washington regimen [10].

Kleinert program

In the 1960s, Kleinert and others introduced an early controlled passive motion protocol using a dorsal protective splint (wrist, 30° flexion and

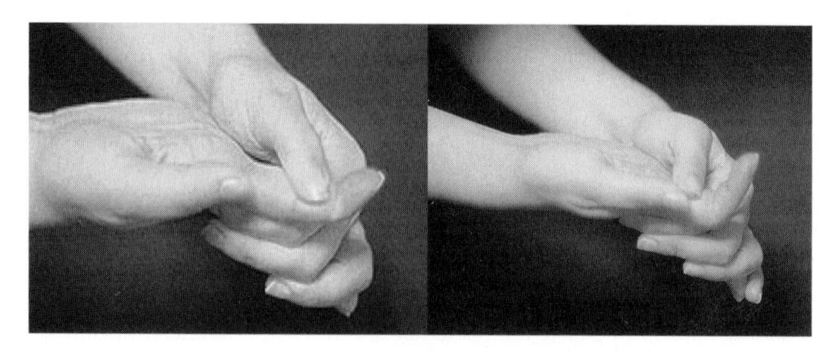

Fig. 2. FDP and FDS blocking exercises.

Table 1
Immobilization program

0 to 3–4 weeks	3–4 weeks	4–6 weeks	6–8 weeks
∘ Cast or dorsal protective splint in wrist and MCP joint flexion and IP joint full extension	∘ Dorsal protective splint replaces cast ∘ Splint modified to bring wrist to neutral ∘ Hourly: 10 repetitions of passive digital flexion and extension with wrist at 10° extension ∘ Hourly: 10 repetitions of active tendon gliding exercises	∘ Dorsal blocking splint discontinued ∘ Gentle blocking exercises initiated 10 repetitions, 4–6 times daily added to passive flexion and tendon gliding	∘ Gentle resistive exercise begins and progresses gradually

MCP, 30°–40° flexion) with elastic traction from the fingernail to the volar forearm (Fig. 3).

The elastic flexion pull acts as the repaired flexor tendon unit without flexor muscle contraction. Active extension of the digit is performed to the limits of the dorsal blocking splint. Because of flexion contractures at the proximal interphalangeal (PIP) joint and loss of active distal interphalangeal (DIP) motion, two modifications became standard: a palmar pulley was added to improve DIP flexion, and at night the elastic traction is detached and the fingers strapped into extension within the splint to prevent PIP joint flexion contractures. Table 2 outlines the basic Kleinert protocol.

Duran program

In the 1970s Duran and Houser [11] introduced a controlled passive motion protocol using a similar dorsal protective splint without elastic traction. The program was designed in response to their measurement that 3–5 mm of tendon glide would prevent restrictive adhesion in zone II. Passive DIP extension with PIP and MCP joint flexion was found to glide the FDP away from the FDS suture sites. Passive PIP joint extension with MCP and DIP flexed glides both tendons away from the injury site. Table 3 outlines the basic Duran protocol.

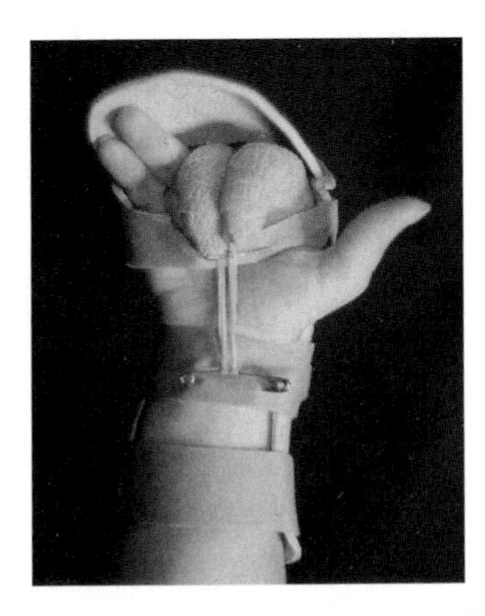

Fig. 3. Kleinert splint with palmar pulley.

Early active motion

Since the late 1980s and early 1990s early active motion protocols developed in response to experimental and clinical studies that demonstrate beneficial effects of early (as early as 24 hours postoperative) active motion [12,13]. Early active motion protocols depend on strong repair techniques [14]. The force application during rehabilitation must be less than the tensile strength of the repair to prevent gapping or rupture. Combined metacarpophalangeal (MP) flexion and wrist extension has been found to produce the least tension on the repaired site and to allow the most differential excursion between FDS and FDP on a repaired tendon [15,16] Cadaver studies using tenodesis motion showed the following tendon excursions: FDS, 15.2 mm; FDP, 19.8 mm; and FDS-P, 4.6 mm.

Strickland introduced an early active motion protocol (Indiana Hand Center) for a four-strand repair with an epitendinous suture (Table 4) [17]. The Indiana protocol incorporates the tenodesis motion within a hinged splint that allows for 30° of wrist extension. Good patient motivation and comprehension and controlled edema and minimal wound complications are required [18].

There are protocols that incorporate early active motion exercises while using a Kleinert

Table 2
Kleinert program

0–3 days	0–4 weeks	4–6 weeks	6–8 weeks
○ Dorsal protective splint applied with wrist and MCP joints in flexion and IP joints in full extension; elastic traction from fingernail, through palmar pulley, to volar forearm ○ Velcro strap to allow night release of elastic traction, splinting IPs in full extension	○ Hourly active extension to limits of splint, followed by flexion with elastic traction only ○ Wound and scar management and education	○ Dorsal protective splint discontinued, sometimes replaced with wrist cuff and elastic traction ○ Night protective splint to prevent flexion contracture ○ Active wrist and gentle active fisting initiated unless signs of minimal adhesions ○ At 6 weeks blocking exercises begin	○ Progressive resistive exercises begin

type dorsal blocking splint. Evans developed a program for the repair with a conventional modified Kessler and epitendinous suture with a two-strand core [19]. The program includes a dorsal blocking splint with wrist in 30° flexion, MCP joints in 45° flexion, and IP joints in full extension. The splint includes four-finger elastic traction with palmar pulley during the day and full IP extension at night. The active motion component of the program is performed only with therapist participation, until 3 weeks, when the patient is permitted to perform them without supervision. For zone I repairs, Evans includes a second dorsal digital splint extending the length of P2 and P3 maintaining the DIP joint in 40°–45° of flexion with no dynamic traction [20].

Silfverskiöld and May designed a program for a modified Kessler repair and epitendinous circumferential cross-stitch [21]. The dorsal blocking splint holds the wrist in neutral, MCP joints at 50°–70° flexion, and the IP joints in full extension. All fingertips have elastic traction through a palmar pulley. Active extension/passive flexion with elastic traction and passive flexion to the distal palmar crease are performed 10 times hourly. During passive flexion, light active muscle contraction is allowed for 2–3 seconds. Active motion is performed only under therapy or surgeon supervision for the first 4 weeks. At 4 weeks the splint is removed and unassisted active flexion and extension are initiated. Gentle resistive flexion begins at 6 weeks, and at 8 weeks progressive resistive exercises begin.

Even with the advances of early motion rehabilitation programs after a primary flexor tendon repair, getting good to excellent results in active functional PIP and DIP joint motion remains a clinical challenge for hand therapy clinicians. Each patient with a repaired flexor tendon presents a unique set of challenges requiring an individualized approach to rehabilitation. Karen Pettengill promotes that institution of and progression to an active mobilization program depends on the extent of injury, repair technique, patient compliance, patient general health, and tendon response. In general, if good tendon excursion is achieved quickly, "keep the brakes on"; if poor tendon excursion,

Table 3
Duran program

0–3 days	0–4.5 weeks	4.5–5.5 weeks	5.5 weeks	7.5 weeks
○ Dorsal Protective splint applied with wrist in 20° flexion, MCP joints in ~50° flexion, IP joints full extension	○ Hourly exercises within the splint: ○ 10 repetitions passive DIP extension with PIP and MCP flexion ○ 10 repetitions passive PIP extension with MCP and DIP joint flexion	○ Splint replaced by wrist cuff with elastic flexion traction from fingernail to cuff ○ Continue active extension/passive flexion	○ Wrist cuff discontinued ○ Blocking and fisting exercises initiated	○ Light resistive exercises with putty ○ Splinting to correct any joint or extrinsic flexor tightness

Table 4
Early active motion program (Strickland/Indiana Hand Center)

0–3 days	0–4 weeks	4 weeks	5 weeks	6 weeks	8 weeks	14 weeks
Dorsal blocking splint with wrist in 20° flexion, MCP joints in 50° flexion Tenodesis splint allowing 30° wrist extension and full wrist flexion, maintaining MCP joints in 50° flexion (a single hinge splint with a detachable extension block can also be used)	Duran passive motion performed 15 times every 2 hours Tenodesis exercises within hinged splint 15 times every 2 hours	Dorsal blocking splint removed during exercise but continued for protection Tenodesis exercises continue Instruction to avoid simultaneous wrist and finger extension	Active IP flexion with MCP extension followed by full digital extension	Blocking exercises begin if active tip to distal palmar crease is more than 3 cm Passive extension can begin at 7 weeks	Progressive resistive exercises initiated	Unrestricted use of hand

"accelerate!" (Karen M. Pettengill, MS, OTR/L, CHT, personal communication, May 2004).

Instead of advocating a "sweeping postoperative regimen or protocol without allowances for individual physiologic tissue or biological responses," Groth [22] proposes a methodic rehabilitation model that progresses the patient based on force application and individual tissue response through her thorough literature review. Groth's "pyramid of progressive force application" places the exercise with the lowest level of force on the bottom, with a total of eight progressions to the top of the pyramid where the load is the highest. The bottom five levels are with wrist protection, the top three without. The progression from lowest to highest is as follows: passive protected digital extension, place and hold finger flexion, active composite fist, hook and straight fist, isolated joint motion, resistive composite fist, resistive hook and straight fist, resistive isolated joint motion. Groth details internal tendon loads, tendon excursion amounts, and clinical application information for each of the progressive levels. A flexion lag grade becomes the basis for systematic and tailored application of motion stress to the repaired tendon. Adhesions are absent if less than or equal to a 5° discrepancy exist between active and passive flexion. Adhesions are responsive if there is greater than or equal to a 10% resolution of lag between therapy sessions. And adhesions are considered unresponsive if there is less than or equal to 10% resolution of active lag between therapy sessions. If the flexion lag is determined to be unresponsive, the load application increases one level up the pyramid. For example, active composite fist exercises might begin as early as week 2 if the active lag is determined to be unresponsive. If a lag never occurs, this exercise is delayed until 8 weeks postsurgery. Groth's model can be used with any existing protocol and is not limited to zone, type of suture repair, or time sequence. Groth cites two case studies based on her model; both of the patients were discharged with excellent results based on Strickland's formula and classification system.

Clinical problem solving is of utmost importance for the hand therapy clinician in progressing a patient with a primary flexor tendon repair [18]. The future of good to excellent functional outcomes through rehabilitation after a primary repair to the flexor tendon system is based on science and art. Functional outcomes do not depend on following a prescribed protocol, but on progressing each patient individually with the available evidence-based information and on observation of the individual's healing response. More experimental research and clinical outcome studies are critical to the continued advancement of rehabilitation after a primary flexor tendon repair. Through experimental cadaver studies, Mass has concluded that using a locked cruciate four-strand repair is as strong as the modified Becker repair (>60 N), has a lower work of flexion, and is easier to perform [23]. Clinical studies to determine functional outcomes after such repairs are underway to support his findings. Appropriate patients begin immediate early active gentle fisting with therapist supervision with the wrist positioned in neutral to −30° extension and MP joint extension limited to 60° flexion (Fig. 4).

Rehabilitation after flexor tendon reconstruction

When a primary repair of the flexor tendons is not an option, staged tendon reconstruction becomes the treatment of choice. The following outlines rehabilitation after flexor tendon reconstruction using passive and active tendon implants.

Passive tendon implant

Stage I

Therapy goals during stage I are maximum passive motion, correction of flexion contractures, and a viable gliding bed. A dorsal protective splint is worn for 3 weeks with wrist positioned in 30° flexion, MCP joints flexed to 60°, and splint extending 2 cm beyond the fingertips. Gentle passive flexion/active extension and light finger

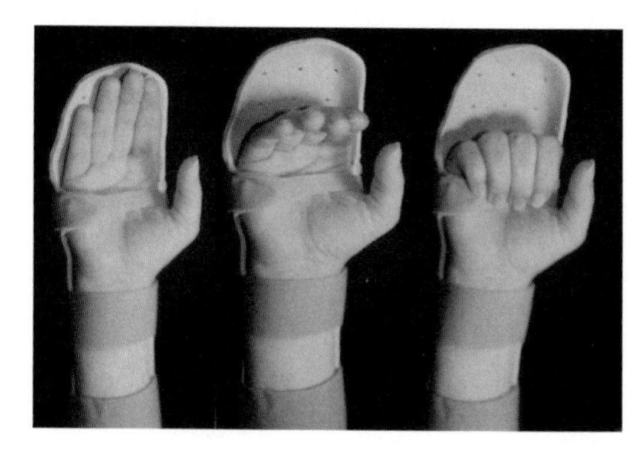

Fig. 4. Immediate gentle active fisting and active extension to limits of splint.

trapping, 10 repetitions each, 4 times a day are initiated the first week. PIP joint flexion contractures must be addressed immediately with a dorsal digital extension splint within the dorsal protective splint. Synovitis must be avoided carefully through instructing the patient not to be overly aggressive. At 3 weeks the dorsal blocking splint is discontinued and buddy taping begins.

Stage II

A dorsal blocking splint with identical positioning as the stage I splint is applied. Full IP joint extension must be allowed within the splint. Gentle passive flexion of each IP joint is performed hourly. At 4 weeks the dorsal protective splint is replaced by a wrist cuff with elastic traction. The traction should allow full IP joint extension with the wrist in neutral. At rest the repaired finger is maintained in flexion. The wrist cuff is removed at 6 weeks and light activity is allowed. Blocking and tendon-gliding exercises are initiated. Contracture control continues. At 8 weeks, progressive resistive exercises begin.

Early protected active motion can be considered if the tendon graft is fixed with strong techniques, the gliding bed is in good post-surgical condition, and the patient is known to be motivated and compliant.

Active tendon implant

Stage I

Therapy begins the day after surgery with a dorsal blocking splint and passive flexion exercises. At 2 weeks elastic traction is added. If pulleys were reconstructed, they must be protected using a pulley ring made from thermoplastic material or Velcro, and during flexion exercises the patient must apply pressure to support the pulley. IP flexion contracture control begins the first postoperative week. Soft foam squeezing begins at week 3 and light putty squeezing after 4 weeks. At week 6 the dorsal protective splint is replaced with the wrist cuff with elastic traction. By 8 weeks progressive strengthening begins.

Stage II

After removal of the tendon implant and insertion of the tendon graft, the same dorsal blocking splint is applied. Early motion with elastic traction begins on day 1. Ten repetitions every waking hour of passive flexion/active digital extension are performed by the patient. Gentle passive flexion is performed 10 times, several times a day. Therapy is similar to after stage I; however, because early pain-free gliding usually occurs, the progression of the program may have to be slowed to protect the tendon junctures [24].

Rehabilitation after tenolysis

Tenolysis, the surgical release of adherent tendons, is indicated for patients whose post-repair progress has plateaued with a significant difference between passive and active range of motion measurements. Tenolysis is considered only if a patient is highly motivated and presents with soft and supple tissues, good passive range of motion, and good strength [25]. Thorough

Box 1. Tenolysis program

Edema control: within 24 hours, bulky dressing removed and light compressive dressing applied.
Active and passive extrinsic stretching: active wrist and digital flexion followed by active wrist and digital extension for maximum FDS and FDP excursion, every waking hour.
Active and passive tendon gliding: composite fist, hook fist, full digital extension for maximum differential tendon glide between FDS and FDP (Fig. 5) every waking hour.
Blocking exercises: independent blocking at the PIP joint and DIP joint for maximum mechanical advantage of tendon pull-through, every waking hour.
Isolated PIP joint blocking: for independent contraction of FDS without motor help from FDP, every waking hour (Fig. 6).
Splinting: static extension splinting between exercises and at night recommended.
Progressive resistance exercises: begins at approximately 6 weeks postoperatively.
Wound and scar management throughout rehabilitation process.
Adjunct therapy: modalities including neuromuscular electrical stimulation (NMES), ultrasound, and so on.

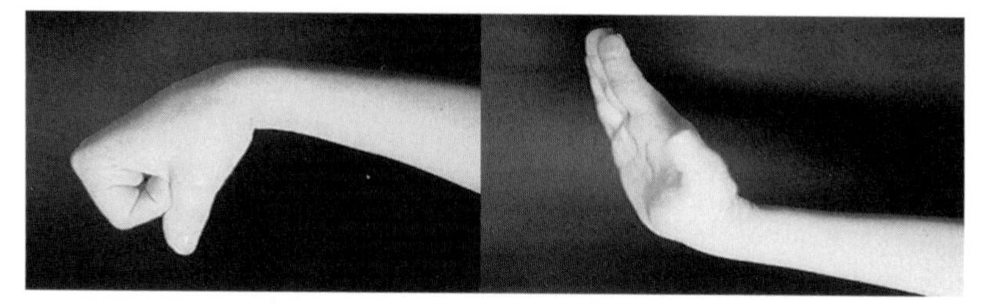

Fig. 5. Extrinsic stretching for maximum FDS and FDP glide.

information must be obtained from the surgeon at the time of referral, including the active and passive range of motion achieved during surgery, vascularity, any additional procedures that might have been done, and prognosis. Rehabilitation depends on poor or good tendon integrity based on the referral information obtained. Tendons of poor integrity have an increased likelihood of rupture and require protective splinting and a controlled range of motion program. Cannon and Strickland advocate a frayed exercise program that includes place and hold exercises that place less tensile loading on the lysed tendon than active range of motion [26]. Tendons of good integrity begin therapy immediately, summarized as follows (Box 1) [27].

Summary

Flexor tendon rehabilitation after injury and surgical intervention has progressed over the last several decades. This evolution has left a vast amount of information for the hand therapy clinician. The hand therapist treating a primary flexor tendon repair can easily feel daunted, confused, and apprehensive because of the sheer amount of information before him or her, which may lead to patient treatment with a textbook or cookbook approach. This article outlines the history of flexor tendon programs and their evidenced-based development so that the clinician can approach each patient individually and progress them with a personalized, tailored approach in close communication with the surgeon. Successful flexor tendon rehabilitation's end-result is functional hand motion and strength. As experimental studies on improved surgical techniques continue to develop, more clinical research to support rehabilitation techniques that lead to good hand function results are necessary.

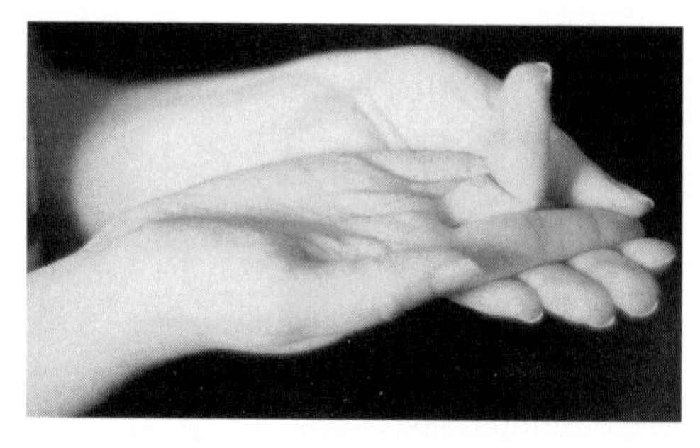

Fig. 6. Isolated PIP joint blocking for isolation of FDS contraction.

References

[1] Robert Collyer. 1823–1912. English-born American orator.

[2] Bunnell S. Repair of nerves and tendons of the hand. J Bone Joint Surg 1928;10:1.

[3] Stewart KM, van Strien G. Postoperative management of flexor tendon injuries. In: Hunter JM, Mackin EJ, Callahan AD, editors. Rehabilitation of the hand. 4th edition. St. Louis: CV Mosby; 2002. p. 439.

[4] Collins DC, Schwarze L. Early progressive resistance following immobilization of flexor tendon repairs. J Hand Ther 1991;4:111–6.

[5] Strickland JW. Development of flexor tendon surgery: twenty-five years of progress. J Hand Surg 2000;25A:214–35.

[6] Freehan LM, Beauchene JG. Early tensile properties of healing flexor tendons: early controlled passive motion versus postoperative immobilization. J Hand Surg 1990;15A:63–8.

[7] Gelberman RH, Vandeberg JS, Manske PR, Akeson WH. The early stages of flexor tendon healing: a morphologic study of the first fourteen days. J Hand Surg [Am] 1985;10:776–84.

[8] Zhao C, Amadio PC, Zobitz ME, An K. Sliding characteristics of tendon repair in canine flexor digitorum profundus tendons. J Orthop Res 2001;19:580–6.

[9] Stein T, Ali A, Hamman J, Mass DP. A randomized biomechanical study of zone II human flexor tendon

repairs analyzed in an in vitro model. J Hand Surg 1998;23:1046–51.

[10] Dovelle A, Heeter P. The Washington regimen: rehabilitation of the hand following flexor tendon injuries. Phys Ther 1989;69:1034.

[11] Duran RJ, House RG. Controlled passive motion following flexor tendon repairs in zones 2 and 3. In: American Academy of Orthopedic Surgeons: Symposium on Tendon Surgery in the Hand. St. Louis: CV Mosby Co.; 1975.

[12] Iwuagwu FC, McGrouther DA. Early response in tendon injury: the effect of loading. Plast Reconstr Surg 1998;102(6):2064–71.

[13] Evans RB, Thompson DE. The application of force to the healing tendon. J Hand Ther 1993;6(4): 266–84.

[14] Strickland JW. Flexor tendon injuries: II. Operative treatment. J Am Acad Orthop Surg 1995;3:55–62.

[15] Savage R. The influence of wrist position on the minimum force required for active movements of the interphalangeal joints. J Hand Surg 1988;13B: 262–8.

[16] Cooney WP, Lin GT, An KN. Improved tendon excursion following flexor tendon repair. J Hand Ther 1989;2(2):102–6.

[17] Strickland JW, Cannon NM. Flexor tendon repair—Indiana method. Indiana Hand Center Newsletter 1993;1:1–19.

[18] Skirven TM. Rehabilitation after tendon injuries in the hand. Hand Surg 2002;7(1):47–59.

[19] Evans RB. Early active motion following flexor tendon repair. In: Berger RA, Weiss AP, editors. Hand surgery. Philadelphia: Lippincott and Williams; 2003.

[20] Evans R. A study of the zone I flexor tendon injury and implications for treatment. J Hand Ther 1990; 3:133.

[21] Silfverskiöld KL, May EJ. Flexor tendon repair in zone 2 with a new suture technique and an early mobilization program combining passive and active motion. J Hand Surg 1994;19A:53–60.

[22] Groth GN. Pyramid of progressive force exercises to the injured flexor tendon. J Hand Ther 2004;17(1): 31–42.

[23] Angeles JG, Heminger H, Mass DP. Comparative biomechanical performances of 4-strand core suture repairs for zone II flexor tendon lacerations. J Hand Surg 2002;27A:508–17.

[24] Hunter JM, Taras JS, Mackin EJ, Maser SA, Culp RW. Staged flexor tendon reconstruction using passive and active tendon implants. In: Hunter JM, Mackin EJ, Callahan AD, editors. Rehabilitation of the hand. 4th edition. St. Louis: CV Mosby; 1995. 447–514.

[25] Schneider LH, Berger-Feldscher S. Tenolysis: dynamic approach to surgery and therapy. In: Hunter JM, Mackin EJ, Callahan AD, editors. Rehabilitation of the hand. 4th edition. St. Louis: CV Mosby; 463–72.

[26] Cannon NM, Strickland JW. Therapy following flexor tendon surgery. Hand Clin 1985;1:147.

[27] Cannon NM. Enhancing flexor tendon glide through tenolysis...and hand therapy. J Hand Ther 1989;2(2).

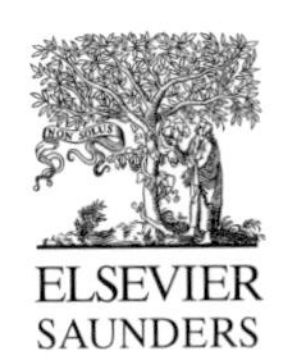

ELSEVIER
SAUNDERS

Hand Clin 21 (2005) 267–273

HAND
CLINICS

The Future of Flexor Tendon Surgery

Jeffrey Luo, MD[a,c,*], Daniel P. Mass, MD[a], Craig S. Phillips, MD[b], T.C. He, MD, PhD[c]

[a]*Orthopaedic Surgery and Rehabilitation Medicine, Department of Surgery, University of Chicago Hospitals, 5841 South Maryland Avenue, MC 3079, Chicago, IL 60637, USA*
[b]*Reconstructive Hand and Upper Extremity Surgery, Microvascular Surgery, The Illinois Bone and Joint Surgery, 2401 Ravine Way, Glenview, IL 60025, USA*
[c]*Molecular Oncology Laboratory, Department of Surgery, The University of Chicago Medical Center, 5841 South Maryland Avenue, MC 3079, Chicago, IL 60637, USA*

Restoration of hand function following flexor tendon laceration has been one of the most difficult problems in hand surgery. As recently as the 1960s, tendons lacerated in "no man's land" routinely were entirely removed and later grafted to allow for a smooth tendinous unit [1]. Although this remained the standard of care for many decades, reports began emerging that challenged the dominance of secondary repair [2–4]. These investigators suggested that immediate suture fixation of the lacerated tendon yielded better results than secondary free tendon grafting. Coupled with the development of primary tendon repair were various rehabilitation protocols that allowed for early motion of the post-repair tendon [5,6]. Gradually the philosophy of primary tendon repair became accepted and practiced.

The difficulties in regaining normal hand function after injury stem from considerations unique to the flexor tendon system. First of all, injuries that lacerate the tendon also tend to compromise the nutritional systems, either by allowing leakage of the synovial fluid or by direct trauma to the vincula. Next, the trauma caused by the surgery itself must not be discounted, because adhesions form in proportion to tendon manipulation and trauma at the time of surgery [7]. Finally, not only does the continuity of tendon fibers need to be restored, but also the gliding mechanism between the lacerated tendon and the surrounding structures. Like most other tissues, tendons heal by deposition of scar tissue into the site of the laceration. Although this initial scar tissue is vital to restoring the continuity of the tendon unit, however, proliferation of this same scar can in fact be harmful to the gliding mechanism that is the function of the tendon. This problem is compounded by the fibro-osseous tunnel found in zone II of the flexor tendon system, where scarring leads to adhesions between the tendon and the surrounding tunnel and prevents proper tendon excursion. Primary tendon repairs therefore can fail from inadequate healing at the site of injury. Unlike other injuries, repairs also can fail when there is too much healing that leads to loss of motion, contracture formation, and ultimately loss of function.

In the last 30 years, significant strides have been made such that recovery of good to excellent function can be expected in approximately 80% of good tendon repairs with an early motion protocol. These advances have been made possible by the enormous amount of basic research that has improved understanding of flexor anatomy, kinesiology, biologic response to injury and repair, mechanical characteristics of the various suture repair techniques, and effects of early motion on tendon healing and strength. As a result of these investigations, general principles have been established for the repair of flexor tendons. These principles include the use of nonabsorbable braided core sutures, epitendinous suture repair, equal tension across all strands, and motion at the repair site to promote stronger (but not faster) repair. In addition, complementary research has

* Corresponding author
E-mail address: jeffrey.luo@uchospitals.edu (J. Luo).

0749-0712/05/$ - see front matter
doi:10.1016/j.hcl.2005.01.001

advanced the development of postoperative rehabilitation protocols that prevent adhesion formation and protect the integrity of the tendon while improving the tensile strength of the repair tissue.

The vast majority of the research to date has focused on the mechanical aspects of tendon repair and healing, including surgical techniques and rehabilitation protocols. This groundwork is largely responsible for the significant improvement in patient function and satisfaction. Unfortunately postoperative scarring and adhesion formation are still frequent and disappointing outcomes; this may be because of shortcomings in the current approach to flexor tendon repair. The focus of research and the clinical principles that have stemmed from the research are based on increasing strength of the repair to allow for decreased protection at the operative site. This then permits more aggressive postoperative motion that in theory minimizes adhesions. Even the best technical repairs coupled with optimal rehabilitation, however, still do not lead to universally good to excellent results. Recently only incremental improvements have been made in outcomes, because each of the different variables of tendon repair is in turn optimized. These limited clinical results suggest that more needs to be done to improve patient outcomes. It is conceivable and probable, therefore, that new biologic strategies may be a useful adjunct to further improve current clinical outcomes.

Biology of flexor tendon repairs

Research on the healing of tendons after injury has provided insight into the biology of tendon regeneration [8]. Like many other connective tissues, tendon healing has been characterized by three sequential phases: inflammation, fibroblastic or reparative, and remodeling [9–12]. The injury and the surgical treatment damage blood vessels, which leads to the formation of a fibrin clot. Platelets trapped within the clot release various cytokines, such as platelet-derived growth factor (PDGF) and transforming growth factor beta (TGF-β). This cytokine rich environment then attracts inflammatory cells from surrounding tissue, which in turn phagocytize necrotic tissue and clot [9]. In the next stage, fibroblastic cells proliferate and lay down the components of the new extracellular matrix. Finally, in the remodeling phase the newly produced collagen fibers become organized in parallel and linear bundles running along the axis of the tendon.

Further research has uncovered a dual mechanism of repair that is unique to the intrasynovial environment of flexor tendons. The first is the extrinsic mechanism, in which fibroblasts and inflammatory cells from the periphery and synovium promote repair of the tendon. In contrast, the intrinsic mechanism involves the fibroblast population that is within the tendon and epitenon. This difference leads to two distinct responses to injury [13–15]. The extrinsic mechanism seems to be activated earlier than the intrinsic mechanism [14]. This may explain why the synovial sheath is more reactive than the tendon in the early stages after injury [13]. Furthermore, the fibroblasts from the synovial sheath are more active than those from the tendon, with a greater capacity to degrade the extracellular matrix [14]. Finally, increased extrinsic activity leads to increased collagen deposition and a decreased level of collagen organization [15,16]. These studies suggest that extrinsic healing promotes adhesion and scar formation between the tendon and the surrounding fibro-osseous structures.

It follows, therefore, that efforts should be directed at suppressing the extrinsic pathway, thereby curtailing adhesion formation. Simultaneously, enhancing the intrinsic pathway promotes tendon healing. The difficulty is that the healing response observed clinically is a combination of these two concurrent mechanisms. Furthermore, such fine manipulation is neither fully understood nor possible at this time. The concepts do provide a valuable framework with which to understand new biologic approaches to augmenting tendon healing.

Biologic advances

The cellular processes underlying tendon healing have been well described and have become well understood. The next frontier is comprehension of the healing process at the molecular and genetic levels. Each of these three levels, the cellular, the molecular, and the genetic, offers unique approaches to improving clinical outcomes.

Cell-based strategies

Cell-based strategies incorporate one or both of two compatible techniques: mesenchymal stem cells (MSCs) and tissue engineering. MSCs are progenitor cells that have the ability to differentiate into various types of specialized cells, including myocytes, chondrocytes, lipocytes, and of course, tenocytes or tendon fibroblasts [17]. They reside in bone marrow, fat, muscle, and skin, and can be harvested from each of these tissue types. Although the fibroblastic cells that appear during tendon healing are from mesenchymal stem cells, the source of these stem cells has not been elucidated yet [18]. Mesenchymal stem cells offer a viable alternative because of their pluripotential abilities: besides the ability to differentiate into tendon fibroblasts, the MSCs also produce extracellular matrix and secrete growth factors that are vital to beginning the cascade of cellular events needed for tendon healing.

Tissue engineering refers to the ability to construct new tissues, in this case flexor tendons, in an ex vivo environment. Efforts are centered about the use of a tissue scaffold onto which cells (ie, MSCs) are placed. These scaffolds, typically biodegradable polymers, provide a matrix that allows cell adhesion and growth in a three-dimensional conformation, allowing for high density cell suspensions simulating normal cell architecture. This conformation allows for better cell spacing with the subsequent formation of extracellular matrix and release of growth factors.

Although this technique has been applied to many tissue types, including bone and cartilage, its use in reconstructing flexor tendons has not yet been studied extensively. Cao used these tissue engineering techniques to bridge flexor tendon defects in a hen model [19]. Tenocytes harvested from adult Leghorn hens were expanded in vitro and then mixed with unwoven polyglycolic acid fibers to form a cell-scaffold construct in the shape of a tendon. The constructs were wrapped with intestinal submucosa for mechanical strength and then cultured for 1 week before in vivo implantation into a 3–4-cm defect created in the second flexor digitorum profundus tendon. By 14 weeks the investigators noted that the collagen bundles had become longitudinally aligned, with good interface healing to normal tendon. Also, biomechanical analysis showed that the engineered tendon gained 83% of the normal tendon tensile strength. Furthermore, the polymer scaffold and the submucosa construct did not elicit a significant immune response and contributed only minimally to the final tensile strength achieved by the engineered tendon.

To avoid harvesting autologous flexor tendon cells, Chen et al used autologous dermal fibroblasts in a similar cell-scaffold construct [20]. Fibroblasts were isolated and cultured from skin pieces and then implanted onto a polyglycolic acid scaffold and placed in a 3-cm flexor tendon defect in a pig model. They noted near normal histology and 50% of normal tensile strength. Taken together these studies suggest one future approach to reconstructing flexor tendon injuries. These techniques are especially appealing for use in cases in which a tendon defect needs to be spanned. Furthermore, they sidestep the current debate over the use of intrasynovial versus extrasynovial tendons for use in grafting [21,22]. They do have one weakness that may delay clinical adoption. Cell-based strategies require cells to be isolated and cultured before implantation. This necessitates a staged procedure for repair of an injury, rather than harvesting autograft at the initial procedure.

Despite possible shortcomings with cell-based strategies, tissue engineering likely will play a role in future reconstructive techniques. As understanding of molecular medicine increases, various cytokines, growth factors, and extracellular matrix molecules have been found to play a critical role in tendon healing. The goal of molecular approaches is to reduce scarring and improve healing by modulating the timing and delivery of these factors. The usefulness of a cell scaffold is an exciting advancement and plays an integral role in delivery of molecular and gene therapy products to the zone of injury.

Molecular medicine

Molecular approaches to augmenting tendon healing focus on the complex interplay of cytokines or growth factors and extracellular matrix molecules. Cytokines, a diverse group of soluble proteins and peptides, modulate the functional activities of individual cells and tissues. These proteins also mediate interactions between cells directly and regulate processes taking place in the extracellular environment. They are an ideal way to modulate the effects of the extrinsic healing pathway by targeting adhesion formation.

Before the current era of molecular medicine, researchers investigated different means of reducing the effects of extrinsic healing. Initially, various mechanical barriers were placed between the healing tendon and sheath, including silicone [23], hydroxyapatite and alumina [24], and polyethylene [25]. Other researchers attempted chemical modulation of the inflammatory reaction to reduce adhesion formation. Agents included corticosteroids [26], ibuprofen [27,28], 5-fluorouracil [29], and hyaluronic acid [30,31], among many others. These investigations have yielded varying degrees of adhesion reduction, but none have led to any changes in clinical practice.

Current knowledge of the biology of tendon healing has led to promising advances in molecular modulation of adhesion formation. Initial work has focused on identifying cytokines or growth factors that play a role in the healing tendon [32], including TGF-β [33–35], PDGF [36,37], basic fibroblast growth factor (b-FGF) [36,38,39], and insulin-like growth factor (IGF) [40,41]. Many of these cytokines have specific effects during tissue repair. For example, the principle effects of b-FGF include fibroblast chemotaxis and initiation of angiogenesis. Similarly, IGF has been shown to stimulate matrix components, such as proteoglycan and collagen, while also increasing DNA synthesis and cell proliferation [40].

TGF-β is a cytokine that is secreted by all major cell types involved in the healing process, including macrophages, lymphocytes, degranulating platelets, endothelial cells, and fibroblasts. TGF-β increases fibroblast and macrophage recruitment and proliferation, promotes angiogenesis, and regulates the transcription of multiple matrix proteins, including collagen, fibronectin, matrix-degrading proteases and their inhibitors, and glycosaminoglycans [33]. As such, it has been implicated in scar formation following injury or surgery [34,42] and even the pathogenesis of excessive scar formation [43]. Attempts at perioperative modulation of TGF-β levels with neutralizing antibodies [35] have yielded promising initial results in reduction of adhesions and increased flexion range of motion [43].

Further research into the roles of the various cytokines will allow the identification and ultimately the manipulation of cytokines at the site of repair. Although the specific roles of each cytokine are being discovered only now, there is already promising evidence that strategies that attempt to modulate cytokine expression can indeed reduce adhesion formation. Specific cytokines could be added to the site of injury to inhibit excessive scar formation directly or to suppress the activity of a different cytokine, such as TGF-β, that might otherwise cause adhesions. As appealing as this concept is, there are still numerous obstacles to be overcome. Cytokines are involved in a complex interaction with multiple other receptors, promoters, and cytokines. Appropriate application of a cytokine to augment tissue healing therefore would require knowledge of specific reaction conditions, such as ideal concentration, timing of application, and effect on downstream targets. These limitations will be overcome by further research into cytokine biology.

Gene therapy

Gene therapy at its most basic level refers to the treatment of a disorder by introducing specific engineered genes into a patient's cells. In many ways it is not distinct from the previous discussions of cell-based and molecular medicine, because the therapeutic genes selected are often the same ones as those identified by molecular techniques. Gene therapy is based on the same understanding of flexor tendon biology, but diverges from previous techniques by interacting with target cells at the genetic level.

Although first conceived as a systemic treatment for hereditary single-gene defects [44], localized gene therapy is well suited for flexor tendon repair because of the ability to deliver genes to a discrete site. Also, transient expression is a desirable benefit and is readily available with existing gene transfer techniques. In addition, it has the ability to deliver multiple genes and to regulate their expression temporally and quantitatively. Gene therapy in flexor tendon regeneration thus has the unique ability to deliver multiple gene products to precise anatomic locations at elevated levels for an appropriate duration.

Gene delivery can be accomplished by using viral vectors or nonviral means. Nonviral approaches include delivery of naked DNA/plasmids by direct injection, liposome-mediated transfection, particle-mediated delivery (eg, gene gun), and microseeding [45–48]. These techniques often are less costly and are able to sustain gene expression, as compared with direct delivery of recombinant proteins. The use of nonviral vectors, however, is restricted by their low efficiency of gene transfer compared with viral vectors, although some studies are attempting to overcome this limitation.

Gene transfer mediated by viral vectors represents the most common approach in gene therapy studies. There are five major types of viral vectors, including adenovirus, herpes virus, retrovirus, adeno-associated virus, and lentivirus [44]. Of note, adenoviral vectors mediate the highest level of transgene production [49]. As a result, most previous work in flexor tendon regeneration has used adenovirus vectors, with only a small number of studies using retroviral vectors. The disadvantages of viral techniques include cellular toxicity and immunogenicity.

In addition to the selection of proper gene delivery vehicles, it is equally important to choose an appropriate route of gene delivery. In the case of flexor tendon healing, local gene delivery is the method most desired. There are two main strategies in local gene therapy: direct delivery (in vivo) and transplantation of genetically modified tendon fibroblasts or mesenchymal stem cells (MSC) (cell-based or ex vivo). The in vivo approach tends to be straightforward, faster, and less costly, whereas the ex vivo method theoretically is safer and more effective, because genetic manipulations take place outside the patient's body. Both methods currently are used for flexor tendon research.

The authors and other investigators recently have focused on the role of bone morphogenetic proteins (BMP) in the healing of flexor tendons [50–52]. BMPs belong to the TGF-β superfamily and are active growth factors in musculoskeletal development. BMPs 13 and 14 have been shown in the authors' laboratory to be the most tenogenic of the known BMPs in inducing the tendon marker scleraxis, and the authors believe these two BMPs to hold the greatest promise in promoting tendon healing. Currently the authors are evaluating the ability of in vivo adenovirus-mediated delivery of BMP-13 to improve healing in flexor tendon lacerations. It is conceivable that a cocktail of biologic factors will significantly enhance the healing of tendon injuries in the near future.

Summary

Clinical outcomes following flexor tendon repair have made significant improvements in the last 50 years. In that time standard treatment has evolved from secondary grafting to primary repair with postoperative rehabilitation protocols. Unfortunately, excellent results are not yet attained universally following treatment. Improving understanding of tendon healing at the cellular, molecular, and genetic levels will likely enable surgeons to modulate the normal repair process. We now look toward biologic augmentation of flexor tendon repairs to address the problems of increasing tensile strength while reducing adhesion formation following injury and operative repair.

References

[1] Bunnell S. Repair of tendons in the fingers and description of two new instruments. Surg Gynecol Obstet 1918;26:103–10.
[2] Kessler I, Nissim F. Primary repair without immobilization of flexor tendon division within the digital sheath. An experimental and clinical study. Acta Orthop Scand 1969;40(5):587–601.
[3] Verdan CE. Primary repair of flexor tendons. Am J Orthop 1960;42A:647–57.
[4] Verdan C. Practical considerations for primary and secondary repair in flexor tendon injuries. Surg Clin N Am 1964;44:951–70.
[5] Lister GD, Kleinert HE, Kutz JE, Atasoy E. Primary flexor tendon repair followed by immediate controlled mobilization. J Hand Surg [Am] 1977;2(6): 441–51.
[6] Strickland JW, Glogovac SV. Digital function following flexor tendon repair in zone II: a comparison of immobilization and controlled passive motion techniques. J Hand Surg [Am] 1980;5(6):537–43.
[7] Potenza AD. Critical evaluation of flexor-tendon healing and adhesion formation within artificial digital sheaths. J Bone Joint Surg [Am] 1963;45: 1217–33.
[8] Beredjiklian PK. Biologic aspects of flexor tendon laceration and repair. J Bone Joint Surg [Am] 2003;85A(3):539–50.
[9] Gelberman RH, Vandeberg JS, Manske PR, Akeson WH. The early stages of flexor tendon healing: a morphologic study of the first fourteen days. J Hand Surg [Am] 1985;10(6 Pt 1):776–84.
[10] Manske PR, Gelberman RH, Lesker PA. Flexor tendon healing. Hand Clin 1985;1(1):25–34.
[11] Gelberman RH. Flexor tendon physiology: tendon nutrition and cellular activity in injury and repair. Instr Course Lect 1985;34:351–60.
[12] Gelberman RH, Manske PR, Akeson WH, Woo SL, Lundborg G, Amiel D. Flexor tendon repair. J Orthop Res 1986;4(1):119–28.
[13] Khan U, Edwards JC, McGrouther DA. Patterns of cellular activation after tendon injury. J Hand Surg [Br] 1996;21(6):813–20.
[14] Khan U, Occleston NL, Khaw PT, McGrouther DA. Differences in proliferative rate and collagen lattice contraction between endotenon and synovial fibroblasts. J Hand Surg [Am] 1998;23(2):266–73.
[15] Matthews P, Richards H. Factors in the adherence of flexor tendon after repair: an experimental study in the rabbit. J Bone Joint Surg [Br] 1976;58(2): 230–6.
[16] Nyska M, Porat S, Nyska A, Rousso M, Shoshan S. Decreased adhesion formation in flexor tendons by topical application of enriched collagen solution—a histological study. Arch Orthop Trauma Surg 1987;106(3):192–4.
[17] Caplan AI, Bruder SP. Mesenchymal stem cells: building blocks for molecular medicine in the 21st century. Trends Mol Med 2001;7(6):259–64.
[18] Caplan AI. The mesengenic process. Clin Plast Surg 1994;21(3):429–35.
[19] Cao Y, Liu Y, Liu W, Shan Q, Buonocore SD, Cui L. Bridging tendon defects using autologous

tenocyte engineered tendon in a hen model. Plast Reconstr Surg 2002;110(5):1280–9.

[20] Chen B, Ding X, Liu F, et al. Tissue engineered tendon with skin fibroblasts as seed cells: a preliminary study. Zhonghua Yi Xue Za Zhi 2002;82(16): 1105–7.

[21] Seiler JG III, Chu CR, Amiel D, Woo SL, Gelberman RH. The Marshall R. Urist Young Investigator Award. Autogenous flexor tendon grafts. Biologic mechanisms for incorporation. Clin Orthop 1997; 345:239–47.

[22] Leversedge FJ, Zelouf D, Williams C, Gelberman RH, Seiler JG III. Flexor tendon grafting to the hand: an assessment of the intrasynovial donor tendon—a preliminary single-cohort study. J Hand Surg [Am] 2000;25(4):721–30.

[23] Eskeland G, Eskeland T, Hovig T, Teigland J. The ultrastructure of normal digital flexor tendon sheath and of the tissue formed around silicone and polyethylene implants in man. J Bone Joint Surg [Br] 1977;59(2):206–12.

[24] Siddiqi NA, Hamada Y, Ide T, Akamatsu N. Effects of hydroxyapatite and alumina sheaths on postoperative peritendinous adhesions in chickens. J Appl Biomater 1995;6(1):43–53.

[25] Austin RT, Walker F. Flexor tendon healing and adhesion formation after Sterispon wrapping: a study in the rabbit. Injury 1979;10(3):211–6.

[26] Kapetanos G. The effect of the local corticosteroids on the healing and biomechanical properties of the partially injured tendon. Clin Orthop 1982;163: 170–9.

[27] Kulick MI, Brazlow R, Smith S, Hentz VR. Injectable ibuprofen: preliminary evaluation of its ability to decrease peritendinous adhesions. Ann Plast Surg 1984;13(6):459–67.

[28] Kulick MI, Smith S, Hadler K. Oral ibuprofen: evaluation of its effect on peritendinous adhesions and the breaking strength of a tenorrhaphy. J Hand Surg [Am] 1986;11(1):110–20.

[29] Khan U, Kakar S, Akali A, Bentley G, McGrouther DA. Modulation of the formation of adhesions during the healing of injured tendons. J Bone Joint Surg [Br] 2000;82(7):1054–8.

[30] Salti NI, Tuel RJ, Mass DP. Effect of hyaluronic acid on rabbit profundus flexor tendon healing in vitro. J Surg Res 1993;55(4):411–5.

[31] Wiig M, Abrahamsson SO, Lundborg G. Tendon repair—cellular activities in rabbit deep flexor tendons and surrounding synovial sheaths and the effects of hyaluronan: an experimental study in vivo and in vitro. J Hand Surg [Am] 1997;22(5):818–25.

[32] Evans CH. Cytokines and the role they play in the healing of ligaments and tendons. Sports Med 1999;28(2):71–6.

[33] Roberts AB, Sporn MB. Transforming growth factor-β. In: Clark RAF, editor. The molecular and cellular biology of wound repair. New York: Plenum Press; 1995. p. 275–308.

[34] Chang J, Most D, Stelnicki E, et al. Gene expression of transforming growth factor beta-1 in rabbit zone II flexor tendon wound healing: evidence for dual mechanisms of repair. Plast Reconstr Surg 1997; 100(4):937–44.

[35] Zhang AY, Pham H, Ho F, Teng K, Longaker MT, Chang J. Inhibition of TGF-beta-induced collagen production in rabbit flexor tendons. J Hand Surg [Am] 2004;29(2):230–5.

[36] Duffy FJ Jr, Seiler JG, Gelberman RH, Hergrueter CA. Growth factors and canine flexor tendon healing: initial studies in uninjured and repair models. J Hand Surg [Am] 1995;20(4):645–9.

[37] Nakamura N, Shino K, Natsuume T, et al. Early biological effect of in vivo gene transfer of platelet-derived growth factor (PDGF)-B into healing patellar ligament. Gene Ther 1998;5(9):1165–70.

[38] Chan BP, Chan KM, Maffulli N, Webb S, Lee KK. Effect of basic fibroblast growth factor. An in vitro study of tendon healing. Clin Orthop 1997;342: 239–47.

[39] Chang J, Most D, Thunder R, Mehrara B, Longaker MT, Lineaweaver WC. Molecular studies in flexor tendon wound healing: the role of basic fibroblast growth factor gene expression. J Hand Surg [Am] 1998;23(6):1052–8.

[40] Abrahamsson SO. Similar effects of recombinant human insulin-like growth factor-I and II on cellular activities in flexor tendons of young rabbits: experimental studies in vitro. J Orthop Res 1997;15(2): 256–62.

[41] Abrahamsson SO, Lohmander S. Differential effects of insulin-like growth factor-I on matrix and DNA synthesis in various regions and types of rabbit tendons. J Orthop Res 1996;14(3):370–6.

[42] Border WA, Noble NA. Transforming growth factor beta in tissue fibrosis. N Engl J Med 1994; 331(19):1286–92.

[43] Chang J, Thunder R, Most D, Longaker MT, Lineaweaver WC. Studies in flexor tendon wound healing: neutralizing antibody to TGF-beta1 increases postoperative range of motion. Plast Reconstr Surg 2000;105(1):148–55.

[44] Thomas CE, Ehrhardt A, Kay MA. Progress and problems with the use of viral vectors for gene therapy. Nat Rev Genet 2003;4(5):346–58.

[45] Bonadio J, Smiley E, Patil P, Goldstein S. Localized, direct plasmid gene delivery in vivo: prolonged therapy results in reproducible tissue regeneration. Nat Med 1999;5(7):753–9.

[46] Ferry N, Heard JM. Liver-directed gene transfer vectors. Hum Gene Ther 1998;9(14):1975–81.

[47] Park J, Ries J, Gelse K, et al. Bone regeneration in critical size defects by cell-mediated BMP-2 gene transfer: a comparison of adenoviral vectors and liposomes. Gene Ther 2003;10(13):1089–98.

[48] Hoeller D, Petrie N, Yao F, Eriksson E. Gene therapy in soft tissue reconstruction. Cells Tissues Organs 2002;172:118–25.

[49] Gerdes CA, Castro MG, Lowenstein PR. Strong promoters are the key to highly efficient, noninflammatory and noncytotoxic adenoviral-mediated transgene delivery into the brain in vivo. Mol Ther 2000;2(4):330–8.
[50] Helm GA, Li JZ, Alden TD, et al. A light and electron microscopic study of ectopic tendon and ligament formation induced by bone morphogenetic protein-13 adenoviral gene therapy. J Neurosurg 2001;95(2):298–307.
[51] Lou J, Tu Y, Burns M, Silva MJ, Manske P. BMP-12 gene transfer augmentation of lacerated tendon repair. J Orthop Res 2001;19(6):1199–202.
[52] Lou J, Manske PR, Aoki M, Joyce ME. Adenovirus-mediated gene transfer into tendon and tendon sheath. J Orthop Res 1996;14(4):513–7.

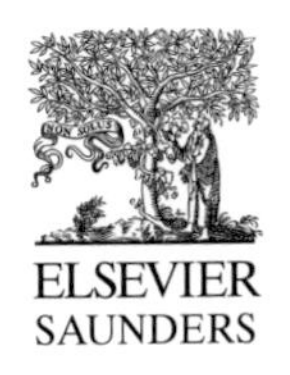

ELSEVIER
SAUNDERS

Hand Clin 21 (2005) 275–278

HAND
CLINICS

Index

Note: Page numbers of article titles are in **boldface** type.

doi:10.1016/S0749-0712(05)00053-3

S

T

V

W